ACP | MKSAP® 17
Medical Knowledge Self-Assessment Program®

Cardiovascular Medicine

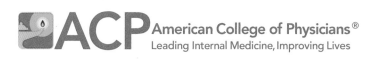

Welcome to the Cardiovascular Medicine Section of MKSAP 17!

In these pages, you will find updated information on risk assessment in cardiovascular disease, diagnostic testing, coronary artery disease, heart failure, arrhythmias, pericardial and myocardial disease, valvular heart disease, and other clinical challenges. All of these topics are uniquely focused on the needs of generalists and subspecialists *outside* of cardiovascular medicine.

The publication of the 17th edition of Medical Knowledge Self-Assessment Program (MKSAP) represents nearly a half-century of serving as the gold-standard resource for internal medicine education. It also marks its evolution into an innovative learning system to better meet the changing educational needs and learning styles of all internists.

The core content of MKSAP has been developed as in previous editions—newly generated, essential information in 11 topic areas of internal medicine created by dozens of leading generalists and subspecialists and guided by certification and recertification requirements, emerging knowledge in the field, and user feedback. MKSAP 17 also contains 1200 all-new, psychometrically validated, and peer-reviewed multiple-choice questions (MCQs) for self-assessment and study, including 120 in Cardiovascular Medicine. MKSAP 17 continues to include *High Value Care* (HVC) recommendations, based on the concept of balancing clinical benefit with costs and harms, with links to MCQs that illustrate these principles. In addition, HVC Key Points are highlighted in the text. Also highlighted, with blue text, are *Hospitalist*-focused content and MCQs that directly address the learning needs of internists who work in the hospital setting.

MKSAP 17 Digital provides access to additional tools allowing you to customize your learning experience, including regular text updates with practice-changing, new information and 200 new self-assessment questions; a board-style pretest to help direct your learning; and enhanced custom-quiz options. And, with MKSAP Complete, learners can access 1200 electronic flashcards for quick review of important concepts or review the updated and enhanced version of Virtual Dx, an image-based self-assessment tool.

As before, MKSAP 17 is optimized for use on your mobile devices, with iOS- and Android-based apps allowing you to sync your work between your apps and online account and submit for CME credits and MOC points online.

Please visit us at the MKSAP Resource Site (mksap.acponline.org) to find out how we can help you study, earn CME credit and MOC points, and stay up to date.

Whether you prefer to use the traditional print version or take advantage of the features available through the digital version, we hope you enjoy MKSAP 17 and that it meets and exceeds your personal learning needs.

On behalf of the many internists who have offered their time and expertise to create the content for MKSAP 17 and the editorial staff who work to bring this material to you in the best possible way, we are honored that you have chosen to use MKSAP 17 and appreciate any feedback about the program you may have. Please feel free to send us any comments to mksap_editors@acponline.org.

Sincerely,

Philip A. Masters, MD, FACP
Editor-in-Chief
Senior Physician Educator
Director, Content Development
Medical Education Division
American College of Physicians

Cardiovascular Medicine

Committee

Andrew Wang, MD, Section Editor[2]
Professor of Medicine
Director, Cardiovascular Disease Fellowship Program
Division of Cardiology
Duke University Medical Center
Durham, North Carolina

Howard H. Weitz, MD, MACP, Associate Editor[1]
Professor of Medicine
Director, Jefferson Heart Institute
Director, Division of Cardiology
Vice-Chairman, Department of Medicine
Sidney Kimmel Medical College at Thomas Jefferson
    University
Philadelphia, Pennsylvania

Jeffrey S. Berger, MD, MS[2]
Assistant Professor of Medicine (Cardiology and
    Hematology)
Assistant Professor of Surgery (Vascular Surgery)
Director of Cardiovascular Thrombosis
New York University School of Medicine
New York, New York

Heidi M. Connolly, MD[1]
Professor of Medicine
Mayo Clinic College of Medicine
Rochester, Minnesota

W. Schuyler Jones, MD[2]
Assistant Professor of Medicine
Division of Cardiology
Duke University Medical Center and Durham Veterans
    Affairs Medical Center
Durham, North Carolina

Andrew M. Kates, MD[2]
Associate Professor of Medicine
Director, Cardiovascular Fellowship Program
Washington University School of Medicine
St. Louis, Missouri

Jonathan P. Piccini, MD, MHS[2]
Associate Professor of Medicine
Division of Cardiology
Duke University Medical Center
Duke Clinical Research Institute
Durham, North Carolina

Donna Polk, MD, MPH[2]
Program Director, Cardiovascular Medicine Fellowship
Brigham and Women's Hospital
Boston, Massachusetts

Stuart D. Russell, MD[2]
Associate Professor of Medicine
Chief, Heart Failure and Transplantation
Johns Hopkins School of Medicine
Baltimore, Maryland

Paul Sorajja, MD[1]
Director, Center for Valve and Structural Heart Disease
Senior Consulting Cardiologist
Program Director, Structural Heart Interventional
    Fellowship
Minneapolis Heart Institute at Abbott Northwestern Hospital
Minneapolis, Minnesota

Editor-in-Chief

Philip A. Masters, MD, FACP[1]
Director, Clinical Content Development
American College of Physicians
Philadelphia, Pennsylvania

Director, Clinical Program Development

Cynthia D. Smith, MD, FACP[2]
American College of Physicians
Philadelphia, Pennsylvania

Cardiovascular Medicine Reviewers

Joel S. Karliner, MD[1]
Kent A. Kirchner, MD, FACP[1]
Mark E. Pasanen, MD, FACP[1]
Michael W. Peterson, MD, FACP[1]
Ileana L. Piña, MD, MPH[2]
Mark D. Siegel, MD, FACP[1]

Cardiovascular Medicine ACP Editorial Staff

Jackie Twomey[1], Staff Editor
Margaret Wells[1], Director, Self-Assessment and Educational
    Programs
Becky Krumm[1], Managing Editor

ACP Principal Staff

Patrick C. Alguire, MD, FACP[2]
Senior Vice President, Medical Education

Sean McKinney[1]
Vice President, Medical Education

Margaret Wells[1]
Director, Self-Assessment and Educational Programs

Becky Krumm[1]
Managing Editor

Valerie A. Dangovetsky[1]
Administrator

Ellen McDonald, PhD[1]
Senior Staff Editor

Katie Idell[1]
Digital Content Associate/Editor

Megan Zborowski[1]
Senior Staff Editor

Randy Hendrickson[1]
Production Administrator/Editor

Linnea Donnarumma[1]
Staff Editor

Susan Galeone[1]
Staff Editor

Jackie Twomey[1]
Staff Editor

Kimberly Kerns[1]
Administrative Coordinator

---

1. Has no relationships with any entity producing, marketing, reselling, or distributing health care goods or services consumed by, or used on, patients.

2. Has disclosed relationship(s) with any entity producing, marketing, reselling, or distributing health care goods or services consumed by, or used on, patients.

Disclosure of Relationships with any entity producing, marketing, reselling, or distributing health care goods or services consumed by, or used on, patients:

Patrick C. Alguire, MD, FACP
Board Member
Teva Pharmaceuticals
Consultantship
National Board of Medical Examiners
Royalties
UpToDate
Stock Options/Holdings
Amgen Inc, Bristol-Myers Squibb, Covidien, GlaxoSmithKline, Stryker Corporation, Zimmer Orthopedics, Teva Pharmaceuticals, Express Scripts, Medtronic

Jeffrey S. Berger, MD, MS
Research Grants/Contracts
AstraZeneca, American Heart Association, Doris Duke Charitable Foundation, National Institutes of Health
Consultantship
Bristol-Myers Squibb, Takeda Pharmaceuticals
Other
Maintenance of Certification: Pri-Med; Planning Committee: American College of Cardiology

W. Schuyler Jones, MD
Other
American Physician Institute
Research Grants/Contracts
AstraZeneca, Bristol-Myers Squibb, American Heart Association, Boston Scientific

Andrew M. Kates, MD
Speakers Bureau
Pfizer, American College of Cardiology, MCE Medical

Jonathan P. Piccini, MD, MHS
Consultantship
Medtronic, Forest Laboratories, Pfizer/Bristol-Myers Squibb, Spectranetics, Johnson & Johnson
Research Grants/Contracts
Janssen Pharmaceuticals, GE Healthcare, Boston Scientific, ARCA Biopharma, ResMed

Ileana L. Piña, MD, MPH
Employment
Montefiore-Einstein Medical Center
Research Grants/Contracts
Duke University/National Institutes of Health
Royalties
UpToDate
Consultantship
Novartis

Donna Polk, MD, MPH
Board Member
American Society of Nuclear Cardiology
Honoraria
American College of Cardiology

Stuart D. Russell, MD
Consultantship
Thoratec, Amgen, SulfaGENIX
Speakers Bureau
American College of Cardiology, Heart Failure Society of America

Cynthia D. Smith, MD, FACP
Stock Options/Holdings
Merck and Co.; spousal employment at Merck

Andrew Wang, MD

Research Grants/Contracts
Abbott Vascular, Edwards Lifesciences, Gilead Sciences,
    American Heart Association
Consultantship
American College of Cardiology Foundation
Other
Expert reviewer for legal case of infective endocarditis

Acknowledgments

The American College of Physicians (ACP) gratefully
acknowledges the special contributions to the development and production of the 17th edition of the Medical
Knowledge Self-Assessment Program® (MKSAP® 17) made
by the following people:

Graphic Design: Michael Ripca (Graphics Technical
Administrator) and WFGD Studio (Graphic Designers).

Production/Systems: Dan Hoffmann (Director, Web
Services & Systems Development), Neil Kohl (Senior
Architect), Chris Patterson (Senior Architect), and Scott
Hurd (Manager, Web Projects & CMS Services).

MKSAP 17 Digital: Under the direction of Steven Spadt,
Vice President, Digital Products & Services, the digital version of MKSAP 17 was developed within the ACP's Digital
Product Development Department, led by Brian Sweigard
(Director). Other members of the team included Dan
Barron (Senior Web Application Developer/Architect),
Chris Forrest (Senior Software Developer/Design Lead),
Kara Kronenwetter (Senior Web Developer), Brad Lord
(Senior Web Application Developer), John McKnight
(Senior Web Developer), and Nate Pershall (Senior Web
Developer).

The College also wishes to acknowledge that many other
persons, too numerous to mention, have contributed to
the production of this program. Without their dedicated
efforts, this program would not have been possible.

MKSAP Resource Site
(mksap.acponline.org)

The MKSAP Resource Site (mksap.acponline.org) is a
continually updated site that provides links to MKSAP 17
online answer sheets for print subscribers; the latest
details on Continuing Medical Education (CME) and
Maintenance of Certification (MOC) in the United States,
Canada, and Australia; errata; and other new information.

ABIM Maintenance of Certification

Check the MKSAP Resource Site (mksap.acponline.org)
for the latest information on how MKSAP tests can be
used to apply to the American Board of Internal Medicine
for Maintenance of Certification (MOC) points.

Royal College Maintenance of Certification

In Canada, MKSAP 17 is an Accredited Self-Assessment
Program (Section 3) as defined by the Maintenance of
Certification (MOC) Program of The Royal College of
Physicians and Surgeons of Canada and approved by
the Canadian Society of Internal Medicine on December
9, 2014. Approval extends from July 31, 2015 until July
31, 2018 for the Part A sections. Approval extends from
December 31, 2015 to December 31, 2018 for the Part B
sections.

Fellows of the Royal College may earn three credits per
hour for participating in MKSAP 17 under Section 3.
MKSAP 17 also meets multiple CanMEDS Roles, including that of Medical Expert, Communicator, Collaborator,
Manager, Health Advocate, Scholar, and Professional.
For information on how to apply MKSAP 17 Continuing
Medical Education (CME) credits to the Royal College
MOC Program, visit the MKSAP Resource Site at
mksap.acponline.org.

The Royal Australasian College of Physicians CPD Program

In Australia, MKSAP 17 is a Category 3 program that may
be used by Fellows of The Royal Australasian College
of Physicians (RACP) to meet mandatory Continuing
Professional Development (CPD) points. Two CPD credits are awarded for each of the 200 *AMA PRA Category 1
Credits*™ available in MKSAP 17. More information about
using MKSAP 17 for this purpose is available at the MKSAP
Resource Site at mksap.acponline.org and at www.racp.
edu.au. CPD credits earned through MKSAP 17 should be
reported at the MyCPD site at www.racp.edu.au/mycpd.

Continuing Medical Education

The American College of Physicians (ACP) is accredited
by the Accreditation Council for Continuing Medical
Education (ACCME) to provide continuing medical education for physicians.

The ACP designates this enduring material, MKSAP 17,
for a maximum of 200 *AMA PRA Category 1 Credits*™.
Physicians should claim only the credit commensurate
with the extent of their participation in the activity.

Up to 21 *AMA PRA Category 1 Credits*™ are available
from July 31, 2015, to July 31, 2018, for the MKSAP 17
Cardiovascular Medicine section.

Learning Objectives

The learning objectives of MKSAP 17 are to:

- Close gaps between actual care in your practice and preferred standards of care, based on best evidence
- Diagnose disease states that are less common and sometimes overlooked or confusing
- Improve management of comorbid conditions that can complicate patient care
- Determine when to refer patients for surgery or care by subspecialists
- Pass the ABIM Certification Examination
- Pass the ABIM Maintenance of Certification Examination

Target Audience

- General internists and primary care physicians
- Subspecialists who need to remain up-to-date in internal medicine and in areas outside of their own subspecialty area
- Residents preparing for the certification examination in internal medicine
- Physicians preparing for maintenance of certification in internal medicine (recertification)

Earn "Instantaneous" CME Credits Online

Print subscribers can enter their answers online to earn instantaneous Continuing Medical Education (CME) credits. You can submit your answers using online answer sheets that are provided at mksap.acponline.org, where a record of your MKSAP 17 credits will be available. To earn CME credits, you need to answer all of the questions in a test and earn a score of at least 50% correct (number of correct answers divided by the total number of questions). Take any of the following approaches:

1. Use the printed answer sheet at the back of this book to record your answers. Go to mksap.acponline.org, access the appropriate online answer sheet, transcribe your answers, and submit your test for instantaneous CME credits. There is no additional fee for this service.

2. Go to mksap.acponline.org, access the appropriate online answer sheet, directly enter your answers, and submit your test for instantaneous CME credits. There is no additional fee for this service.

3. Pay a $15 processing fee per answer sheet and submit the printed answer sheet at the back of this book by mail or fax, as instructed on the answer sheet. Make sure you calculate your score and fax the answer sheet to 215-351-2799 or mail the answer sheet to Member and Customer Service, American College of Physicians, 190 N. Independence Mall West, Philadelphia, PA 19106-1572, using the courtesy envelope provided in

your MKSAP 17 slipcase. You will need your 10-digit order number and 8-digit ACP ID number, which are printed on your packing slip. Please allow 4 to 6 weeks for your score report to be emailed back to you. Be sure to include your email address for a response.

If you do not have a 10-digit order number and 8-digit ACP ID number or if you need help creating a user name and password to access the MKSAP 17 online answer sheets, go to mksap.acponline.org or email custserv@acponline.org.

Disclosure Policy

It is the policy of the American College of Physicians (ACP) to ensure balance, independence, objectivity, and scientific rigor in all of its educational activities. To this end, and consistent with the policies of the ACP and the Accreditation Council for Continuing Medical Education (ACCME), contributors to all ACP continuing medical education activities are required to disclose all relevant financial relationships with any entity producing, marketing, re-selling, or distributing health care goods or services consumed by, or used on, patients. Contributors are required to use generic names in the discussion of therapeutic options and are required to identify any unapproved, off-label, or investigative use of commercial products or devices. Where a trade name is used, all available trade names for the same product type are also included. If trade-name products manufactured by companies with whom contributors have relationships are discussed, contributors are asked to provide evidence-based citations in support of the discussion. The information is reviewed by the committee responsible for producing this text. If necessary, adjustments to topics or contributors' roles in content development are made to balance the discussion. Further, all readers of this text are asked to evaluate the content for evidence of commercial bias and send any relevant comments to mksap_editors@acponline.org so that future decisions about content and contributors can be made in light of this information.

Resolution of Conflicts

To resolve all conflicts of interest and influences of vested interests, the American College of Physicians (ACP) precluded members of the content-creation committee from deciding on any content issues that involved generic or trade-name products associated with proprietary entities with which these committee members had relationships. In addition, content was based on best evidence and updated clinical care guidelines, when such evidence and guidelines were available. Contributors' disclosure information can be found with the list of contributors' names and those of ACP principal staff listed in the beginning of this book.

Hospital-Based Medicine

For the convenience of subscribers who provide care in hospital settings, content that is specific to the hospital setting has been highlighted in blue. Hospital icons (🄷) highlight where the hospital-based content begins, continues over more than one page, and ends.

High Value Care Key Points

Key Points in the text that relate to High Value Care concepts (that is, concepts that discuss balancing clinical benefit with costs and harms) are designated by the HVC icon (**HVC**).

Educational Disclaimer

The editors and publisher of MKSAP 17 recognize that the development of new material offers many opportunities for error. Despite our best efforts, some errors may persist in print. Drug dosage schedules are, we believe, accurate and in accordance with current standards. Readers are advised, however, to ensure that the recommended dosages in MKSAP 17 concur with the information provided in the product information material. This is especially important in cases of new, infrequently used, or highly toxic drugs. Application of the information in MKSAP 17 remains the professional responsibility of the practitioner.

The primary purpose of MKSAP 17 is educational. Information presented, as well as publications, technologies, products, and/or services discussed, is intended to inform subscribers about the knowledge, techniques, and experiences of the contributors. A diversity of professional opinion exists, and the views of the contributors are their own and not those of the American College of Physicians (ACP). Inclusion of any material in the program does not constitute endorsement or recommendation by the ACP. The ACP does not warrant the safety, reliability, accuracy, completeness, or usefulness of and disclaims any and all liability for damages and claims that may result from the use of information, publications, technologies, products, and/or services discussed in this program.

Publisher's Information

Unauthorized Use of This Book Is Against the Law

MKSAP 17 ISBN: 978-1-938245-18-3
(Cardiovascular Medicine) ISBN: 978-1-938245-19-0

Printed in the United States of America.

For order information in the United States or Canada call 800-523-1546, extension 2600. All other countries call 215-351-2600, (M-F, 9 AM – 5 PM ET). Fax inquiries to 215-351-2799 or email to custserv@acponline.org.

Errata

Errata for MKSAP 17 will be available through the MKSAP Resource Site at mksap.acponline.org as new information becomes known to the editors.

Table of Contents

Cardiovascular Medicine High Value Care Recommendations

The American College of Physicians, in collaboration with multiple other organizations, is engaged in a worldwide initiative to promote the practice of High Value Care (HVC). The goals of the HVC initiative are to improve health care outcomes by providing care of proven benefit and reducing costs by avoiding unnecessary and even harmful interventions. The initiative comprises several programs that integrate the important concept of health care value (balancing clinical benefit with costs and harms) for a given intervention into a broad range of educational materials to address the needs of trainees, practicing physicians, and patients.

HVC content has been integrated into MKSAP 17 in several important ways. MKSAP 17 now includes HVC-identified key points in the text, HVC-focused multiple choice questions, and, for subscribers to MKSAP Digital, an HVC custom quiz. From the text and questions, we have generated the following list of HVC recommendations that meet the definition below of high value care and bring us closer to our goal of improving patient outcomes while conserving finite resources.

High Value Care Recommendation: A recommendation to choose diagnostic and management strategies for patients in specific clinical situations that balance clinical benefit with cost and harms with the goal of improving patient outcomes.

Below are the High Value Care Recommendations for the Cardiovascular Medicine section of MKSAP 17.

- Current guidelines do not support the use of high-sensitivity C-reactive protein (hsCRP) evaluation in the general population, but hsCRP testing may be used in intermediate-risk patients in whom choice of therapy may be affected by reclassification of risk.
- There is currently no role for the routine measurement of Lp(a) lipoprotein levels, homocysteine levels, or evaluation of lipid particle size as these tests are expensive and no studies to date have shown that treatment targeted to these levels affects outcomes.
- The evaluation of subclinical disease with coronary artery calcium scoring may be appropriate to further risk stratify intermediate-risk patients but is not a component of routine risk assessment.
- Aspirin should not routinely be given to patients with diabetes mellitus who are at low cardiovascular risk (men younger than 50 years and women younger than 60 years

without other major risk factors such as hypertension or tobacco use) (see Item 88).
- Stress testing is most efficacious in patients with an intermediate pretest probability of coronary artery disease (10%-90%), because it is these patients who, by the result of their stress test, can be reclassified into higher or lower risk categories.
- Exercise electrocardiographic testing is recommended as the initial test of choice in patients who are able to exercise with a normal baseline electrocardiogram and an intermediate pretest probability of coronary artery disease based on age, sex, and symptoms (see Item 87).
- Measurement of coronary artery calcium should be limited to a select group of asymptomatic patients with an intermediate Framingham risk score (10%-20%) in whom results will influence treatment strategy because of its associated cost and radiation exposure.
- Routine yearly imaging evaluation of structural heart disease in asymptomatic patients is usually not indicated.
- Patients with grade 1 or 2 midsystolic murmurs who are asymptomatic with no associated findings and those with continuous murmurs suggestive of a venous hum or mammary souffle do not warrant echocardiographic evaluation.
- For stable angina pectoris, percutaneous coronary intervention is reserved for patients with refractory symptoms while on optimal medical therapy, those who are unable to tolerate optimal medical therapy owing to side effects, or those with high-risk features on noninvasive imaging.
- Clinical practice guidelines do not recommend the routine use of ECG monitoring, stress testing, or anatomic testing (coronary CT angiography or invasive angiography) in asymptomatic patients after percutaneous coronary intervention or coronary artery bypass graft surgery.
- Routine stress testing is not currently recommended for asymptomatic patients following an acute coronary syndrome who are not entering a cardiac rehabilitation program.
- Evaluation of unusual causes of heart failure should not be performed routinely but should be performed when there are suggestions of specific diseases by history or physical examination findings (see Item 116).
- In patients with chronic heart failure who are clinically stable, annual or more frequent follow-up echocardiography rarely provides therapeutic or diagnostic benefit and is not recommended.
- Patients hospitalized for heart failure who are scheduled for a follow-up appointment within 1 week after discharge

have a reduced risk of future heart failure hospitalization (see Item 34).

- Patients with asymptomatic, mild aortic stenosis or regurgitation require echocardiography every 3 to 5 years.
- Asymptomatic patients with moderate aortic regurgitation should be evaluated clinically on a yearly basis and have echocardiography performed every 1 to 2 years, but they do not require medical or surgical intervention (see Item 59).
- Patients with asymptomatic, severe aortic stenosis with preserved left ventricular function may be managed with close clinical follow-up and echocardiography every 6 to 12 months and should not undergo valve replacement (see Item 20).
- Patients with an asymptomatic bicuspid aortic valve should undergo surveillance transthoracic echocardiography yearly if the aortic root or ascending aortic diameter is greater than 4 cm (see Item 97).
- Infective endocarditis prophylaxis should be limited to those with a prosthetic cardiac valve; a history of infective endocarditis; unrepaired cyanotic congenital heart disease or repaired congenital heart defect with prosthesis or shunt (≤6 months post-procedure) or residual defect; or valvulopathy following cardiac transplantation.
- Antibiotic prophylaxis to prevent bacterial endocarditis is not recommended for nondental procedures, including transesophageal echocardiography and genitourinary or gastrointestinal procedures, in the absence of active infection (see Item 25).
- There is no indication for patent foramen ovale closure or for antiplatelet therapy in asymptomatic patients, and randomized trials do not support patent foramen ovale closure to reduce risk of recurrent stroke or migraine.
- A small atrial septal defect (pulmonary-to-systemic blood flow ratio [Qp:Qs] <1.5:1) with no associated symptoms or right heart enlargement can be followed clinically.
- A small membranous ventricular septal defect without left heart enlargement, pulmonary hypertension, recurrent endocarditis, or valve regurgitation can be observed clinically (see Item 45).

- Screening of asymptomatic patients for abnormalities of the thoracic aorta should be reserved for patients with underlying vascular pathology (such as Marfan or Ehlers-Danlos syndrome), a bicuspid aortic valve, or a family history of aortic disease.
- Invasive imaging of the aorta by angiography is rarely necessary for the diagnosis of acute disease; it should be reserved for patients in whom a percutaneous intervention is planned.
- Diuretics, particularly in high doses, will exacerbate the propensity towards dynamic left ventricular outflow tract obstruction and, therefore, should be avoided in patients with hypertrophic cardiomyopathy (see Item 5).
- When an atrial septal aneurysm is identified incidentally, no further evaluation, medical treatment, or intervention is needed (see Item 10).
- Influenza vaccine should be administered to patients with established cardiovascular disease to reduce the risk of future cardiovascular events (see Item 13).
- Accelerated idioventricular rhythm is a common complication following coronary reperfusion and does not require intervention when it occurs within 24 hours of reperfusion (see Item 42).
- Routine screening for coronary artery disease in asymptomatic patients with diabetes mellitus does not reduce mortality (see Item 65).
- Supervised exercise therapy can effectively treat claudication, with increases in pain-free walking time and maximal walking time, and is recommended as part of the initial treatment regimen for intermittent claudication (see Item 84).
- Asymptomatic first-degree atrioventricular block with bifascicular block does not require pacemaker implantation (see Item 109).
- Patients with acute pericarditis who do not have high-risk features (fever, leukocytosis, acute trauma, abnormal cardiac biomarkers, immunocompromise, oral anticoagulant use, large pericardial effusions, or evidence of cardiac tamponade) can be managed medically on an outpatient basis with close clinical follow-up (see Item 114).

Cardiovascular Medicine

Epidemiology and Risk Factors

Overview

In the United States, the mortality rate from cardiovascular disease (CVD), including heart disease, stroke, peripheral vascular disease, hypertension, and heart failure has steadily declined over the past decade—33% from 1999 to 2009, likely as a result of better prevention and acute care efforts. Nonetheless, CVD is the leading killer of both men and women, and although mortality of CVD is decreasing, CVD prevalence is increasing. By 2030, according to the American Heart Association's Heart Disease and Stroke Statistics, more than 40% of the U.S. population is projected to have some form of CVD. More than one in three American adults currently have some form of CVD, and the prevalence increases from more than 10% in those aged 20 to 39 years to more than 70% in those aged 60 to 79 years. Based on data from the Framingham Heart Study, two out of three men and one out of two women will develop CVD in their lifetime. Despite the decreasing mortality, hospitalizations for cardiovascular-related diseases have steadily continued to rise. There were nearly 6 million hospital discharges for cardiovascular-related diseases in 2009, with an estimated cost of $312.6 billion.

The prevalence of heart failure continues to rise, with a predicted prevalence in the United States of 25% by 2030. It is estimated that 5.1 million Americans older than 20 years have a diagnosis of heart failure. Currently, the incidence is 1/100 annually in those older than 65 years. Most of these patients have a history of hypertension. Both systolic dysfunction and diastolic dysfunction are associated with the development of symptomatic heart failure, and the prevalence of heart failure with preserved ejection fraction (diastolic dysfunction) is increasing. Mortality in heart failure is quite high—nearly 50% mortality at 5 years.

Cardiovascular Disease in Women

Since 1984, the number of deaths from CVD has been greater for women than men and highest among black women. More than 400,000 women died of CVD in 2009, 51% of all CVD deaths. Women have a higher mortality rate after myocardial infarction: 26% in women versus 19% in men older than 45 years. The death rate for women with heart failure is higher than among men, although women are often older. Incidence of and mortality from stroke is highest among women, with the highest among black women.

Women have a higher prevalence of risk factors for CVD, including elevated cholesterol levels, diabetes mellitus, hypertension, and inactivity. Only tobacco use is higher among men.

More women present with angina than men, but women often have other symptoms in addition to chest pain. Women have "atypical" symptoms more frequently than men, including nausea, shortness of breath, and unusual fatigue. More than two thirds of women who die suddenly from coronary heart disease either did not recognize the symptoms or had no previous symptoms. Women undergo fewer revascularization procedures than men, with 25% of coronary artery bypass surgeries and nearly 33% of percutaneous coronary interventions occurring in women.

Ethnicity and Cardiovascular Disease

The prevalence of CVD and risk factors in the United States vary by ethnicity. American Indians and Alaska Natives have the highest rate of heart disease (12.7%), followed by whites (11.1%), blacks or African Americans (10.7%), Hispanics or Latinos (8.6%), and Asians (7.4%). Peripheral arterial disease affects nearly 8.5% of Americans older than 40 years, and prevalence is highest among older persons, non-Hispanic blacks, and women. The population most affected by heart failure is African Americans, at a rate of 4.6/1000 person-years, followed by Hispanic, white, and Chinese Americans.

Cardiovascular risk factors also vary among ethnicities. Blacks have the highest rate of hypertension, at 33.4% (higher in black women), followed by American Indians or Alaska Natives (25.8%), whites (23.3%), Hispanics or Latinos (22.2%), and Asians (18.7%). Blacks have the highest prevalence of two or more cardiovascular risk factors (48.7%). The prevalence of risk factors is increased with decreasing levels of education and income. Obesity and lack of physical activity are highest among Hispanic/Latino adults and non-Hispanic blacks.

Environmental influences on cardiovascular risk factors are changing the prevalence of CVD in certain populations. In countries with previously low rates of CVD, rates of disease are increasing with the adoption of Western eating habits and increasing tobacco use. With declining rates of infant mortality and death from infectious diseases, the influence of urbanization and change in traditional lifestyles are resulting in increasing rates of CVD.

Genetics in Cardiovascular Disease

Family history of premature (male <45 years; female <55 years) coronary artery disease (CAD) significantly increases risk of CVD. Having a parent with premature CAD doubles risk of myocardial infarction in men and increases risk in women by 70%. CAD in a sibling increases risk by 50%. Genetic predisposition as well as shared environment may contribute to increased risk in family members. Although prediction models based on the genetics of CVD are not yet available, research continues at a rapid pace.

Lifestyle Risk Factors

As much as 90% of the risk for myocardial infarction has been attributed to modifiable risk factors, with elevated cholesterol levels, smoking, and psychosocial stressors accounting for a significant portion of the attributable risk. The attributable risk for myocardial infarction is highest for cholesterol levels, followed by current smoking, psychosocial stressors, diabetes, hypertension, abdominal obesity, no alcohol intake, inadequate exercise, and irregular consumption of fruits and vegetables.

Elevated cholesterol levels increase the risk of CVD, and multiple studies have shown that reductions in cholesterol levels, particularly LDL cholesterol, reduce risk. Nearly 14% of adults older than 20 years have total cholesterol levels greater than 240 mg/dL (6.21 mmol/L); approximately 6% of adults are estimated to have undiagnosed hypercholesterolemia. Elevated LDL cholesterol and low HDL cholesterol levels are independent risk factors for CVD. For every 1% decrease in LDL cholesterol level, there is a corresponding 1% decrease in risk for coronary artery disease. The risk reduction is even greater with changes in HDL cholesterol, with a risk reduction of 2% to 3% for every 1% increase in HDL cholesterol level. However, randomized clinical trials evaluating pharmacologic therapies that raise HDL cholesterol levels in patients with well-treated LDL cholesterol levels have not shown reduction in clinical endpoints. Long-standing guidelines (Adult Treatment Panel III [ATP III]) have provided treatment goals for LDL and non-HDL cholesterol levels based on cardiovascular risk factors and Framingham risk score. In 2013, the American College of Cardiology and the American Heart Association (ACC/AHA) published revised guidelines that treat lipid blood levels according to cardiovascular risk, rather than LDL cholesterol targets (see MKSAP 17 General Internal Medicine, Dyslipidemia).

The use of tobacco has declined over the past few decades, but despite this decline, in 2011, more than 21.3% of men, 16.7% of women, and 18% of high school students were smokers. The rates were highest among American Indian/Alaska Natives and non-Hispanic black males and lowest among Hispanic females. Tobacco use increases the risk of CVD, including coronary heart disease, stroke, and peripheral vascular disease, for which smoking is a major risk factor, and increases CVD mortality by 2 to 3 times. The risk of coronary artery disease is increased by 25% in women who smoke. Smoking increases the risk of stroke by 2 to 4 times. Secondhand smoke is also a risk factor for CVD, increasing the risk by 25% to 30%. Smoking cessation substantially reduces cardiovascular risk within 2 years, and this risk returns to the level of a nonsmoker within 5 years. Efforts to assess smoking status and provide assistance with cessation should be made at every encounter (see MKSAP 17 General Internal Medicine, Routine Care of the Healthy Patient).

Nearly one in three adults in the United States older than 20 years has hypertension, and the rates are equal among men and women. Nearly 30% of adults older than 20 years have pre-hypertension (systolic blood pressure 120-139 mm Hg; diastolic blood pressure 80-89 mm Hg). The rates increase with age, with a prevalence greater than 70% in persons older than 65 years. Treatment of hypertension reduces risk for cardiovascular events, including stroke, and reduces end-organ damage such as heart failure and kidney disease. Although the prevalence of blood pressure control (that is, blood pressure within recommended ranges) has improved in the United States from less than 30% two decades ago (1988-1994), it still is only 50% (2007-2008).

Sedentary lifestyle, poor diet, and obesity contribute to increased cardiovascular risk and increased risk for diabetes. Nearly one third of all U.S. adults report no leisure time activity, and less than 30% of high school students engaged in 60 minutes of daily physical activity; this rate was lowest among girls. Between 1971 and 2004, total energy consumption increased by 22% in women and 10% in men. Average fruit and vegetable consumption was 2.4 to 4 servings daily (recommended, >5 daily) and was lowest among blacks. The increased caloric intake coupled with decreased physical activity has led to an increased incidence of obesity. More than two thirds of the American population older than 20 years are overweight (BMI 25-29.9) with more than one third obese (BMI >30). In children and adolescents between the ages of 2 and 19 years, nearly 33% are obese or overweight and 17% of these children are obese.

Psychosocial stressors are an important contributor to cardiovascular risk. These include depression, anger, and anxiety, and are associated with worse outcomes. Depression has been associated with higher risk for cardiovascular events, and psychosocial stressors also affect the course of treatment and adherence to healthy lifestyles after an event. Awareness of these factors and appropriate therapies may improve outcomes in these individuals.

Impaired glucose control is a significant component of the metabolic syndrome, which is characterized by elevated glucose, central obesity, low HDL cholesterol, elevated triglycerides, and high blood pressure. More than 34% of adults older than 20 years meet the criteria for metabolic syndrome (three of the five components). The presence of metabolic syndrome is associated with an increased risk of CVD. This risk increases with an increased number of components and also appears to be higher among women. The National Diabetes Prevention Program found that in persons at high risk for diabetes, improved food choices and at least 150 minutes of exercise weekly led to 5% to 7% weight loss and reduced the risk of developing diabetes by 58%, but no interventions have shown a reduction in CVD events to date.

- Elevated cholesterol levels, smoking, and psychosocial stressors are the greatest modifiable risk factors for cardiovascular disease.

Specific Risk Groups

Diabetes Mellitus

The presence of diabetes mellitus is associated with increased cardiovascular risk, particularly among women. Persons with diabetes have a 2 to 4 times increased risk of CVD, with more than two thirds of those with diabetes eventually dying of heart disease. The risk of stroke is increased 1.8- to 6-fold in persons with diabetes. The presence of diabetes in those older than 65 years is nearly 27%. In those aged 12-19 years, the prevalence of diabetes and prediabetes is increasing, from 9% to 23% from 1999-2007. Diabetes is often undiagnosed, and is frequently diagnosed at the time of an acute event such as myocardial infarction. Appropriate treatment of cardiovascular risk factors in persons with diabetes is associated with reduced cardiovascular risk. The most recent cholesterol guidelines recommend moderate- or high-intensity statin therapy in patients aged 40 to 75 years with diabetes. Patients with diabetes aged 40 to 75 years with a 10-year atherosclerotic cardiovascular disease (ASCVD) risk greater than or equal to 7.5% should receive high-intensity statin therapy because of their increased risk. In patients with diabetes in this age group with a 10-year risk below 7.5%, moderate-intensity statin therapy is recommended.

Chronic Kidney Disease

Chronic kidney disease (CKD) is associated with higher cardiovascular mortality, and more patients with kidney disease will die of CVD than will go on to have end-stage kidney disease requiring dialysis. Chronic kidney disease shares many of the same risk factors for CVD such as hypertension, diabetes, and smoking. The exact etiology of the high death rate in patients with CKD is uncertain and may be related to a higher incidence of fatal arrhythmias, lack of adequate therapies at the time of an acute cardiovascular event, or multi-organ changes related to kidney failure.

Systemic Inflammatory Conditions

Patients with systemic inflammatory conditions, such as systemic lupus erythematosus (SLE) and rheumatoid arthritis, have an increased risk of CVD. Most deaths in persons with SLE and nearly 40% of deaths in those with rheumatoid arthritis are cardiovascular and, in particular, heart failure related. The risk of CVD increases with the duration of the underlying inflammatory condition. The risk of CVD increases from two times that of the general population to three times after 10 years' duration of rheumatoid arthritis. The increased atherosclerotic burden is likely a result of both the inflammatory process of the systemic disease, including a prothrombotic state, as well as the presence of traditional cardiovascular risk factors.

Calculating Cardiovascular Risk

Cardiovascular risk scores should be utilized to stratify patients for appropriate prevention targets. Traditionally, the Framingham risk score has been used to estimate the 10-year risk of a major cardiovascular event (myocardial infarction or coronary death). An online Framingham risk calculator is available at http://cvdrisk.nhlbi.nih.gov/calculator.asp. Using this method, a 10-year risk of ASCVD of less than 10% is considered low risk, 10% to 20% is classified as intermediate risk, and above 20% is designated as high risk. Age is the component that drives most of the risk, with increasing age reflected in increased risk. The Framingham risk score underestimates risk in women and minority populations. In an effort to account for the underestimation in women, the Reynolds risk score was developed, which is a sex-specific score for both men and women that includes family history and high-sensitivity C-reactive protein (hsCRP) levels (www.reynoldsriskscore.org).

The Pooled Cohort Equations are a new risk assessment instrument developed from multiple community-based cohorts (including the Framingham study) that includes a broader range of variables than the Framingham score when evaluating 10-year ASCVD risk. Its use as a primary risk assessment tool was recommended in the 2013 ACC/AHA Guideline on Assessment of Cardiovascular Risk. The ACC/AHA CV risk calculator includes age, sex, race, total and HDL cholesterol levels, systolic blood pressure, blood pressure–lowering medication use, diabetes status, and smoking status. Using this method, a 10-year risk of ASCVD of below 5% is considered low risk, 5% to below 7.5% is classified as intermediate risk, and 7.5% or above is designated as high risk. The new risk calculator can be accessed at http://my.americanheart.org/professional/StatementsGuidelines/PreventionGuidelines/Prevention-Guidelines_UCM_457698_SubHomePage.jsp.

- Cardiovascular risk scores should be utilized to stratify patients for appropriate prevention targets; risk assessment tools include the Framingham risk score, the Reynolds risk score, and the American College of Cardiology/American Heart Association's cardiovascular risk calculator based on the Pooled Cohort Equations.

Emerging Risk Factors

Because atherosclerotic disease is thought to be in part an inflammatory process, hsCRP measurement has been investigated for enhancing risk prediction. Current guidelines do not support the use of hsCRP evaluation in the general population. However, hsCRP testing may be used in intermediate-risk patients (Framingham 10-year risk score of 10%-20%) in whom choice of therapy may be affected by reclassification of risk. Elevated hsCRP levels should be rechecked within 2 weeks, and other potential causes of infection or inflammation should be ruled out. Although statin therapy has been shown to lower hsCRP levels, therapy targeting hsCRP alone is not appropriate as patients should be treated according to cardiovascular risk.

Although elevated levels of Lp(a) lipoprotein and homocysteine have been associated with elevated cardiovascular risk, these tests should not be routinely performed. Interventions to reduce homocysteine levels with folic acid supplementation have not been shown to reduce cardiovascular events. Although epidemiologic evidence supports the association between elevated levels of Lp(a) lipoprotein and cardiovascular events, to date no trials have shown that treatment to lower Lp(a) lipoprotein levels lowers risk. There is currently no role for the evaluation of lipid particle size and number. No studies to date have shown that treatment targeted to particle size and number affects outcomes.

The evaluation of subclinical disease with coronary artery calcium (CAC) scoring may be appropriate to further risk stratify intermediate-risk patients but is not a component of routine risk assessment. Evidence of calcification of coronary vessels is indicative of atherosclerotic disease, but the absence of calcification does not rule out the presence of soft plaque.

KEY POINTS

HVC   • Current guidelines do not support the use of high-sensitivity C-reactive protein (hsCRP) evaluation in the general population, but hsCRP testing may be used in intermediate-risk patients in whom choice of therapy may be affected by reclassification of risk.

HVC   • There is currently no role for the routine measurement of Lp(a) lipoprotein levels or homocysteine levels or evaluation of lipid particle size as these tests are expensive and no studies to date have shown that treatment targeted to these levels affects outcomes.

HVC   • The evaluation of subclinical disease with coronary artery calcium scoring may be appropriate to further risk stratify intermediate-risk patients but is not a component of routine risk assessment.

Aspirin for Primary Prevention

Aspirin is a powerful agent for both primary and secondary prevention of coronary artery disease. Aspirin for secondary prevention is discussed under Coronary Artery Disease. For primary prevention of myocardial infarction, data suggest that there is greater benefit in men, particularly those older than 45 years. For women, benefit outweighs risk of aspirin therapy after the age of 65 years. Between the ages of 55 and 65 years, the risk of stroke is reduced in women on aspirin therapy. Guidance for using aspirin for primary prevention of myocardial infarction and stroke is provided in **Table 1** and **Table 2**.

It is important to balance the benefits of aspirin therapy with the risks of gastrointestinal (GI) bleeding. The risk of serious bleeding is greatly increased in patients with a history of GI ulcers and who use NSAIDs, and these factors should be considered when assessing the benefits and harms of using aspirin in the individual patient.

Aspirin should not be routinely given to patients with diabetes who are at low risk for CVD (men <50 years and women <60 years with no major additional CVD risk factors; 10-year CVD risk <5%). It is reasonable to give low-dose aspirin to adults with diabetes and no previous history of vascular disease who are at increased CVD risk (10-year Framingham risk >10%) and without increased risk for bleeding.

KEY POINTS

• In men ages 45 to 79 years, aspirin for primary prevention of myocardial infarction is recommended if the benefit of treatment outweighs the risk of gastrointestinal bleeding.

• In women ages 55 to 79 years, aspirin for primary prevention of stroke is recommended if the benefit of treatment outweighs the risk of gastrointestinal bleeding.

• Aspirin should not be routinely given to patients with diabetes who are at low risk; that is, men younger than 50 years and women younger than 60 years with no major additional cardiovascular risk factors.   HVC

TABLE 1. Use of Aspirin for Primary Prevention of Cardiovascular Disease	
Patient Category	**Recommendation**
Men age 45-79 years	Aspirin recommended when potential benefit of reduction in MI outweighs risk of GI bleeding
Women age 55-79 years	Aspirin recommended when potential benefit of reduction in ischemic stroke outweighs risk of GI bleeding
Men/women age >80 years	Insufficient evidence for primary prevention
Men age <45 years, women age <55 years	Aspirin not recommended for prevention of MI in men or stroke in women

GI = gastrointestinal; MI = myocardial infarction.

Adapted with permission from U.S. Preventive Services Task Force. Aspirin for the prevention of cardiovascular disease: U.S. Preventive Services Task Force recommendation statement. Ann Intern Med. 2009 Mar 17;150(6):396-404. [PMID: 19293072]

TABLE 2. Risk Level at Which CHD Events Prevented Exceed GI Harms in Patients Taking Daily Aspirin for Primary Prevention

Men		Women	
10-Year CHD Risk[a]		**10-Year Stroke Risk[b]**	
Age 45-59 years	≥4%	Age 55-59 years	≥3%
Age 60-69 years	≥9%	Age 60-69 years	≥8%
Age 70-79 years	≥12%	Age 70-79 years	≥11%

CHD = coronary heart disease; GI = gastrointestinal.

[a]Risk factors for CHD include age, diabetes mellitus, total cholesterol level, HDL cholesterol level, blood pressure, and smoking. CHD risk estimation tool: http://cvdrisk.nhlbi.nih.gov/calculator.asp. (Note: This is the Framingham risk score.)

[b]Risk factors for ischemic stroke include age, high blood pressure, diabetes mellitus, smoking, history of cardiovascular disease, atrial fibrillation, and left ventricular hypertrophy.

NOTE: This table applies to adults who are not taking NSAIDs and who do not have upper GI pain or a history of GI ulcers.

Adapted with permission from U.S. Preventive Services Task Force. Aspirin for the prevention of cardiovascular disease: U.S. Preventive Services Task Force recommendation statement. Ann Intern Med. 2009 Mar 17;150(6):396-404. [PMID: 19293072]

Diagnostic Testing in Cardiology

Clinical History and Physical Examination

The initial step in evaluating for heart disease is a thorough history and physical examination. Specifically, a careful exploration of changes in functional status, associated symptoms, and the timing and nature of symptoms will help focus the assessment and guide selection of appropriate testing, if indicated.

Cardiovascular testing provides both diagnostic and prognostic information and its use should be guided by symptoms, the level of risk for heart disease, and whether outcomes may be altered by interventions based on testing results.

Diagnostic Testing for Atherosclerotic Coronary Disease

Cardiac Stress Testing

Patients are referred for stress testing to establish the diagnosis of coronary artery disease (CAD) most often because of new onset of or a change in symptoms. The utility of stress testing should be interpreted in the context of the pretest likelihood of disease. Those with low probability of disease, such as younger patients, have a higher incidence of false-positive tests and may undergo unnecessary testing without changing patient outcomes. Those with a high probability of disease should proceed directly to an invasive diagnostic strategy, such as cardiac catheterization, because the risk of a false-negative result and missed diagnosis is too high. Furthermore, a negative test in a high-risk patient would not significantly change the post-test probability of CAD, and therefore would not change management. Stress testing is most clinically appropriate in patients with an intermediate risk of CAD. It is these patients who, by the result of their

stress test, can be reclassified into higher or lower risk categories. Stress testing also has important prognostic value for predicting the risk of myocardial infarction and death in selected patients. For example, in patients with a previous history of CAD and worsening cardiac symptoms, stress testing is helpful to assess for possible recurrent or progressive disease. However, although the leading cause of death in patients with diabetes mellitus is cardiovascular disease, routine stress testing in asymptomatic patients with diabetes has not been shown to reduce mortality.

The modalities able to detect cardiac ischemia are highly dependent on the degree of impairment of coronary blood flow. The earliest changes with mild stenosis are perfusion changes detectable only with highly sensitive modalities, such as nuclear or cardiac magnetic resonance (CMR) imaging. With progressive coronary occlusion, diastolic dysfunction followed by systolic dysfunction may be seen by imaging studies such as echocardiography. Only when there is significant coronary stenosis will electrocardiographic (ECG) changes be seen and symptoms occur.

The many different types of tests to diagnose CAD can be broadly categorized as assessing either functional or anatomic evidence of ischemia. Functional studies evaluate for obstructive CAD from evidence of ECG changes, myocardial perfusion abnormalities, or wall motion abnormalities, usually under stress conditions. Anatomic studies assess percentage stenosis of the coronary vessels at rest, which can be visualized by single-photon emission CT (SPECT), PET/CT scan, or CMR imaging study. These imaging modalities may also be used to quantify infarction size and assess myocardial viability. More specific signs of ischemia such as reduced regional contractility can be assessed by echocardiography or MRI.

Testing modalities for suspected CAD are summarized in **Table 3**. In intermediate-risk patients who are able to exercise and have a normal baseline ECG, the initial type of stress testing should be exercise stress testing. The additional prognostic information available with exercise, including functional

TABLE 3. Diagnostic Testing for Coronary Artery Disease

Diagnostic Test	Utility	Advantages	Limitations
Exercise Stress Testing			
Exercise ECG	Initial diagnostic test in most patients with suspected CAD	Data acquired on exercise capacity, blood pressure and heart rate response, and provoked symptoms	Not useful when baseline ECG is abnormal (LVH, LBBB, paced rhythm, WPW syndrome, >1 mm ST-segment depression)
Stress echocardiography	Recommended when baseline ECG is abnormal or when information on a particular area of myocardium at risk is needed	Exercise data acquired along with imaging for wall motion abnormalities to indicate ischemia	Image quality is suboptimal in some patients but can be improved with microbubble transpulmonary contrast
		Allows evaluation of valve function and pulmonary pressures	Image interpretation is difficult when baseline wall motion abnormalities are present
		Relatively portable and less costly than nuclear protocols	Diagnostic accuracy decreases with single-vessel disease or delayed stress image acquisition
		Entire study is completed in <1 h	
Nuclear SPECT perfusion	Recommended when baseline ECG is abnormal or when information on a particular area of myocardium at risk is needed With LBBB, conduction delay in the septum may cause false-positive abnormality; this can be improved with the use of vasodilator stress	Gating (image acquisition coordinated with the cardiac cycle), use of higher energy agents such as technetium, and techniques used to correct for attenuation provide improved specificity Late reperfusion imaging allows evaluation of myocardial viability if thallium is used	Attenuation artifacts can be caused by breast tissue or diaphragm interference Radiation exposure
Pharmacologic Stress Testing			
Dobutamine echocardiography	Recommended in patients who cannot exercise Recommended when information on an area of myocardium at risk is needed	Because the patient is supine, images are acquired continuously, allowing the test to be stopped as soon as ischemia is evident	Dobutamine contraindications are severe baseline hypertension, unstable angina, and arrhythmias β-Blockers must be withheld before the test
Vasodilator nuclear perfusion (adenosine, dipyridamole, regadenoson)	Recommended in patients who cannot exercise May minimize septal abnormalities frequently seen with nuclear perfusion scanning in patients with LBBB	Vasodilator stress testing may minimize effect of β-blockade on perfusion defect size Can image sooner after myocardial infarction with vasodilator stress	Contraindications are bronchospastic airway disease, theophylline use, sick sinus syndrome, and high-degree AV block Caffeine must be withheld 24 hours before the test Adenosine or dipyridamole may cause chest pain, dyspnea, or flushing Radiation exposure
Dobutamine nuclear perfusion	Recommended in patients who cannot exercise and have contraindications to vasodilators Recommended when information on an area of myocardium at risk is needed	Has comparable sensitivity and specificity to exercise or vasodilator perfusion imaging for diagnosis of myocardial ischemia	Dobutamine contraindications are severe baseline hypertension, unstable angina, and arrhythmias β-Blockers should be withheld before the test Radiation exposure
PET/CT	Provides best perfusion images in larger patients Provides data on myocardial perfusion, function, and viability	Study duration is shorter and radiation dose is lower than conventional nuclear perfusion imaging Absolute myocardial blood flow can be measured Can be combined with CAC scoring	Not widely available More expensive than other imaging modalities Used with pharmacologic stress only (no exercise protocol) Radiation exposure

(Continued on the next page)

TABLE 3. Diagnostic Testing for Coronary Artery Disease *(Continued)*

Diagnostic Test	Utility	Advantages	Limitations
Other Tests			
Coronary angiography	Provides anatomic diagnosis of the presence and severity of CAD	Percutaneous revascularization can be performed following diagnostic study	Invasive Risks of vascular access and radiocontrast exposure (kidney dysfunction, allergy, bleeding) Radiation exposure
CAC testing	CAC testing is reasonable in asymptomatic patients at intermediate risk for CAD	CAC scores are predictive of cardiovascular risk in selected patients	Does not provide data on coronary luminal narrowing Radiation exposure
Coronary CT angiography	Identifies anomalous coronary arteries Useful for selected patients with intermediate risk for CAD	Coronary artery vessel lumen and atherosclerotic lesions can be visualized in detail	Requires high-resolution (64-slice) CT instruments Does not provide detailed images of distal vessel anatomy Catheterization will be needed if intervention is planned Ability to quantify lesion severity can be limited by significant calcification Radiation and radiocontrast exposure
CMR imaging	Gadolinium-enhanced images identify viable and infarcted myocardium Identifies anomalous coronary arteries	Accurate test for myocardial viability	Some patients experience claustrophobia May be contraindicated in patients with pacemaker, ICD, or other implanted device Gadolinium is contraindicated in kidney failure Sinus rhythm and a slower heart rate are needed for improved image quality Limited availability and expertise

AV = atrioventricular; CAC = coronary artery calcium; CAD = coronary artery disease; CMR = cardiac magnetic resonance; ECG = electrocardiography; ICD = implantable cardioverter-defibrillator; LBBB = left bundle branch block; LVH = left ventricular hypertrophy; SPECT = single-photon emission CT; WPW = Wolff-Parkinson-White.

H CONT.

capacity and heart rate and blood pressure response, can be utilized in prediction models such as the Duke treadmill score, which factors development of symptoms, degree of ST-segment depression, and exercise duration to provide incremental prognostic information for 5-year mortality risk. Heart rate recovery is another powerful predictor; patients with a heart rate drop of less than 12/min in the first minute after cessation of exercise have a higher mortality rate.

Ischemia is identified on the basis of the development of 1 mm or greater of horizontal or downsloping ST depression with exercise (**Figure 1**), but the coronary territory involved cannot be localized based on the ECG changes alone. Ideally, patients should exercise for 6 to 12 minutes to provide adequate time for development of maximal metabolic demand. Although achieving 85% of the age-predicted maximal heart rate (PMHR) is considered adequate for diagnosis of ischemia, as heart rate and blood pressure are the major determinants

of myocardial oxygen demand, patients should continue to exercise until limited by symptoms. Achieving a rate pressure product (heart rate × systolic blood pressure) of at least 25,000 is also considered an adequate workload, as this measure reflects left ventricular myocardial performance. A standard Bruce protocol increases the speed and grade of the treadmill every 3 minutes, and patients who have poor functional capacity and cannot achieve at least the first stage of the Bruce protocol (5 metabolic equivalents [METs]) have significantly higher all-cause mortality. Stress tests should be terminated when the patient has exerted maximal effort and achieved at least 85% PMHR, the patient requests to stop or experiences significant anginal or other physical symptoms, or when other adverse markers develop, such as exertional hypotension, significant hypertension, ST-segment elevation or significant ST-segment depression, or ventricular or supraventricular arrhythmias.

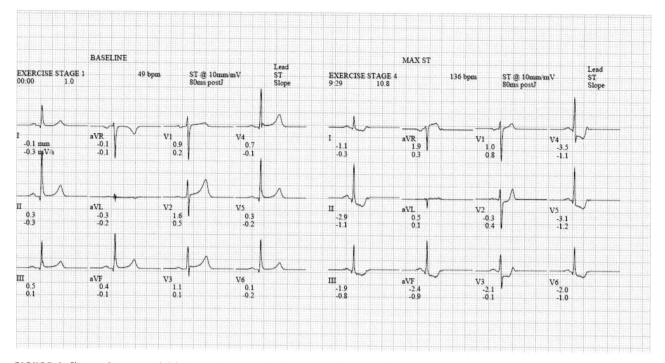

FIGURE 1. Electrocardiogram recorded during exercise stress testing. The presence of 2-mm downsloping ST-segment depressions in leads I, II, III, and aVF, and leads V$_3$ through V$_6$ indicates ischemia.

The decision about whether to keep a patient on cardiac medications during stress testing should be individualized based on the clinical question being addressed. If the stress test is being performed to establish the diagnosis of CAD, medications such as β-blockers and nitrates should be withheld for at least 24 hours before the test. If the stress test is being performed to evaluate symptoms or to define prognosis in a patient with known disease, the patient should remain on current therapy to determine if ischemia is present on the current regimen.

There are several indications for stress testing with additional imaging with either echocardiography, CMR imaging, or perfusion imaging with SPECT or PET/CT. These include inability to exercise, baseline ECG abnormalities, and conditions in which exercise is contraindicated. Patients with abnormal baseline ECGs that interfere with the interpretation of the exercise ECG (for example, left bundle branch block [LBBB], left ventricular hypertrophy with ST-segment abnormalities, or a paced rhythm) should undergo stress imaging to identify obstructive CAD. In addition, stress testing with imaging may be helpful to elucidate a diagnosis in patients with indeterminate results on treadmill testing. Patients with right bundle branch block (RBBB), bifascicular block, or who are on digoxin can undergo exercise stress testing, but ST segments may be more difficult to interpret or may produce false-positive results. Patients with severe aortic stenosis, abdominal aortic aneurysm, severe hypertension, or uncontrolled arrhythmias should not exercise; rather, these patients should undergo pharmacologic stress testing with vasodilators. Patients who are unable to exercise should undergo pharmacologic stress testing with imaging. In addition, in patients with LBBB undergoing nuclear stress testing, a pharmacologic stressor should be used even if

the patient is able to exercise because of the potential for a false-positive test owing to a septal perfusion abnormality that may occur with exercise. The choice of imaging modality should be based on local expertise and patient characteristics.

In stress testing with adjunctive imaging, baseline images are obtained and compared with images obtained after either exercise or pharmacologic stress (**Table 4**). Exercise invokes ischemia as the epicardial vessels become unable to maintain adequate flow related to myocardial oxygen demand via autoregulation, and ischemia develops distal to the obstruction. Dobutamine, like exercise, increases myocardial oxygen demand and elicits ischemia because of insufficient perfusion to the affected myocardium. Vasodilators, such as regadenoson or adenosine, produce hyperemia and a flow disparity between myocardium supplied by the stenotic vessel (in which the distal vasculature is already maximally dilated) as compared with the myocardium supplied by unobstructed vessels. In addition to identifying the presence of disease, perfusion imaging can define the location and extent of reduced perfusion and provide additional prognostic information compared with ECG stress testing alone. These imaging modalities may also be used to quantify infarction and assess myocardial viability. The additional information and impact on patient care obtained with imaging must be balanced with the additional costs, time, and exposure to radiation or contrast agents incurred.

Exercise stress echocardiography is performed with either supine ergometry or treadmill testing. Supine ergometry allows for continuous imaging during exercise, whereas with treadmill testing, images need to be obtained immediately after exercise, and any delay can reduce the accuracy of the information obtained. New regional wall motion abnormalities seen on

TABLE 4. Interpretation of Stress Testing with Imaging

Stress SPECT

At Rest	After Stressor	Interpretation
Normal	Normal	Normal, no ischemia
Normal	Perfusion defect	Normal function at rest, ischemia after stress
Perfusion defect	Perfusion defect	Infarct
Normal	LV dilation	Small or no distinct zone of ischemia, possible balanced ischemia or multivessel CAD

Stress Echocardiography

At Rest	After Stressor	Interpretation
Normal	Normal	Normal, no ischemia
Normal	Wall motion abnormality	Normal function at rest, ischemia with stress
Abnormal	Abnormal	Infarct
Normal	LV dilation	Small or no distinct zone of ischemia, possible balanced ischemia or multivessel CAD

CAD = coronary artery disease; LV = left ventricle; SPECT = single-photon emission CT.

the echocardiogram following exercise indicate areas of ischemia (see Table 4). Wall motion abnormalities at rest that do not change with exercise usually indicate infarction. Improvement in regional wall motion with low-dose exercise or dobutamine that worsens at higher levels suggests viable but hibernating myocardium. As with perfusion imaging, the extent of wall motion abnormalities provides prognostic information regarding risk of future cardiovascular events.

The sensitivity of stress echocardiography is reduced with single-vessel disease and is dependent on timely imaging. In addition, interpretation can be more subjective than with other modalities, particularly with baseline wall motion abnormalities or systolic dysfunction. A major advantage of stress echocardiography is the ability to obtain additional information, such as changes in pulmonary pressures or changes in valvular function with exercise. At minimum,

stress echocardiography allows assessment of wall motion at rest and at peak or immediately following imaging to assess for obstructive CAD. If the examination is performed to assess dyspnea on exertion or valvular function with exercise, these should be specifically requested in order to be sure that adequate echocardiographic information is obtained. Routine transthoracic echocardiography (TTE) evaluates left and right ventricular size, thickness, and function; valvular morphology and function; diastolic function; and the pericardium. These are not necessarily routinely performed in a stress echocardiogram so if this information is clinically important, it may be necessary to obtain both a TTE and a stress echocardiogram. Dobutamine stress echocardiography is used for patients who cannot exercise and can be particularly useful for evaluation of myocardial viability (**Table 5**) and to evaluate aortic stenosis in patients with a low ejection fraction.

TABLE 5. Interpretation of Myocardial Viability Studies

SPECT Viability Testing		
Initial Study (at rest)	**Rest Study Repeated After 4-24 h (with thallium)**	**Interpretation**
Perfusion defect	Perfusion defect	Fixed defect: infarct, no viability
Perfusion defect	Reperfusion of area	Viable myocardium
PET Viability Testing		
Baseline	**Metabolism**	**Interpretation**
Perfusion defect	Metabolically active	Mismatch indicative of viable myocardium
Echocardiography Viability Testing		
Baseline	**Response to Dobutamine**	**Interpretation**
Wall motion abnormality	Low dose: improvement of function Higher dose: worsening of function	Biphasic response indicative of viable myocardium

SPECT = single-photon emission CT.

CONT.

SPECT imaging takes advantage of the relative differences in blood flow with stress. Radioactive tracer is injected and taken up by the myocardium with blood flow. Images are obtained at rest. Then, with exercise or vasodilator stress, a second injection is given. Tracer is again distributed with blood flow and, therefore, less tracer is taken up in the left ventricular region supplied by a stenotic vessel. This relative difference in flow between stress and rest tomographic images is seen as a perfusion defect and is indicative of CAD (**Figure 2**). Most commonly, technetium-based radiotracers are used. These have a higher energy and provide good image quality. This is particularly useful when there is potential for soft-tissue attenuation that can interfere with interpretation, such as with breast attenuation in women. Thallium is a potassium analogue and can only be taken up by active myocytes. Like technetium, thallium can be used for myocardial perfusion imaging, but because it requires active metabolism, thallium also can be used to assess viability. Myocytes that on initial stress testing appear to be infarcted may slowly take up thallium tracer, identifying them as viable. The benefits of thallium are balanced against higher radiation exposure because of its long half-life.

Myocardial perfusion imaging can quantify the extent and severity of disease and help direct treatment strategies. High-risk features that may be seen on myocardial perfusion imaging include lack of augmentation of post-stress ejection fraction, cavity dilatation, and new wall motion abnormalities. Unlike stress echocardiography, images are not obtained immediately post stress and are often delayed. If there is evidence of a new wall motion abnormality in these delayed images, it signifies a high degree of stenosis.

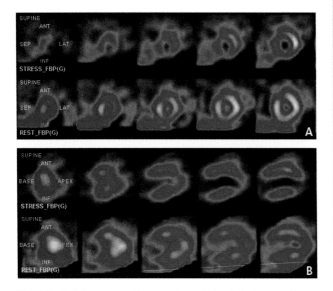

FIGURE 2. Selected images from a nuclear perfusion single-photon emission CT (SPECT) stress study. Short axis views (*panel A*) of the heart with stress (*top row*) and at rest (*bottom row*) show a radiotracer defect in the septum and inferior wall that is filled on the rest images. Long axis views (*panel B*) demonstrate an apical filling defect with stress (*top row*) that is perfused on rest images (*bottom row*).

Like SPECT imaging, cardiac PET can be used to detect ischemia. PET imaging provides improved diagnostic accuracy compared with SPECT and can be particularly useful in patients with nondiagnostic imaging stress tests, obese patients, and patients with diabetes mellitus. Cardiac PET also allows for assessment of peak stress ejection fraction, quantitation of myocardial blood flow, and evaluation of myocardial metabolism. Because some PET radiotracers identify metabolically active myocytes, it is an excellent tool to evaluate for viability. Because cardiac PET uses CT for attenuation correction, limited anatomic information about coronary calcification is also obtained. Because of the short half-life of PET radiotracers, all studies must be performed with vasodilators. The utility of PET/CT scanning is limited by its availability.

CMR imaging can be used for evaluation of myocardial and pericardial disease processes and can be particularly useful for evaluation of infiltrative and inflammatory diseases. It can be utilized to detect the extent and severity of myocardial infarction and viability. Because CMR imaging can be gated, measures of right and left ventricular function can be obtained. Although not widely performed, stress testing with dobutamine to assess wall motion and vasodilators such as adenosine to assess perfusion can be used with CMR imaging to detect ischemia. Limitations of the use of CMR imaging include the length of time needed to acquire images and magnetic interference with cardiac implanted electronic devices. ▣

KEY POINTS

- Stress testing is most efficacious in patients with an intermediate pretest probability of coronary artery disease, because it is these patients who, by the result of their stress test, can be reclassified into higher or lower risk categories. **HVC**

- In patients who are able to exercise and have a normal baseline electrocardiogram, the initial type of stress testing should be exercise stress testing. **HVC**

- Patients with abnormal baseline electrocardiograms (ECGs) that interfere with the interpretation of the exercise ECG (for example, left bundle branch block, left ventricular hypertrophy with ST-segment abnormalities, or a paced rhythm) should undergo stress imaging to identify obstructive coronary artery disease.

Visualization of the Coronary Anatomy

Coronary angiography and coronary CT angiography (CTA) provide anatomic information regarding the coronary vessels (**Figure 3**). Both procedures require iodinated contrast and expose the patient to radiation. Coronary angiography provides a two-dimensional image of the lumen of the vessel filled with contrast. Assessment of the stenotic lesions is made from multiple views of the vessel. Coronary CTA can provide additional information about some of the characteristics of the plaque. If, however, culprit lesions are visualized on coronary CTA, the patient typically requires coronary angiography for

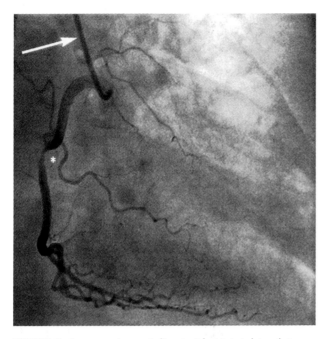

FIGURE 3. Coronary angiogram. Radiocontrast dye is injected via catheter (*arrow*) during coronary angiography, demonstrating 85% to 90% occlusion of the mid right coronary artery (*asterisk*).

better definition of the degree of coronary stenosis. Coronary angiography is also required if coronary revascularization is to be performed. If percutaneous coronary intervention is indicated, it may be performed at the time of a patient's diagnostic catheterization. Coronary angiography may be useful as a diagnostic test in patients who, despite maximal medical therapy, have intolerable ischemic symptoms as long as they are candidates for coronary revascularization. Coronary CTA may be used to rule out CAD in symptomatic patients with an intermediate risk of coronary disease. Other limitations of coronary CTA include poor visualization of distal vessels and artifact from calcification that may limit interpretation.

Suspected coronary anomalies, such as anomalous coronary origins, can be evaluated by coronary CTA, CMR imaging, or coronary angiography. These imaging modalities can help identify those abnormalities that are associated with a higher risk of sudden cardiac death.

Coronary Artery Calcium Scoring

Coronary artery calcium (CAC) scoring provides information regarding the burden of atherosclerotic disease but does not provide information regarding the degree of obstruction it may be causing. CAC scoring can be performed with either electron beam or multi-detector CT, and newer technologic advances limit radiation exposure to the patient. It detects the presence of calcification in the walls of the coronary arteries, which is directly proportional to the degree of plaque burden present. CAC scores are categorized as follows: 0, no disease; 1-99, mild disease; 100-399, moderate disease; and above 400, severe disease. Coronary calcium scores greater than 400 are

associated with a higher incidence of abnormal perfusion on SPECT imaging. Because of its cost and associated radiation exposure, measurement of coronary artery calcium should be limited to a select group of asymptomatic patients with an intermediate Framingham risk score (10%-20%) in whom results will influence treatment strategy. CAC scoring may be useful particularly if the results will influence treatment strategy, such as initiation of lipid-lowering therapy.

KEY POINT

- Measurement of coronary artery calcium should be limited to a select group of asymptomatic patients with an intermediate Framingham risk score (10%-20%) in whom results will influence treatment strategy because of its associated cost and radiation exposure.

Risks of Coronary Diagnostic Testing

In addition to the physical and societal costs of downstream testing that result from inappropriate testing, each of the modalities used for diagnosis and risk stratification carry specific risks. It is important to determine the pretest probability of disease and to focus additional testing appropriately. For example, ordering an exercise stress test in a patient with a low pretest probability of disease may result in a false-positive stress test and additional downstream testing. Obtaining a CAC score in a low-risk patient may lead to additional tests or procedures for an incidental finding on CT.

Exercise testing is associated with a small risk of myocardial infarction or death (1/2500 tests). Exercise stress testing is contraindicated in patients with unstable cardiac conditions, such as uncontrolled cardiac arrhythmias, severe symptomatic aortic stenosis, uncontrolled heart failure, and unstable angina. Pharmacologic stress agents, including dipyridamole, adenosine, and regadenoson, are associated with development of high-degree atrioventricular block and bronchospasm.

Nuclear stress testing, CAC scoring, coronary CTA, and coronary angiography expose the patient to radiation. The amount of exposure is dependent on factors such as the radiotracer used, equipment, operator technique, complexity of procedure performed, and patient characteristics (such as body size).

Various contrast agents are used for CMR imaging (gadolinium), echocardiography (microbubble contrast agents used for enhancement of endocardial borders), coronary CTA, and coronary angiography (nonionic contrast). Nonionic contrast may be associated with hypersensitivity reactions and acute kidney injury whereas gadolinium is associated with the development of nephrogenic fibrosing dermatopathy in patients with chronic kidney disease.

Cardiac catheterization can result in complications from vascular access, injury to the coronary arteries, dissection of the aorta, or disruption of plaque resulting in peripheral emboli and possible stroke. Vascular access complications include retroperitoneal hematoma from bleeding at the groin access site as well as pseudoaneurysm at the arterial puncture

CONT.

site. Both of these complications require prompt recognition and treatment.

Diagnostic Testing for Structural Heart Disease

Diagnostic testing for structural heart disease should be based on a thorough history and physical examination. New murmurs or a change in examination findings or symptoms in a patient with known structural heart disease should prompt further evaluation. Routine yearly imaging evaluation of structural heart disease in asymptomatic patients is usually not indicated. Benign murmurs, such as grade 1/6 or 2/6 midsystolic murmurs, are common with pregnancy, anemia, and other high-flow states, and do not routinely need echocardiographic evaluation.

Imaging modalities used to evaluate structural heart disease are listed in **Table 6**. Evaluation of structural heart disease typically begins with a TTE. TTE provides information about left and right ventricular cavity size, thickness, and function, as well as quantitative information regarding valvular function, diastolic function, and filling pressures. TTE can be used with intravenous agitated saline contrast, normally cleared by the pulmonary circulation, to document the presence of an intracardiac shunt or a patent foramen ovale. Atrial septal defect is suggested by shunting of microbubbles from the right atrium to the left atrium. TTE is a noninvasive procedure and is the preferred imaging modality for evaluating anterior structures of the heart, such as the aortic valve.

Transesophageal echocardiography (TEE) takes advantage of the proximity of the heart to the esophagus for better image quality. The procedure requires sedation and is contraindicated in patients with esophageal strictures or active esophageal varices or bleeding. Complications include esophageal injury and bleeding. TEE is commonly used to evaluate for endocarditis in patients with a high pretest probability; to assess for diagnostic findings or complications of endocarditis (such as abscess); to better visualize valvular pathology, particularly when planning repair; to evaluate specific structures that cannot be well visualized on TTE (such as prosthetic heart valves); to evaluate acute aortic pathologies; and to rule out left atrial thrombus prior to cardioversion (**Figure 4**).

KEY POINTS

HVC • Routine yearly imaging evaluation of structural heart disease in asymptomatic patients is usually not indicated; benign murmurs, such as grade 1/6 or 2/6 midsystolic murmurs, are common with pregnancy, anemia, and other high-flow states and do not routinely need echocardiographic evaluation.

• Evaluation of structural heart disease typically begins with transthoracic echocardiography, which provides information about ventricular cavity size, thickness, and function, as well as quantitative information regarding valvular function, diastolic function, and filling pressures.

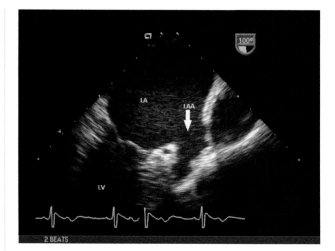

FIGURE 4. Transesophageal echocardiogram. The transducer is posterior to the heart, and the left atrium (*LA*) and left atrial appendage (*LAA, arrow*) are more easily seen than with transthoracic echocardiography, showing absence of thrombus in the appendage. LV = left ventricle.

Diagnostic Testing for Cardiac Arrhythmias

In addition to a careful history and physical examination, the evaluation of a patient with a history of palpitations, presyncope, or syncope in which an arrhythmia is suspected begins with a 12-lead resting ECG. Evidence of preexcitation, ectopic rhythms, atrioventricular block, or intraventricular conduction delay may give insight into the etiology of the symptoms. In patients in whom the presence of structural heart disease is suspected, echocardiography may also be indicated. Because of the intermittent nature of arrhythmias, their diagnosis and documentation can be challenging. Monitoring and diagnostic strategies are based on the frequency of the patient's episodes (**Table 7**, on page 14). Patients with daily symptoms can be evaluated with a 24- or 48-hour ambulatory ECG monitor (Holter monitor), whereas patients with less frequent episodes require other monitoring strategies. For infrequent symptomatic events, an external patient-triggered event recorder can capture the arrhythmia, provided the event lasts long enough for the patient to record it. A looping event recorder captures several seconds of the ECG signal prior to the device being triggered and is useful when episodes are accompanied by syncope or presyncope. For very infrequent events, an implanted loop recorder may be warranted.

Exercise testing is also frequently employed in patients with a suspected or known arrhythmia. Treadmill exercise testing is an important tool for evaluating chronotropic response, ischemia, and exercise-induced or adrenergically induced arrhythmia.

Once a patient is diagnosed with an arrhythmia or arrhythmia-prone cardiovascular condition, diagnostic electrophysiology testing can be helpful for both risk stratification and treatment (such as catheter ablation). Selection of these diagnostic tests is dependent upon the particular patient and the diagnostic concerns, and most patients with arrhythmias do not require an electrophysiology study.

TABLE 6. Diagnostic Testing for Structural Heart Disease

Diagnostic Test	Major Indications	Advantages	Limitations
Transthoracic echocardiography	Heart failure Cardiomyopathy Valve disease Congenital heart disease Pulmonary hypertension Aortic disease Pericardial disease	Accurate diagnosis of presence and severity of structural heart disease Quantitation of LV size and function, pulmonary pressures, valve function, and intracardiac shunts Widely available, portable, fast	Operator-dependent data acquisition. Interpretation requires expertise. Variability in instrumentation Image quality limits diagnosis in some patients, may require microbubble contrast agents
Transesophageal echocardiography	Endocarditis Prosthetic valve dysfunction Aortic disease Left atrial thrombus	High-quality images, especially of posterior cardiac structures Most accurate test for endocarditis evaluation, prosthetic valves, and left atrial thrombus	Requires esophageal intubation, typically with conscious sedation
Three-dimensional echocardiography	Mitral valve disease ASD (percutaneous ASD closure)	Improved tomographic imaging Used during cardiac procedures for device placement Improved assessment of LV global/regional systolic function	Adjunct to two-dimensional imaging Limited availability and expertise
Radionuclide angiography (MUGA)	Evaluation of LV systolic function	Quantitative EF measurements Accurate for serial LVEF measurements with cardiotoxic drugs	Radiation exposure No data on other cardiac structures
Cardiac catheterization (left and right)	Congenital heart disease Coronary artery disease Valve assessment Shunt assessment	Direct measurement of intracardiac pressures, gradients, and shunts Contrast angiography provides visualization of complex cardiac anatomy Allows percutaneous intervention for structural heart disease	Invasive Radiation and radiocontrast exposure Images not tomographic, limiting evaluation of complex three-dimensional anatomy
Coronary CT angiography	Coronary artery disease Congenital heart disease	Visualization of complex cardiac anatomy High-resolution tomographic images	Invasive Radiation and radiocontrast exposure Image acquisition improved with sinus rhythm and slower heart rate
CMR imaging	Congenital heart disease Aortic disease Myocardial disease (infiltrative disease, myocarditis, hypertrophic cardiomyopathy) RV cardiomyopathy (ARVC) Quantitation of LV mass and function	High-resolution tomographic imaging and blood-flow data Quantitative RV volumes and EF No ionizing radiation or contrast Enables three-dimensional reconstruction of aortic and coronary anatomy	Limited availability and expertise Some patients experience claustrophobia May be contraindicated in patients with pacemaker, ICD, or other implanted devices Gadolinium is contraindicated in kidney failure Sinus rhythm and slower heart rate are needed for improved image quality
Chest CT	Aortic disease Coronary disease Cardiac masses Pericardial disease	High-resolution tomographic images Enables three-dimensional reconstruction of vascular structures	Radiation and radiocontrast exposure

ARVC = arrhythmogenic right ventricular cardiomyopathy; ASD = atrial septal defect; CMR = cardiac magnetic resonance; EF = ejection fraction; ICD = implantable cardioverter-defibrillator; LV = left ventricle; LVEF = left ventricular ejection fraction; MUGA = multi-gated acquisition; RV = right ventricle.

TABLE 7. Diagnostic Tests for Suspected or Known Cardiac Arrhythmias

Diagnostic Test	Utility	Advantages	Limitations
Resting ECG	Initial diagnostic test in all patients	12-lead ECG recorded during the arrhythmia often identifies the specific arrhythmia	Most arrhythmias are intermittent and not recorded on a resting ECG
Ambulatory ECG (Holter monitor)	Frequent (at least daily) asymptomatic or symptomatic arrhythmias	Records every heart beat during a 24- or 48-hour period for later analysis Patient log allows correlation with symptoms	Not helpful when arrhythmia occurs less frequently ECG leads limit patient activities
Exercise ECG	Arrhythmias provoked by exercise	Allows diagnosis of exercise-related arrhythmias Allows assessment of impact of arrhythmia on blood pressure	Physician supervision needed in case a serious arrhythmia occurs Most arrhythmias are not exercise related
Patient-triggered event recorder	Infrequent symptomatic arrhythmias that last more than 1-2 minutes	Small, pocket-sized recorder is held to the chest when symptoms are present Recorded data are transmitted to central monitoring service	Only useful for symptomatic arrhythmias that persist long enough for patient to activate the device Arrhythmia onset not recorded Not useful for syncope or extremely brief arrhythmias
Looping event recorder (wearable)	Infrequent symptomatic brief arrhythmias Syncope	Continuous ECG signal is recorded with the previous 30 seconds to 2 minutes saved when the patient activates the recording mode Arrhythmia onset is recorded	ECG leads limit patient activities Device records only when activated by patient
Implantable loop recorder	Very infrequent asymptomatic or symptomatic arrhythmias	Long-term continuous ECG monitoring with patient-triggered or heart rate-triggered episode storage Specific heart rate or QRS parameters can be set to initiate recording of data	Invasive procedure with minor risks Device must be explanted later
Mobile cardiac outpatient telemetry	Continuous outpatient ECG recording for precise quantification or capture of rare arrhythmia	Auto-triggered and patient-triggered capture of arrhythmia events Up to 96 hours of retrievable memory	ECG leads limit patient activities Resource intensive
Electrophysiology study	Used for both inducing, identifying, and clarifying mechanism of arrhythmia as well as potential treatment (catheter ablation)	The origin and mechanism of an arrhythmia can be precisely defined	Invasive procedure with some risk Some arrhythmias may not be inducible, particularly if the patient is sedated

ECG = electrocardiogram.

Coronary Artery Disease
Stable Angina Pectoris
Diagnosis and Evaluation

The most common manifestation of coronary artery disease (CAD) is stable angina pectoris: chest pain, pressure, or discomfort that develops with exertion and is relieved with rest.

Symptoms often occur when the burden of atheromatous plaque results in fixed coronary stenosis and limitation of blood flow, leading to an imbalance between myocardial oxygen supply and demand. When patients with cardiovascular risk factors present with chest pain, the location of the pain, quality of symptoms (sharp/dull, transient/persistent, occurring at rest/with exertion), and the age and sex of the patient can help to differentiate stable angina pectoris from other causes of chest pain, such as gastrointestinal, musculoskeletal, or pulmonary causes. These factors are also used to determine a patient's pretest likelihood of CAD (**Table 8**).

The decision to perform exercise or pharmacologic stress testing or coronary CT angiography (CTA) is based on the pretest likelihood of CAD, the patient's baseline electrocardiogram (ECG), the patient's ability to exercise, and the patient's comorbid illnesses, such as asthma or emphysema, that would limit pharmacologic testing (**Figure 5**).The selection of tests for evaluating patients with chest pain is discussed in Diagnostic Testing in Cardiology. Stress testing is most useful in patients at intermediate pretest likelihood of CAD (10% to 90%). In patients with low pretest probability, a normal test result only confirms that the patient is low risk, and an abnormal stress test result is most likely a false-positive, possibly leading to more testing (additional stress testing or invasive angiography). In patients with a high pretest likelihood, the use of stress testing for diagnostic purposes is not indicated, as an abnormal test result only confirms the presence of disease and a normal test result is most likely to indicate a false-negative result.

Stress testing in patients with high pretest likelihood can be used to obtain prognostic information, but the results should not affect the initiation of optimal medical therapy. In patients who have been started on medical therapy for CAD, stress testing can be used to determine a patient's response to optimal medical therapy, measure exercise capacity, and evaluate the extent and severity of ischemia.

The development of coronary CTA is an emerging alternative to stress testing, but coronary CTA does not provide important functional information, such as extent of ischemia, reproduction of symptoms, or exercise capacity. Coronary CTA is useful for diagnostic purposes in patients at intermediate risk for CAD if stress testing is contraindicated or revascularization is unlikely to be performed or change management.

The use of invasive coronary angiography in patients with stable angina pectoris is generally limited to those with persistent or progressive life-limiting symptoms while on optimal medical therapy or those with high-risk criteria on noninvasive stress testing or coronary CTA (see Figure 5).

KEY POINTS

- When patients with cardiovascular risk factors present with chest pain, the quality of symptoms, the age, and the sex of the patient can help to differentiate stable angina pectoris from other causes of chest pain.
- Stress testing is most useful in patients at intermediate **HVC** pretest likelihood of coronary artery disease (10% to 90%).

General Approach to Treatment of Stable Angina Pectoris

All patients with ischemic heart disease should be counseled on the importance of risk factor modification, including lifestyle changes, such as smoking cessation, weight management, daily physical activity, and diet modification; as well as control of modifiable risk factors, such as diabetes mellitus, hypertension, and hyperlipidemia. Medical therapy should be initiated in all patients with ischemic heart disease. The combination of risk factor modification and medical therapy is

TABLE 8.	Pretest Likelihoods of Coronary Artery Disease in Low-Risk and High-Risk Symptomatic Patients					
	Pretest Likelihood					
	Nonanginal Chest Pain[a]		**Atypical Angina[b]**		**Typical Angina[c]**	
Age (y)	**Men**	**Women**	**Men**	**Women**	**Men**	**Women**
35	3-35	1-19	8-59	2-39	30-88	10-78
45	9-47	2-22	21-70	5-43	51-92	20-79
55	23-59	4-25	45-79	10-47	80-95	38-82
65	49-69	9-29	71-86	20-51	93-97	56-84

[a]Nonanginal chest pain has one or none of the components for typical chest pain.

[b]Atypical angina has two of the three components for typical angina.

[c]Typical angina has three components: (1) substernal chest pain or discomfort, (2) provoked by exertion or emotional stress, (3) relieved by rest and/or nitroglycerin.

NOTE: Each value represents the percentage with significant coronary artery disease. The first is the percentage for a low-risk, mid-decade patient without diabetes mellitus, smoking, or hyperlipidemia. The second is that of the same-age patient with diabetes mellitus, smoking, and hyperlipidemia. Both high- and low-risk patients have normal results on resting electrocardiography. If ST-T wave changes or Q waves had been present, the likelihood of coronary artery disease would be higher in each entry of the table.

Adapted with permission of Elsevier Science and Technology Journals, from Gibbons RJ, Abrams J, Chatterjee K. ACC/AHA 2002 guideline update for the management of patients with chronic stable angina--summary article: a report of the American College of Cardiology/American Heart Association Task Force on practice guidelines (Committee on the Management of Patients With Chronic Stable Angina). J Am Coll Cardiol. 2003 Jan 1;41(1):159-68. [PMID: 12570960]; permission conveyed through Copyright Clearance Center, Inc.

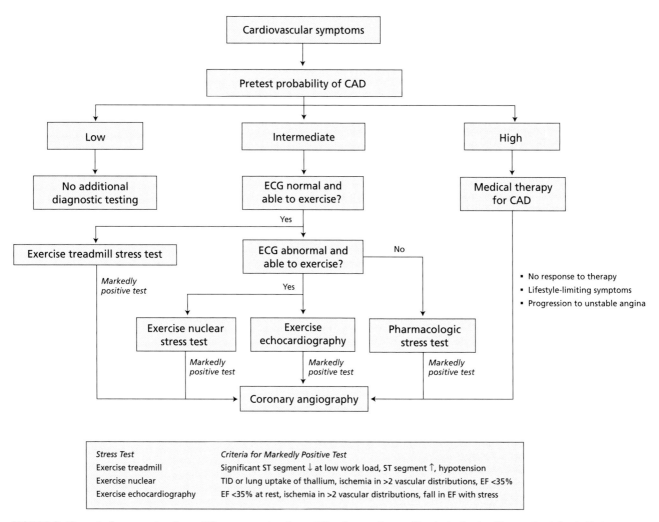

FIGURE 5. Diagnosis of coronary artery disease. CAD = coronary artery disease; ECG = electrocardiogram; EF = ejection fraction; TID = transient ischemic dilation.

referred to as guideline-directed medical therapy (**Figure 6**). Medical therapy is divided into two categories: cardioprotective medications and antianginal medications. Cardioprotective medications improve survival, reduce the occurrence of cardiovascular events, and reduce the progression of systemic atherosclerosis. Antianginal medications vasodilate the coronary vasculature or decrease myocardial oxygen demand, thus reducing the frequency and severity of angina pectoris and improving quality of life.

Cardioprotective Medications

The use of aspirin is associated with a decreased risk of myocardial infarction, stroke, and cardiovascular death in patients with CAD. Aspirin doses of 81 mg to 162 mg daily are recommended in all patients with established CAD unless contraindicated. In patients allergic to aspirin, clopidogrel is recommended as an alternative. The use of newer antiplatelet agents (prasugrel, ticagrelor) as monotherapy has not been tested in patients with stable angina pectoris. Dual antiplatelet therapy (aspirin plus either clopidogrel, prasugrel, or ticagrelor) is currently recommended only following percutaneous coronary intervention (PCI) or an acute coronary event.

Owing to the protective effects of β-blockers, these agents are considered first-line therapy in patients with stable angina pectoris. Dose titration of β-blockers is recommended until the resting heart rate is between 55/min and 60/min. β-Blockers have been associated with fatigue, reduced exercise capacity, symptomatic bradycardia, mood disturbance (depression), and erectile dysfunction. β-Blockers are contraindicated in patients with symptomatic bradycardia, high-grade atrioventricular block, acute decompensated heart failure, and severe reactive airways disease.

ACE inhibitors are indicated in the treatment of patients with stable angina pectoris to reduce cardiovascular and all-cause mortality. This effect on mortality is more profound in patients with concomitant diabetes mellitus and left ventricular systolic dysfunction. Additionally, ACE inhibitors are indicated in patients with concomitant systemic hypertension and proteinuric chronic kidney disease. ACE inhibitors are contraindicated in pregnant women and caution is

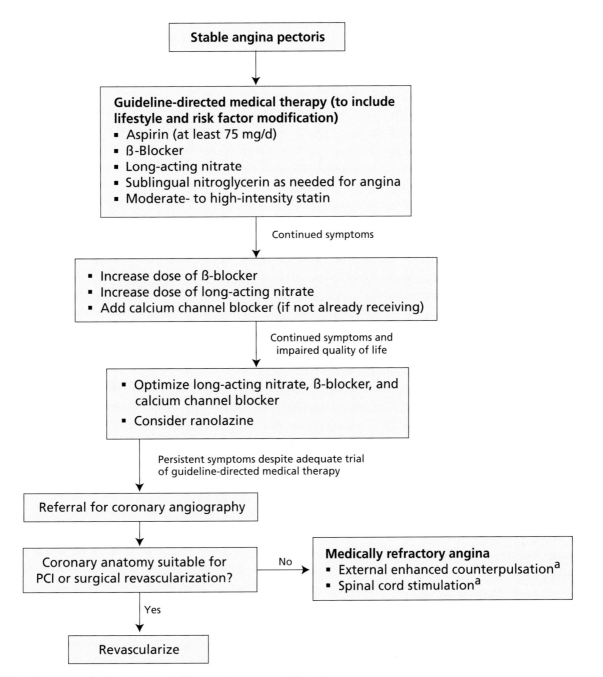

FIGURE 6. Management of stable angina pectoris. PCI = percutaneous coronary intervention.

[a]Not recommended by current guidelines.

Recommendations based on Qaseem A, Fihn SD, Dallas P, Williams S, Owens DK, Shekelle P; Clinical Guidelines Committee of the American College of Physicians. Management of stable ischemic heart disease: summary of a clinical practice guideline from the American College of Physicians/American College of Cardiology Foundation/American Heart Association/American Association for Thoracic Surgery/Preventive Cardiovascular Nurses Association/Society of Thoracic Surgeons. Ann Intern Med. 2012 Nov 20;157(10):735-43. [PMID: 23165665]

advised in patients with advanced chronic kidney disease. Angiotensin receptor blockers are considered acceptable alternatives in patients who are allergic to or intolerant of ACE inhibitors.

Statins have been shown to reduce the risk of myocardial infarction and death in patients with chronic ischemic heart disease by 25% to 30%. The reduction in cardiovascular events is proportional to the degree of LDL cholesterol reduction; however, statins have been proved to be beneficial in patients regardless of cholesterol level. New cholesterol management guidelines recommend the use of moderate- to high-intensity statins for all patients with (1) LDL cholesterol level of 190 mg/dL (4.92 mmol/L) or greater; (2) diabetes mellitus; or (3) greater than 7.5% estimated 10-year risk of atherosclerotic cardiovascular disease (ASCVD). Management of statin therapy is discussed in MKSAP 17 General Internal Medicine.

According to Advisory Committee on Immunization Practices (ACIP) guidelines, all persons aged 6 months or older should have an annual influenza vaccination. In addition, patients at risk for cardiovascular disease warrant influenza vaccination as a preventive measure for cardiovascular disease.

The use of selenium, chromium, β-carotene, vitamin C, vitamin E, and estrogen has not been associated with improved cardiovascular outcomes and is not recommended in patients with ischemic heart disease.

Antianginal Medications

Medications to reduce the frequency and severity of angina pectoris comprise β-blockers, nitrates, calcium channel blockers, and ranolazine.

β-Blockers and nitrates are first-line antianginal agents. In addition to their cardioprotective effects, β-blockers improve angina pectoris by reducing heart rate, myocardial contractility, and blood pressure, resulting in reduced myocardial oxygen demand. Nitrates improve myocardial oxygen supply and reduce myocardial oxygen demand by their effects on coronary and systemic vasodilation, respectively. Nitrates have not been proved to reduce the frequency of cardiovascular events (myocardial infarction, death). Two categories of nitrates are indicated for patients with stable angina pectoris: sublingual or spray nitroglycerin (for emergency use) and topical or oral nitroglycerin (for chronic, daily use). The use of daily nitrates requires periodic nitrate-free intervals (typically at night) to avoid the development of tolerance. The most frequent adverse effect of nitrates is headache. The use of either short- or long-acting nitrates is contraindicated in patients who take phosphodiesterase 5 (PDE-5) inhibitors for erectile dysfunction (sildenafil, vardenafil, tadalafil) owing to the potentiation of hypotension when these drugs are used together.

Calcium channel blockers are second-line therapy in patients with stable angina pectoris who are intolerant of β-blockers or who have continued symptoms on β-blockers and nitrates. All calcium channel blockers cause systemic and coronary vasodilation, and nondihydropyridine calcium channel blockers (diltiazem, verapamil) reduce the heart rate. Because of their vasodilatory properties, calcium channel blockers are first-line agents for the management of patients with Prinzmetal (variant) angina pectoris. The most common adverse effects of calcium channel blockers are peripheral edema, dizziness, constipation, and bradycardia. Calcium channel blockers are contraindicated in patients with left ventricular systolic dysfunction or advanced atrioventricular block.

Ranolazine is a selective inhibitor of the late inward sodium channel in the myocardium. It is generally reserved for patients who remain symptomatic with the use of β-blockers, nitrates, and calcium channel blockers. Ranolazine is an effective antianginal medication; however, its use is limited by cost and adverse effects such as dizziness, headache, nausea, and constipation. Ranolazine should be used with caution in patients with advanced kidney or liver disease and in those taking medications that are potent inhibitors of the CYP3A4 pathway. Examples of strong inhibitors of the CYP3A4 pathway include ketoconazole, clarithromycin, tacrolimus, and cyclosporine.

KEY POINTS

- Aspirin or clopidogrel (if aspirin-allergic) is recommended in all patients with established coronary artery disease unless contraindicated; the use of newer antiplatelet agents (prasugrel, ticagrelor) as monotherapy has not been tested in patients with stable angina pectoris.
- All patients with stable angina pectoris should receive a statin and a β-blocker.
- ACE inhibitors are indicated in the treatment of stable angina pectoris, particularly in patients with concomitant diabetes mellitus and left ventricular systolic dysfunction.

Coronary Revascularization

Decision to Revascularize

In patients with stable angina pectoris whose symptoms are not improved with optimal medical therapy, invasive angiography is warranted to define coronary artery anatomy and prepare for revascularization via PCI or coronary artery bypass graft surgery (CABG). All patients should be counseled on the risks, benefits, and alternatives to angiography and revascularization before diagnostic angiography is pursued.

In patients found to have significant CAD on angiography that would benefit from revascularization, multiple factors are considered in deciding which technique (PCI or CABG) would be best for the patient. These include the degree of left ventricular systolic dysfunction, whether the patient has had a prior CABG, and the patient's ability to adhere to a medication treatment regimen. The SYNTAX score is an anatomic scoring system based on the results of angiography that quantifies lesion complexity in patients with multi-vessel and/or left main coronary artery disease and is useful in helping predict the outcome of different revascularization strategies. The development of appropriate use criteria (AUC), a collection of clinical scenarios that mimic frequently encountered patient presentations, has assisted clinicians in making treatment decisions for patients with all forms of ischemic heart disease.

Percutaneous Coronary Intervention

PCI has not been shown to be superior to optimal medical therapy in patients with stable angina pectoris for reduction of cardiovascular endpoints such as mortality and myocardial infarction. However, PCI has been associated with improvement in quality of life by reducing the severity and frequency of angina. Current guidelines recommend that diagnostic angiography and PCI be reserved for patients with refractory symptoms while on optimal medical therapy, those who are unable to tolerate optimal medical therapy owing to side effects, or those with high-risk features on noninvasive exercise and imaging tests.

Coronary Artery Bypass Graft Surgery

The use of CABG in patients with stable angina is generally indicated only for those who remain symptomatic with optimal medical therapy and have specific angiographic findings (either left main disease or multivessel disease with involvement of the proximal left anterior descending artery), concomitant reduced systolic function, or diabetes mellitus. CABG is typically performed via median sternotomy incision and institution of cardiopulmonary bypass; however, recent advances with off-pump CABG allow patients to avoid the need for cardiopulmonary bypass. Off-pump CABG is associated with adverse event and graft patency rates similar to traditional CABG. This less invasive procedure may be more suitable for patients with significant comorbid medical conditions as it may reduce operative risk and shorten hospital and recovery times, but definitive proof is lacking.

After Revascularization

The long-term goals of therapy for ischemic heart disease are to maximize quality of life and exercise function and minimize morbidity and mortality. Clinical practice guidelines do not recommend the routine use of ECG monitoring, stress testing, or anatomic testing (coronary CTA or invasive angiography) in asymptomatic patients after PCI or CABG.

All patients with stable angina pectoris who undergo PCI or CABG should be treated with aspirin (81-162 mg/d) indefinitely. In patients who undergo PCI, dual antiplatelet therapy (aspirin plus clopidogrel) is recommended for at least 1 month after bare metal stent (BMS) implantation and at least 1 year after drug-eluting stent (DES) implantation, although extended use can be considered on an individual basis if a patient's

ischemic risk is high and bleeding risk is low (**Table 9**). A major risk with premature discontinuation of dual antiplatelet therapy is the occurrence of stent thrombosis, a complication with high morbidity and mortality.

In patients who undergo CABG, preoperative cardioprotective and antianginal medications should be continued indefinitely. The benefit of cardioprotective medications (aspirin, β-blockers, ACE inhibitors, statins) is greatest in patients with high-risk features such as reduced left ventricular systolic function, prior myocardial infarction, chronic kidney disease, or diabetes.

KEY POINTS

- Percutaneous coronary intervention improves angina symptoms and quality of life in patients with stable angina pectoris but does not increase survival or reduce future cardiovascular events.

- For stable angina pectoris, percutaneous coronary **HVC** intervention is reserved for patients with refractory symptoms while on optimal medical therapy, those who are unable to tolerate optimal medical therapy owing to side effects, or those with high-risk features on noninvasive imaging.

- Clinical practice guidelines do not recommend the **HVC** routine use of ECG monitoring, stress testing, or anatomic testing (coronary CT angiography or invasive angiography) in asymptomatic patients after percutaneous coronary intervention or coronary artery bypass graft surgery.

- In patients with stable angina pectoris who undergo percutaneous coronary intervention, dual antiplatelet therapy (aspirin plus clopidogrel) is recommended for at least 1 month after bare metal stent implantation and at least 1 year after drug-eluting stent implantation.

TABLE 9. Duration of Dual Antiplatelet Therapy[a]				
Condition	**No Stent**	**Bare Metal Stent**	**Drug-Eluting Stent**	**CABG**
Stable angina pectoris	Clopidogrel, only if aspirin is contraindicated	Clopidogrel 1 month	Clopidogrel 1 year	Not indicated[b]
UA/NSTEMI	Clopidogrel or ticagrelor 1 year	Clopidogrel, prasugrel, or ticagrelor At least 4 weeks, up to 1 year	Clopidogrel, prasugrel, or ticagrelor 1 year	Clopidogrel or ticagrelor 1 year
STEMI	Clopidogrel or ticagrelor 1 year	Clopidogrel, prasugrel, or ticagrelor At least 4 weeks, up to 1 year	Clopidogrel, prasugrel, or ticagrelor 1 year	Clopidogrel or ticagrelor 1 year

CABG = coronary artery bypass grafting; NSTEMI = non-ST-elevation myocardial infarction; STEMI = ST-elevation myocardial infarction; UA = unstable angina.

[a]Dual antiplatelet therapy consists of aspirin and another antiplatelet agent, with aspirin taken indefinitely unless contraindicated.

[b]Preliminary data suggest clopidogrel improves patency of bypass grafts after CABG.

NOTE: Extended dual antiplatelet therapy can be considered if the risk-benefit ratio is favorable.

Acute Coronary Syndromes

General Considerations

Acute coronary syndrome (ACS) encompasses ST-elevation myocardial infarction (STEMI) and non–ST-elevation acute coronary syndromes (NSTE-ACSs), which comprise non–ST-elevation myocardial infarction (NSTEMI) and unstable angina (UA) (**Figure 7**). The pathophysiology of ACS is most commonly characterized by plaque rupture (75% of cases) and plaque erosion (25% of cases). STEMI is caused by a complete occlusion of an epicardial coronary artery by thrombus at the site of plaque disruption and is defined by the presence of ischemic chest pain (or an equivalent) and the presence of greater than 1-mm ST-segment elevation in two or more consecutive leads or new left bundle branch block on ECG. ST-segment depression in two or more precordial leads (V_1 through V_4) may indicate transmural posterior injury. In UA and NSTEMI, the occlusion is incomplete. NSTE-ACSs are characterized by the presence of ischemic chest pain (or an equivalent), the notable absence of ST-segment elevation on ECG, and the presence of either ST-segment depression or T-wave inversion on ECG. In NSTEMI, cardiac biomarkers (serum creatine kinase MB and troponin) are abnormal, whereas in UA, cardiac biomarkers are normal.

Because the affected artery is completely occluded in STEMI, its diagnosis and treatment are markedly different from those of UA or NSTEMI. For this reason, an initial ECG is imperative in all patients presenting with symptoms consistent with ischemic chest pain, and once diagnosis of STEMI occurs, emphasis is placed on immediate reperfusion of the vessel via thrombolytic therapy or PCI. Patients with ischemic chest pain but without ST-segment elevation on initial ECG are typically classified as having NSTE-ACS and then undergo laboratory testing for cardiac biomarkers. Because these patients do not have an ECG consistent with complete occlusion of a coronary artery and because this group of patients is heterogeneous, risk stratification should occur prior to consideration of coronary angiography and subsequent coronary revascularization with PCI or CABG.

ST-Elevation Myocardial Infarction

Recognition

Optimal management and improved outcomes in patients with STEMI depend on early recognition and institution of reperfusion therapy with either thrombolysis or primary PCI (**Figure 8**). Over the past decade, various systems-based interventions have proved effective in increasing the percentage of patients diagnosed at the time of hospital presentation, reducing the time required to reperfuse an occluded blood vessel with either thrombolysis or PCI and reducing transfer time to a facility capable of thrombolysis or PCI.

STEMI is diagnosed clinically based on the initial ECG and the presence of ischemic chest pain. Several conditions should be considered in the differential diagnosis at the time of presentation, particularly acute aortic dissection, pulmonary embolism, and pericarditis. A focused history should be taken to determine the patient's quality and duration of symptoms, risk factors for CAD, prior history of PCI or CABG, and bleeding risk as it pertains to reperfusion therapy. Physical examination is imperative to evaluate for conditions that mimic STEMI, including acute aortic dissection (asymmetric arm pressures) and pericarditis (pericardial rub). Physical examination should also look for signs of STEMI complications, such as hypotension (ventricular wall rupture, cardiogenic shock) and heart murmur (acute mitral regurgitation). Finally, the physical examination is important to assess for factors that may influence treatment options (gastrointestinal bleeding, neurologic deficits, heart failure, coagulopathy).

Reperfusion

Reperfusion for patients with STEMI occurs primarily via thrombolytic therapy and primary PCI. Despite early success with thrombolytic therapy, some studies suggest that 30% to 50% of patients receiving thrombolysis do not achieve complete reperfusion. Factors that must be considered when deciding to administer thrombolysis or perform primary PCI include the availability of a PCI-capable facility, time from onset of

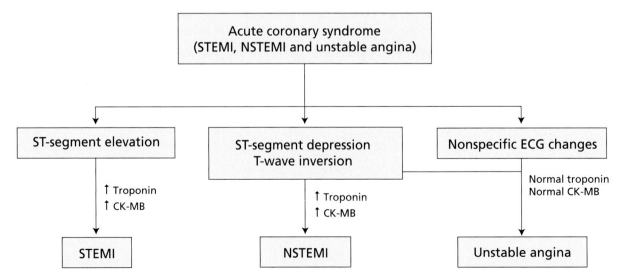

FIGURE 7. Diagnosis of acute coronary syndromes. CK-MB = creatine kinase MB; ECG = electrocardiographic; NSTEMI = non–ST-elevation myocardial infarction; STEMI = ST-elevation myocardial infarction.

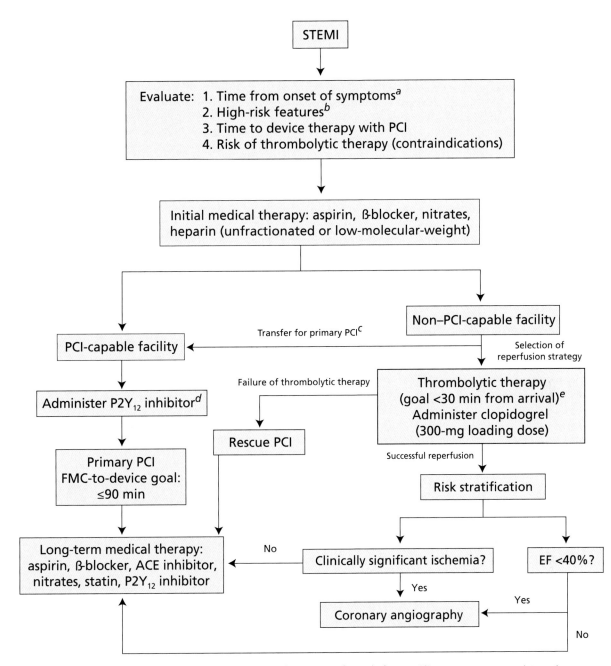

FIGURE 8. Management of ST-elevation myocardial infarction. EF = ejection fraction; FMC = first medical contact; PCI = percutaneous coronary intervention; STEMI = ST-elevation myocardial infarction.

[a]If 4 or more hours have elapsed since symptom onset, PCI is preferred.

[b]High-risk features such as cardiogenic shock and heart failure favor PCI.

[c]FMC-to-device ("door-to-balloon") goal for patients being transferred for primary PCI is as soon as possible and ≤120 minutes.

[d]P2Y$_{12}$ inhibitors: clopidogrel, prasugrel, ticagrelor.

[e]STEMI patients presenting to a hospital without PCI capability and who cannot be transferred to a PCI center and undergo PCI within 120 minutes of first medical contact ("door-to-balloon time") should be treated with thrombolytic therapy within 30 minutes of hospital presentation ("door-to-needle time") as a systems goal unless thrombolytic therapy is contraindicated.

O'Gara PT, Kushner FG, Ascheim DD, et al; American College of Cardiology Foundation/American Heart Association Task Force on Practice Guidelines. 2013 ACCF/AHA guideline for the management of ST-elevation myocardial infarction: a report of the American College of Cardiology Foundation/American Heart Association Task Force on Practice Guidelines. Circulation. 2013 Jan 29;127(4):e362-425. Erratum in: Circulation. 2013 Dec 24;128(25):e481. [PMID: 23247304] symptoms to presentation, the presence of high-risk features, and relative or absolute contraindications to thrombolytic therapy (**Table 10**). The preferred method of reperfusion is primary PCI, especially for patients presenting to hospitals with onsite PCI facilities. Because many patients with STEMI present to hospitals without onsite PCI facilities, a treatment algorithm is typically in place to emergently transfer patients to a PCI-capable facility or administer full-dose thrombolytic therapy. Even when thrombolytic therapy is administered, treatment guidelines recommend that patients be transferred to a PCI-capable facility because of the potential for thrombolytic failure.

In patients who undergo primary PCI, the time from patient presentation to device delivery (balloon inflation or thrombectomy catheter activation) is a major determinant of improved outcomes observed in primary PCI when compared with thrombolysis. Several studies have demonstrated superior efficacy of transfer for primary PCI versus thrombolytic therapy; however, observational studies have reported that patients often experience delays in transfer for primary PCI that exceed 1 hour. When PCI cannot be readily achieved within 120 minutes, thrombolytic therapy is recommended in those patients without contraindications. Regional and national efforts have improved these transfer procedures to include the ability of emergency medical services (EMS) to perform ECG in the field, immediate transfer of patients to PCI-capable facilities when STEMI is recognized, and improved communication between non-PCI facilities and PCI facilities.

Table 11 shows the characteristics of the most commonly used thrombolytic agents that are currently available. Although life-threatening bleeding events, such as intracerebral hemorrhage, are rare, they carry an extremely high mortality rate (50%-60%). Patients treated with thrombolytic therapy should

TABLE 10. Contraindications to Thrombolytic Therapy for ST-Elevation Myocardial Infarction
Absolute Contraindications
Any previous intracerebral hemorrhage
Known cerebrovascular lesion (e.g., arteriovenous malformation)
Ischemic stroke within 3 months
Suspected aortic dissection
Active bleeding or bleeding diathesis (excluding menses)
Significant closed head or facial trauma within 3 months
Relative Contraindications
History of chronic, severe, poorly controlled hypertension
Severe uncontrolled hypertension on presentation (SBP >180 mm Hg or DBP >110 mm Hg)[a]
History of ischemic stroke (>3 months), dementia, or known intracranial pathology
Traumatic or prolonged (>10 minutes) CPR or major surgery (<3 weeks)
Recent (within 2-4 weeks) internal bleeding
Noncompressible vascular puncture site
For streptokinase/anistreplase: previous exposure (>5 days) or previous allergic reaction to these agents
Pregnancy
Active peptic ulcer disease
Current use of anticoagulants: the higher the INR, the higher the bleeding risk

CPR = cardiopulmonary resuscitation; DBP = diastolic blood pressure; SBP = systolic blood pressure.

[a]Thrombolytic therapy can be considered if SBP can be reduced to <140 mm Hg and DBP to <90 mm Hg with initial medical therapy.

TABLE 11. Characteristics of Thrombolytic Agents Used in the Treatment of STEMI				
Characteristic	**Streptokinase**	**Alteplase**	**Reteplase**	**Tenecteplase**
Dose	1.5 million units over 30-60 min	Up to 100 mg in 90 min[a]	10 units × 2 (30 min apart) each over 2 min	30-50 mg[a]
Bolus administration	No	No	Yes	Yes
Allergic reaction possible on repeat exposure	Yes	No	No	No
TIMI flow grade 2/3[b]	~55%	~75%	~83%	~83%
Rate of intracerebral hemorrhage	~0.4%	~0.4-0.7%	~0.8%	~0.9%
Fibrin specificity	None	+++	+	++++

STEMI = ST-elevation myocardial infarction.

[a]Based on body weight.

[b]TIMI flow grade 2/3 refers to mildly impaired flow through the coronary artery involved in the myocardial infarction. The higher the percentage of TIMI 2/3 flow, the more effective the thrombolytic agent.

Adapted from Boden WE, Eagle K, Granger CB. Reperfusion strategies in acute ST-segment elevation myocardial infarction: a comprehensive review of contemporary management options. J Am Coll Cardiol. 2007;50(10):917-929. [PMID: 17765117] be closely observed clinically for symptom resolution and reperfusion arrhythmias, especially an accelerated idioventricular rhythm (AIVR); AIVR is considered a benign rhythm when it occurs within 24 hours of reperfusion. A repeat ECG should be obtained 60 minutes after thrombolysis to determine if ST-segment resolution has occurred.

Thrombolytic failure occurs in approximately 30% of patients, and typically presents with failure to fully resolve chest pain or improve ST-segment elevation by 50%; some patients may show hemodynamic instability or ventricular arrhythmias. In these circumstances, rescue PCI is indicated. Rescue PCI is associated with improved cardiovascular outcomes when compared with conservative medical therapy in patients with failure of thrombolytic therapy. Facilitated PCI is the administration of full- or half-dose thrombolytic therapy (with or without a glycoprotein IIb/IIIa inhibitor) followed by planned, immediate PCI. Adverse events (especially bleeding) have limited the safety and overall use of facilitated PCI.

Medical Therapy

At the time of initial presentation, all patients with STEMI should be given a 325-mg loading dose of aspirin, supplemental oxygen, therapy to improve symptoms (nitrates, analgesics), therapy to reduce infarct size (β-blockers, ACE inhibitors), and antithrombotic therapy (antiplatelet agents, anticoagulants). Aspirin should be administered immediately; however, the administration of other agents should not delay the plan to reperfuse the infarct-related artery.

In many patients with STEMI, control of chest pain can be achieved with sublingual or intravenous nitrates. Morphine and other opioid analgesics are also effective for reducing chest pain by decreasing the body's sympathetic response to STEMI. Caution should be used in patients with inferior STEMI and evidence of right ventricular infarction because nitrates and analgesics can lead to reduced preload and significant hypotension.

In the treatment of STEMI, β-blockers are recommended at the time of initial presentation except in patients with evidence of heart failure, hypotension, bradycardia, advanced atrioventricular block, or other contraindications to β-blockers. Intravenous metoprolol is the most widely used β-blocker for STEMI treatment; it is dosed in 5-mg increments every 5 minutes, for a total dose of 15 mg. Following reperfusion, an oral β-blocker is recommended to reduce myocardial oxygen demand and reduce mortality.

ACE inhibitors should be administered after reperfusion in all patients without contraindications (systolic blood pressure <90 mm Hg, advanced kidney dysfunction, hyperkalemia). Angiotensin receptor blockers may be substituted in patients who are allergic or intolerant to ACE inhibitors.

The use of antiplatelet agents in the setting of STEMI has changed over the past decade with the availability of several new agents. Aspirin remains a mainstay in the treatment of ACS and should be administered to all patients unless allergic or intolerant. Platelet P2Y$_{12}$ receptor inhibitors impair platelet aggregation, and this effect is additive to aspirin. Available agents include clopidogrel, ticagrelor, and prasugrel. Clopidogrel has been the most widely studied, and its use with concomitant thrombolytic therapy and primary PCI is associated with improved outcomes and no apparent increase in the risk of bleeding. For patients for whom primary PCI for treatment of STEMI is planned, both ticagrelor and prasugrel demonstrated superior efficacy when compared with clopidogrel; however, very few patients in these studies were treated with thrombolytic therapy, and little evidence exists to recommend the use of either ticagrelor or prasugrel in patients receiving thrombolytic therapy. Dual antiplatelet therapy should be continued in STEMI patients for a full year, regardless of intervention or stent used; however, if dual antiplatelet therapy cannot be maintained for a full year (for example, because of bleeding, need for surgery, or problems with adherence) and the patient has a bare metal stent implanted, a minimum of 4 weeks of dual antiplatelet therapy is advised.

Platelet glycoprotein IIb/IIIa inhibitors (abciximab, tirofiban, eptifibatide) further inhibit platelet aggregation and impair platelet activation. They are useful in patients with STEMI who undergo primary PCI; however, the use of glycoprotein IIb/IIIa inhibitors should be reserved for administration in the catheterization laboratory rather than up-front in the emergency department owing to the increased risk of bleeding and no clear benefit when administered prior to primary PCI. Routine glycoprotein IIb/IIIa inhibitor use in patients who receive thrombolytic treatment without PCI is controversial and not currently recommended.

The choice of anticoagulant for treatment of STEMI is dependent on the reperfusion strategy available for the patient. Unfractionated heparin (UFH) has been thoroughly studied in patients receiving thrombolytic agents, and its use is associated with a reduced incidence of reocclusion of the infarct-related artery. Low-molecular-weight heparin (LMWH) has also been associated with improved outcomes in patients who receive thrombolytic therapy. In patients undergoing primary PCI, the use of UFH is favored over LMWH owing to the ability to monitor the degree of anticoagulation (by measurement of activated clotting times). When a heparin-based strategy is utilized for primary PCI, guidelines recommend the concomitant administration of a glycoprotein IIb/IIIa inhibitor. Recent studies of bivalirudin, a direct thrombin inhibitor, have shown that its use at the time of primary PCI is associated with a similar rate of ischemic events (death, myocardial infarction, stroke, stent thrombosis) and fewer bleeding events when compared with a heparin plus glycoprotein IIb/IIIa inhibitor. In general, therapies that reduce bleeding complications may improve survival but with concern for greater risk of nonfatal ischemic events, such as early stent thrombosis.

In patients with diabetes mellitus who present with STEMI, plasma glucose levels should be maintained below 180 mg/dL (10.0 mmol/L) while avoiding hypoglycemia. Intravenous insulin has been tested in multiple trials, but neither intravenous insulin nor glucose-insulin-potassium infusions are recommended currently.

Complications of STEMI

The most common complications during the early management period after STEMI are arrhythmias, heart failure, and vascular access issues in patients who undergo primary PCI. As many as 75% of patients with STEMI have an arrhythmia during hospitalization, including atrial and ventricular arrhythmias, sinus bradycardia (after inferior wall myocardial infarction), atrioventricular block, and sinus tachycardia (after anterior wall myocardial infarction). Approximately 10% to 15% of patients have atrial fibrillation or flutter during hospitalization, and this is associated with poorer long-term outcomes. The presence of atrial fibrillation or heart block is often transient in patients with inferior wall myocardial infarction and suggestive of more extensive infarction in patients with anterior wall myocardial infarction. Ventricular arrhythmias (ventricular tachycardia, ventricular fibrillation) that occur in the first 24 hours after STEMI diagnosis do not typically affect prognosis, require antiarrhythmic medications, or require defibrillator implantation. The occurrence of recurrent ventricular arrhythmias later in hospitalization is associated with a larger infarct and higher short- and long-term morbidity and mortality. In patients with persistent high-degree atrioventricular block or symptomatic bradycardia, placement of a temporary transcutaneous or transvenous pacemaker may be needed to determine reversibility or benefit of permanent pacemaker implantation.

The severity of heart failure (ranging from asymptomatic left ventricular systolic dysfunction to cardiogenic shock) is dependent on the extent of myocardial infarction, severity of obstructive CAD, time from symptom onset to reperfusion, and patient-specific factors (age, comorbid conditions). Patients who develop cardiogenic shock after STEMI often have more extensive left ventricular infarction and an elevated inpatient mortality rate greater than 60%, thus prompting aggressive medical therapy and hemodynamic support with intra-aortic balloon counterpulsation. The initiation of therapy to reduce preload (diuretics) and afterload (nitrates, ACE inhibitors) is indicated in all patients with symptoms of heart failure; however, caution is advised if systolic blood pressure is less than 90 mm Hg or kidney dysfunction exists.

Vascular access complications include hematoma, pseudoaneurysm, arteriovenous fistula, and retroperitoneal hemorrhage.

Mechanical complications in STEMI patients (**Table 12**) are much less frequent in the reperfusion era. Right ventricular infarction, which most commonly results from occlusion of the proximal right coronary artery, should be considered in all patients with inferior wall myocardial

TABLE 12. Potential Mechanical Complications of Myocardial Infarction

Complication	Physical Examination Findings	Electrocardiography Findings	Echocardiography Findings	Pulmonary Artery Catheter Findings
Right ventricular infarction	Hypotension, jugular venous distention, clear lung fields	>1 mm ST-segment elevation in leads V_3R and V_4R	Dilated right ventricle with reduced systolic function	Elevated right atrial and right ventricular pressures, low wedge pressure
Extensive left ventricular infarction	Systolic blood pressure <90 mm Hg	Extensive ST-segment elevation, usually in anterior leads	Severe left ventricular systolic dysfunction	CI <2.0 L/min/m², wedge pressure >18 mm Hg
Ventricular septal defect	Holosystolic murmur along left sternal border, often with thrill	Nonspecific; approximately 50% of ventricular septal defects occur in anterior wall MI	High-velocity left-to-right systolic jet within ventricular septum, systolic turbulence on right ventricle side of ventricular septum	Prominent, large v waves in wedge pressure tracing; step-up in oxygen saturation from right atrium to right ventricle
Papillary muscle rupture	Holosystolic murmur at left sternal border and apex, may radiate to axillae; pulmonary edema	Usually associated with inferior and inferior-posterior wall MI	Flail mitral valve leaflet with attached mass (papillary muscle head), severe mitral regurgitation	Prominent, large v waves in wedge pressure tracing
Left ventricular free wall rupture	Hypotension, jugular venous distention, distant heart sounds	Nonspecific; pulseless electrical activity	Diffuse or localized pericardial effusion with tamponade; discrete wall motion abnormality; defect in myocardium may be seen	Equalization of diastolic pressures, CI <2.0 L/min/m²

CI = cardiac index; MI = myocardial infarction.

infarction and hypotension. Right ventricular infarction leads to decreased pulmonary blood flow and left atrial return, decreased preload, and impaired filling of the left ventricle. This results in the triad of hypotension, clear lung examination, and elevated jugular venous pressure. Diagnosis is often made clinically and can be confirmed by either ECG (leads V_4R through V_6R) or echocardiography (often used to exclude other causes of cardiogenic shock). Treatment consists of reperfusion, aggressive volume resuscitation, and the use of inotropes (dopamine or dobutamine) until right ventricular function improves (often 2 to 3 days after myocardial infarction).

A ventricular septal defect is an infrequent complication of STEMI. It manifests as hemodynamic compromise in the setting of a new loud holosystolic murmur and often a palpable thrill 3 to 7 days after the initial myocardial infarction. Diagnosis is most commonly made by transthoracic echocardiography. Medical stabilization generally requires the administration of vasopressor agents and placement of an intra-aortic balloon pump. Although surgical mortality is high, inpatient mortality for patients who do not undergo surgery is nearly 100%. Percutaneous ventricular septal defect closure devices are sometimes used in nonsurgical patients, but their use is limited by anatomy and operator expertise.

Mitral regurgitation occurs commonly after STEMI. Mechanisms include severe left ventricular dysfunction with annulus dilatation, worsening of pre-existing mitral regurgitation, and compromise of the mitral apparatus (rupture of papillary muscle or chordae tendineae). Papillary muscle rupture often presents 3 to 7 days after initial myocardial infarction with hemodynamic compromise, pulmonary edema, and a loud systolic murmur. Diagnosis is most often made by transthoracic echocardiography, and transesophageal echocardiography may be required to plan surgical reconstruction. Treatment consists of the administration of vasodilators to reduce afterload and diuretics to decrease preload. If patients become hemodynamically compromised, the administration of vasopressors, placement of an intra-aortic balloon pump, and/or surgical intervention are required.

Left ventricular free wall rupture is the most ominous mechanical complication of STEMI and has a high mortality rate. It often occurs 3 to 7 days after initial myocardial infarction. Risk factors for left ventricular rupture include advanced age, female sex, anterior myocardial infarction, and incomplete reperfusion of STEMI. Patients most commonly present with pericardial tamponade (due to hemopericardium), pulseless electrical activity, and death. Early recognition, emergent pericardiocentesis, and subsequent surgical reconstruction can improve survival.

Left ventricular thrombus occurs in approximately 10% to 20% of patients after anterior myocardial infarction despite reperfusion and aggressive treatment. Transthoracic echocardiography is the most common diagnostic modality, and thrombus is detected as an echo-dense structure, often at the apex of the left ventricle (**Figure 9**). Treatment involves the use of therapeutic warfarin for 3 to 6 months following myocardial infarction to reduce the risk of stroke or systemic embolization. ▪

KEY POINTS

- In patients with ST-elevation myocardial infarction, when percutaneous coronary intervention cannot be readily achieved within 120 minutes, thrombolytic therapy is recommended in the absence of contraindications.

- Patients with ST-elevation myocardial infarction who receive thrombolytic therapy should be transferred to a percutaneous coronary intervention-capable facility because of the potential for thrombolytic failure.

Non-ST-Elevation Acute Coronary Syndromes

The most common pathophysiology of NSTE-ACS is nonocclusive coronary atherosclerosis with or without thrombus formation. The treatment of UA and NSTEMI patients is focused on improvement in epicardial blood flow with medications and revascularization. Because the link between revascularization and clinical outcomes is less clear than in STEMI patients, NSTE-ACS patients should undergo risk stratification prior to invasive treatment.

Risk Stratification

The TIMI risk score is the most commonly used tool for estimating the short-term risk for death and nonfatal myocardial infarction in patients with a NSTE-ACS (**Table 13**). The TIMI risk score is most useful to assist in deciding whether patients will benefit from an early invasive

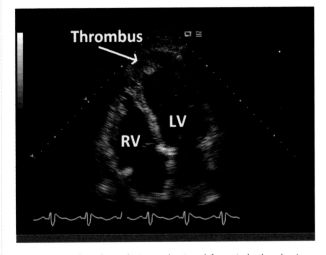

FIGURE 9. Echocardiographic image showing a left ventricular thrombus in a patient with a recent myocardial infarction. LV = left ventricle; RV = right ventricle.

TABLE 13. TIMI Risk Score for Non-ST-Elevation Acute Coronary Syndromes

Prognostic Variables

(1) Age ≥65 years

(2) ≥3 Traditional CAD risk factors[a]

(3) Documented CAD with ≥50% diameter stenosis

(4) ST-segment deviation

(5) ≥2 Anginal episodes in the past 24 hours

(6) Aspirin use in the past week

(7) Elevated cardiac biomarkers (creatine kinase MB or troponin)

TIMI Risk Score (Sum of Prognostic Variables)

0-2 Low risk

3-4 Intermediate risk

5-7 High risk

CAD = coronary artery disease.

[a]Hypertension, hypercholesterolemia, diabetes mellitus, being a current smoker, family history of CAD.

Adapted from Antman EM, Cohen M, Bernink PJ, et al. The TIMI risk score for unstable angina/non-ST elevation MI: a method for prognostication and therapeutic decision making. JAMA. 2000;284(7):835-842. [PMID: 10938172]

treatment strategy (**Figure 10**). The estimated rates of death and nonfatal myocardial infarction also are useful to counsel patients regarding their risk. In patients at low risk (TIMI score of 0-2), practice guidelines recommend an ischemia-guided strategy that utilizes invasive treatment only if medical therapy is ineffective. Patients at higher risk (TIMI score ≥3) are more likely to benefit from an early invasive approach.

Medical Therapy

All patients who present with ischemic chest pain should be treated initially with aspirin, β-blockers, and nitrates. However, compared with STEMI, in which reperfusion is the primary goal of therapy, once the diagnosis of UA or NSTEMI has been established (through the ECG and biomarkers), risk stratification can be used to guide the clinical use of additional therapies (**Table 14**, on pages 28-29). All NSTE-ACS patients should receive a statin and a P2Y$_{12}$ inhibitor (such as clopidogrel). In patients at intermediate or high risk (TIMI score ≥3), additional therapies, such as anticoagulant agents or a glycoprotein IIb/IIIa inhibitor, should be considered.

Antiplatelet Medications

The initial aspirin dose should be 325 mg at the time of presentation for ischemic chest pain. Patients who are allergic to aspirin should be administered clopidogrel at the time of presentation. Although there remains debate about subsequent aspirin dosing based on patient risk and whether revascularization with PCI or CABG occurs, most patients can be treated with a dose of 81 mg daily indefinitely (especially when dual antiplatelet therapy is being used).

Dual antiplatelet therapy (aspirin plus clopidogrel, prasugrel, or ticagrelor) is recommended in all patients with NSTE-ACS, regardless of TIMI risk score, unless an increased risk of bleeding exists (see Table 9). The use of clopidogrel, in addition to aspirin, is the best-studied combination. Clopidogrel should be given as a loading dose (300 mg or 600 mg) at hospital admission and administered as a 75-mg daily dose for at least 1 year regardless of the need for PCI or CABG. Patients with a bare metal stent who cannot tolerate dual antiplatelet therapy for the full year (for example, because of bleeding, need for surgery, or problems with adherence) should remain on the therapy for at least 4 weeks. If CABG is ultimately required, clopidogrel should be discontinued and CABG should be postponed for 5 to 7 days in order to avoid perioperative bleeding.

Two oral P2Y$_{12}$ inhibitors, prasugrel and ticagrelor, have been developed, and when tested, were superior to clopidogrel in UA and NSTEMI patients. Ticagrelor and prasugrel do not require hepatic metabolism, are more potent, and have a faster onset of action when compared with clopidogrel. These agents also should be discontinued 5 to 7 days or more prior to CABG.

Administration of glycoprotein IIb/IIIa inhibitors in patients with NSTE-ACS does not appear to be of net clinical benefit unless high-risk features, such as ongoing angina or evidence of ischemia after the initiation of standard antiplatelet and antianginal medications, reinfarction, or heart failure, are present. However, these agents, in combination with UFH or bivalirudin, are indicated at the time of PCI in patients with NSTE-ACS who ultimately require revascularization. Because of their potent antiplatelet activity, the main adverse effect of glycoprotein IIb/IIIa inhibitors is increased risk of major and minor bleeding events.

Anticoagulant Medications

The use of anticoagulant medications (UFH, LMWH, fondaparinux, and bivalirudin) has been a cornerstone of therapy for NSTE-ACSs for more than three decades. The choice of a particular agent is based on the patient's bleeding risk, TIMI risk score, comorbid conditions (such as chronic kidney disease), plan for an early invasive versus a conservative strategy, timing of coronary angiography, and physician preference.

UFH and LMWH are the most widely used anticoagulants for NSTE-ACSs. In patients in whom an early invasive approach is planned and in patients with chronic kidney disease, UFH is preferred over LMWH. In patients in whom a conservative strategy is planned, both LMWH and fondaparinux have been proved to be safe and effective. Advantages of fondaparinux and LMWH include the ability to dose once or twice daily rather than continuously and no requirement to monitor therapeutic levels. Because of a significantly increased bleeding risk, the use of the anticoagulant bivalirudin is currently not recommended by clinical guidelines other than during PCI or in patients who are allergic to heparin-based products.

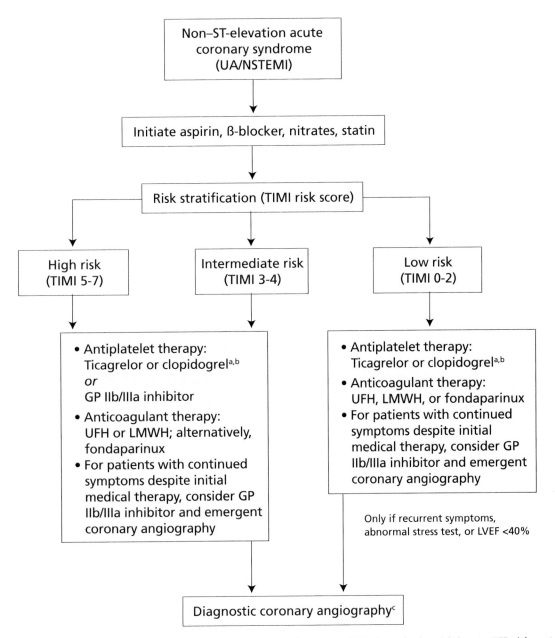

FIGURE 10. Initial management of non-ST-elevation acute coronary syndromes. GP = glycoprotein; LMWH = low-molecular-weight heparin; LVEF = left ventricular ejection fraction; NSTEMI = non-ST-elevation myocardial infarction; UA = unstable angina; UFH = unfractionated heparin.

[a]Clopidogrel or ticagrelor may be dosed at the time of hospital admission and acute coronary syndrome diagnosis.

[b]If coronary artery bypass grafting is required, clopidogrel or ticagrelor should be stopped and surgery delayed for at least 5 days.

[c]If the decision is made to withhold a P2Y$_{12}$ inhibitor until time of angiography and a P2Y$_{12}$ inhibitor is desired, clopidogrel, ticagrelor, or prasugrel can be initiated.

Recommendations based on Amsterdam EA, Wenger NK, Brindis RG, et al; ACC/AHA Task Force Members. 2014 AHA/ACC guideline for the management of patients with non-ST-elevation acute coronary syndromes: executive summary: a report of the American College of Cardiology/American Heart Association Task Force on Practice Guidelines. Circulation. 2014 Dec 23;130(25):2354-94. [PMID: 25249586]

Antianginal Medications

Unless contraindicated, oral β-blockers should be initiated in all patients who present with a NSTE-ACS. Intravenous β-blockers can also be administered; however, caution should be used in patients with heart failure, advanced age, advanced atrioventricular block, and hypotension.

Nitrates that can be administered to NSTE-ACS patients include intravenous, topical, oral, and sublingual formula-tions. Intravenous nitrates are typically used in patients with ongoing chest pain or borderline blood pressure or hemody-namics. In patients without active symptoms, topical and oral formulations should be prescribed in order to prevent recur-rent symptoms. Sublingual nitroglycerin is often prescribed on an as-needed basis for new or worsening angina. All forms of nitrates should be avoided in patients who have taken a PDE-5 inhibitor (such as sildenafil or vardenafil) within 24 hours.

TABLE 14.	Long-Term Medical Therapy for Coronary Artery Disease			
Medication	**Drugs in This Class**	**Dosage**	**Indication**[a]	**Comment**
Antiplatelet Medications				
Aspirin	N/A	75-162 mg/d	All patients, unless intolerant or allergic	
Clopidogrel	N/A	75 mg/d	$P2Y_{12}$ inhibitor in combination with aspirin is indicated in all patients after ACS or PCI	Clopidogrel is recommended as an alternative for patients with intolerance or allergy to aspirin[b]
Prasugrel	N/A	10 mg/d	$P2Y_{12}$ inhibitor in combination with aspirin is indicated in all patients after ACS or PCI	Contraindicated in patients >75 years of age, low body weight (<60 kg [132 lb]), or history of stroke/TIA
Ticagrelor	N/A	90 mg/d	$P2Y_{12}$ inhibitor in combination with aspirin is indicated in all patients after ACS or PCI	More rapid onset of action; does not require first-pass hepatic metabolism; no known genetic polymorphisms. Decreased effectiveness with aspirin dosages ≥100 mg
Cardioprotective Medications				
β-Blockers	Atenolol, metoprolol, carvedilol, nebivolol	Variable	All patients with prior MI or LV systolic dysfunction	Caution is advised in patients with significant obstructive lung disease (e.g., COPD) or advanced atrioventricular block
ACE inhibitors	Benazepril, captopril, enalapril, fosinopril, perindopril, trandolapril, lisinopril, ramipril, quinapril	Variable	All patients with LV systolic dysfunction, hypertension, diabetes, or proteinuric chronic kidney disease	
Angiotensin receptor blockers	Losartan, valsartan, olmesartan, candesartan, irbesartan, telmisartan	Variable	ACE inhibitor–intolerant patients	The use of angiotensin receptor blockers in combination with ACE inhibitors is not well established (class IIb recommendation)
Aldosterone blockade	Spironolactone, eplerenone	Variable	ACS patients with LV systolic dysfunction on therapeutic doses of β-blockers and ACE inhibitors	Caution is advised in patients with significant kidney dysfunction or hyperkalemia
High-intensity statin therapy	Atorvastatin	40-80 mg/d	For all patients with evidence of coronary artery disease and age ≤75 years	
	Rosuvastatin	20-40 mg/d		
Moderate-intensity statin therapy	Atorvastatin	10-20 mg/d	For all patients with evidence of coronary artery disease and age >75 years or otherwise intolerant of high-intensity statin therapy	
	Rosuvastatin	5-10 mg/d		
	Simvastatin	20-40 mg/d		
	Pravastatin	40-80 mg/d		
	Lovastatin	40 mg/d		
	Fluvastatin	40 mg BID		

(Continued on the next page)

TABLE 14. Long-Term Medical Therapy for Coronary Artery Disease *(Continued)*

Medication	Drugs in This Class	Dosage	Indication[a]	Comment
Antianginal Medications				
β-blockers	Atenolol, metoprolol, carvedilol, nebivolol	Variable	All patients with prior MI or LV systolic dysfunction	Caution is advised in patients with significant obstructive lung disease or advanced atrioventricular block
Long-acting nitrates	Isosorbide, transdermal patch, ointment	Variable	Useful for relief of symptoms when maximal, tolerated dose of β-blocker has been achieved[b]	Nitrates are contraindicated in patients taking PDE-5 inhibitors for erectile dysfunction
Short-acting nitrates	Sublingual, spray, or aerosol	Variable	Useful for relief of symptoms, usually prescribed on an as-needed basis	Nitrates are contraindicated in patients taking PDE-5 inhibitors for erectile dysfunction
Calcium channel blockers	Amlodipine, diltiazem, verapamil, nifedipine, nicardipine	Variable	Useful for relief of symptoms when maximal, tolerated dose of β-blocker has been achieved[b]	
Ranolazine	N/A	500-1000 mg BID	Useful for relief of symptoms when maximal, tolerated dose of β-blocker has been achieved[c]	Caution is advised in patients with advanced kidney disease, liver disease, and in those taking potent inhibitors of CYP3A4 pathway

ACS = acute coronary syndrome; BID = twice daily; LV = left ventricular; MI = myocardial infarction; N/A = not applicable; PCI = percutaneous coronary intervention; PDE-5 = phosphodiesterase 5; TIA = transient ischemic attack.

[a]Level of evidence: All are class I, level A, except as noted.

[b]Level of evidence: class I, level B.

[c]Level of evidence: class IIa, level B.

Calcium channel blockers and ranolazine do not have clear indications for use in patients presenting with an ACS. Opioids, such as morphine, may be administered for symptomatic relief of patients with ongoing chest pain, although caution is advised because of their blood pressure–lowering effects.

Lipid-Lowering Medications

The benefits of statin therapy in ACS patients are well established; however, the timing of initiation (hospital admission versus at the time of PCI versus hospital discharge) is less clear. Recent studies suggest that high-intensity dosing of atorvastatin or rosuvastatin is associated with improved 2-year survival after ACS. Current treatment guidelines recommend the initiation of a high-intensity statin in patients at very high cardiovascular risk, including those patients with an ACS.

Invasive Versus Ischemia-Guided Treatment

Once medical therapy has been initiated and risk stratification has occurred, guidelines recommend that patients with a low-risk NSTE-ACS be treated conservatively with an ischemia-guided strategy and that intermediate- to high-risk patients be considered for early invasive treatment. Patients treated with an ischemia-guided strategy should undergo noninvasive stress testing before hospital discharge; coronary angiography and subsequent PCI or CABG should be reserved for those with recurrent symptoms or high-risk features on stress testing. High-risk patients assigned to an early invasive strategy (coronary angiography and subsequent PCI or CABG within 24 hours of initial hospitalization) have been shown to have improved outcomes when compared with high-risk patients treated conservatively. For patients who are appropriate for an early invasive strategy, there is no evidence that very early angiography (<6 hours or at hospital admission) offers incremental benefit.

Clinical guidelines recommend the use of early invasive treatment in NSTE-ACS patients regardless of risk stratification who have recurrent symptoms, hemodynamic instability, or electrical instability.

CABG is often recommended for ACS patients with specific angiographic criteria (that is, left main disease and multivessel CAD with or without proximal left anterior descending stenosis) with concomitant left ventricular systolic dysfunction and/or diabetes mellitus.

- All patients who present with ischemic chest pain should be treated initially with aspirin, β-blockers, and nitrates; once the diagnosis of a non–ST-elevation acute coronary syndrome has been established, risk stratification can be used to guide the clinical use of additional therapies.

- All patients with a non–ST-elevation acute coronary syndrome should receive a statin and dual antiplatelet therapy with aspirin and a $P2Y_{12}$ inhibitor; in patients at intermediate or high risk, additional therapies (anticoagulant agents, glycoprotein IIb/IIIa inhibitor) should be considered.

- Dual antiplatelet therapy is recommended for at least 1 year in all patients with a non–ST-elevation acute coronary syndrome, unless an increased risk of bleeding exists.

- Once medical therapy has been initiated and risk stratification has occurred, guidelines recommend that low-risk patients with a non–ST-elevation acute coronary syndrome be treated conservatively and that intermediate- to high-risk patients be considered for early invasive treatment.

Acute Coronary Syndromes Not Associated with Obstructive Coronary Disease

Although plaque rupture at the site of atherosclerotic plaque deposition is the most common cause of ACS, other disease entities may cause patients to present with chest pain, transient ECG changes, and elevated cardiac biomarkers. The diagnosis of these diseases is generally made once diagnostic coronary angiography has confirmed the absence of obstructive coronary stenoses.

Coronary vasospasm often occurs in normal or near-normal coronary arteries, and spasm can be triggered by the use of illicit drugs, such as cocaine or methamphetamine. In patients who present with ischemic chest pain at rest and transient ST-segment elevation or depression, the diagnosis of vasospasm is often one of exclusion once angiography confirms the absence of obstructive CAD. Vasospasm is most frequently treated with long-term nitrates and calcium channel blockers and avoidance of triggers such as illicit drugs.

Takotsubo cardiomyopathy, often temporally associated with a stressful event, can mimic an ACS with the presence of chest pain, ECG changes, and elevated cardiac biomarkers (see Heart Failure). However, coronary angiography is usually normal or shows only minimal atherosclerotic disease, and left ventriculography is classically defined by the presence of mid-wall and apical wall motion abnormalities with sparing of the basal segments. Treatment is supportive, and more than 95% of patients have resolution of symptoms and recovery of left ventricular function within 7 days.

Owing to the improved sensitivity of troponin assays, other systemic diseases (such as chronic kidney disease, sepsis, and rhabdomyolysis) and cardiac conditions (such as heart failure, atrial fibrillation, and myocarditis) can lead to a diagnosis of ACS without obstructive coronary artery stenosis on coronary angiography. In most cases, the etiology of ACS is presumed to be demand ischemia (myocardial oxygen demand surpasses oxygen supply); it is termed secondary myocardial infarction when cardiac biomarkers are abnormal. Management of these patients typically includes treatment of the underlying condition in addition to medical therapy (aspirin, statin) and preventive measures for heart disease.

Long-Term Care After an Acute Coronary Syndrome

All patients who are diagnosed with an ACS should continue aspirin (81 mg/d) indefinitely. Patients treated medically without PCI should receive an oral $P2Y_{12}$ inhibitor for up to 12 months. The optimal duration of dual antiplatelet therapy in patients with an ACS who undergo PCI with drug-eluting stent implantation is at least 12 months (see Table 9). In patients who undergo PCI with bare metal stent implantation, the duration of dual antiplatelet therapy is at least 4 weeks but up to 12 months as tolerated. In the absence of contraindications, ACE inhibitors and statins should be continued indefinitely in all patients with an ACS. There is evidence of benefit for treatment with a β-blocker for at least 3 years following an ACS, although many clinicians choose to continue these medications indefinitely if they are well tolerated.

Current guidelines recommend that patients who are entering cardiac rehabilitation programs after ACS should undergo routine exercise ECG testing. Routine stress testing is not currently recommended for asymptomatic patients who are not entering a cardiac rehabilitation program. For patients with an ACS who are symptomatic after hospital discharge, the use of stress testing is acceptable and should be determined by the patient's symptoms (for example, unstable angina, stable angina), ability to exercise, and interpretability of ECG.

- Routine stress testing is not currently recommended for **HVC** asymptomatic patients following an acute coronary syndrome who are not entering a cardiac rehabilitation program.

Management of Coronary Artery Disease in Women

Clinical Presentation

Women typically develop ischemic heart disease at a later age in life than men. Unlike men, women present more frequently with stable angina pectoris rather than an ACS or sudden cardiac death. More than 50% of women who present with typical angina are diagnosed with nonobstructive coronary stenoses, and the presence of microvascular disease is thought to be significantly higher in women than in men.

In women presenting with acute myocardial infarction, chest pain remains the predominant symptom; however, the likelihood of atypical symptoms, such as fatigue, dyspnea, nausea, and abdominal complaints, is significantly higher than in men. In women without significant obstruction on invasive angiography, microvascular dysfunction (either endothelium-dependent or endothelium-independent) is thought to be the cause of symptoms.

Evaluation and Treatment

The sensitivity and specificity of noninvasive stress testing for the evaluation of chest pain are lower in women than in men. ST-segment deviation is less accurate in women than in men. Clinical guidelines report an improved diagnostic test accuracy with the use of stress testing with imaging (see Diagnostic Testing in Cardiology). However, no specific diagnostic evaluation guidelines exist for women, and the same guidelines apply to men and women.

In the COURAGE trial, women with stable angina pectoris had reduced overall mortality or nonfatal myocardial infarction with revascularization therapy as compared with men. However, women have a higher complication rate, particularly bleeding and vascular complications, surrounding revascularization procedures. For these reasons, it is recommended that guideline-directed medical therapy be initiated in women prior to consideration for revascularization. In women undergoing PCI, a trend toward fewer such complications has been found with the use of radial rather than femoral arterial access. Overall, treatment guidelines do not currently differ between men and women. The use of estrogen is not recommended to reduce the occurrence of future cardiovascular events in post-menopausal women.

KEY POINTS

- In women presenting with acute myocardial infarction, chest pain remains the predominant symptom; however, atypical symptoms, such as fatigue, dyspnea, nausea, and abdominal complaints, are more likely than in men.

- In women with coronary artery disease, it is recommended that guideline-directed medical therapy be initiated prior to consideration for revascularization; otherwise, treatment guidelines do not currently differ between men and women.

Management of Coronary Artery Disease in Patients with Diabetes Mellitus

Risk and Evaluation

Patients with diabetes mellitus are at increased risk of developing CAD, and cardiovascular mortality is significantly higher in this population. Additionally, patients with diabetes mellitus often do not experience classic angina pectoris and can present with atypical cardiac symptoms, such as dyspnea, nausea, or hyperglycemic symptoms. Sudden cardiac death occurs significantly more frequently in persons with diabetes compared with those without the disease. The diagnostic accuracy of noninvasive stress testing in symptomatic patients with diabetes is similar to that in patients without diabetes; however, the assessment of CAD in asymptomatic persons with diabetes is controversial. Currently, the American Heart Association recommends stress testing in patients with diabetes who are (1) symptomatic, (2) initiating an exercise program, or (3) known to have CAD and have not had a recent (>2 years) stress test.

Invasive Treatment

In patients with diabetes who are candidates for revascularization, the decision to pursue PCI or CABG remains controversial and depends on a multitude of factors, including severity and extent of CAD, the presence of comorbid conditions, and the degree of atherosclerotic narrowing of small, distal vessels. Multiple studies have analyzed outcomes of patients with diabetes undergoing PCI or CABG. Although CABG is generally associated with fewer repeat revascularization procedures, mortality is similar between the two procedures. When a decision is made to pursue PCI, the use of a drug-eluting stent is recommended to reduce the occurrence of target vessel revascularization because of the more extensive coronary artery disease and higher rate of restenosis in patients with diabetes.

Medical Therapy and Secondary Prevention

Aggressive risk factor reduction, control of plasma glucose levels, and medical therapy are essential in patients with diabetes. In most patients with diabetes and CAD, high-intensity statin therapy and antihypertensive treatment with a target blood pressure below 140/90 mm Hg are recommended. Because of the protective renal effects of ACE inhibitors and angiotensin receptor blockers in patients with proteinuric nephropathy, these agents are preferred over other antihypertensive agents, such as thiazide diuretics.

Common medications used for the treatment of diabetes are of special concern in patients with CAD. In a meta-analysis, thiazolidinediones, specifically rosiglitazone, had been associated with an elevated risk of cardiovascular events, especially myocardial ischemia. However, a more recent clinical trial demonstrated no elevated risk of myocardial infarction or death in patients being treated with rosiglitazone when compared with standard-of-care diabetes drugs. The use of metformin at the time of coronary angiography, after myocardial infarction, and in patients with heart failure should be avoided because of a rare but potentially fatal risk of lactic acidosis.

KEY POINT

- In patients with diabetes, stress testing is recommended by the American Heart Association for those who are (1) symptomatic, (2) initiating an exercise program, or (3) known to have coronary artery disease and have not had a recent (>2 years) stress test.

Heart Failure

Pathophysiology of Heart Failure

Heart failure is a complex clinical syndrome in which cardiac output is insufficient for meeting the demands of the body, causing symptoms of exertional dyspnea and fatigue. Approximately one half of patients with heart failure have left ventricular systolic dysfunction, or heart failure with reduced ejection fraction (HFrEF); the other half have normal systolic function, or heart failure with preserved ejection fraction (HFpEF). Regardless of whether left ventricular ejection fraction is reduced or preserved, symptoms of exertional dyspnea and fatigue are the same, and assessment of ejection fraction is required to differentiate between these two entities.

Common causes of HFrEF include hypertension, coronary artery disease, myocarditis, certain drugs (for example, doxorubicin, trastuzumab, cyclophosphamide), and toxins, including alcohol, cocaine, amphetamines, cobalt, and lead. Systemic diseases that may cause HFrEF include hypo- and hyperthyroidism, HIV infection, systemic lupus erythematosus, scleroderma, and neuromuscular diseases such as Duchenne and Becker muscular dystrophy. A high percentage of HFrEF cases are idiopathic. The most common causes of HFpEF are hypertension and coronary artery disease; less common causes include infiltrative diseases such as amyloidosis and hemochromatosis. In general, patients with HFpEF tend to be older, heavier women who have a history of hypertension, coronary disease, and diabetes mellitus.

Although the symptoms of exertional dyspnea and fatigue and hemodynamic abnormalities of reduced stroke volume and elevated ventricular filling pressures are similar between HFpEF and HFrEF, there are significant differences in the pathophysiology between the two disease processes. In patients with HFrEF, the common defect is an abnormality of myocardial contraction. Reduced systolic function results in progressive ventricular dilation. In contrast, patients with HFpEF have similar symptoms but normal systolic contraction and an abnormality in diastolic relaxation. This results in restricted filling and high filling pressures. To maintain a normal cardiac output (heart rate × stroke volume), patients with HFpEF tend to have a higher heart rate. Clinically, because these patients have a very small left ventricular size, they are usually much more sensitive to volume loading than patients with HFrEF.

Diagnosis and Evaluation of Heart Failure

Clinical Evaluation

Approximately half of all heart failure hospital admissions result from HFpEF. There is no difference in mortality between patients with HFpEF and HFrEF. For both groups of patients, there is about a 50% survival rate at 3 years after presenting with symptoms of heart failure.

Classic symptoms of acute heart failure include exertional dyspnea, paroxysmal nocturnal dyspnea, orthopnea, and peripheral edema. In patients with stable chronic heart failure, symptoms are typically similar to those of new-onset heart failure but less intense. A patient may normally sleep on two or three pillows owing to nocturnal dyspnea, but with decompensation will sleep on more pillows or move to sleeping in a recliner. Similarly, a patient at baseline may become short of breath walking up one flight of stairs, but with decompensation may have dyspnea putting on his or her clothes. Patients with previously diagnosed heart failure often do not present with classic findings. These patients may present with increased abdominal girth rather than peripheral edema, or with nausea and anorexia caused by gut edema rather than with exertional dyspnea. Educating patients to weigh themselves daily and report changes in weight or baseline symptoms may reduce heart failure hospital admissions if acted on quickly enough.

The first step in the evaluation of a patient with signs and symptoms of heart failure is a thorough history and physical examination, which should be performed to evaluate for possible causes of heart failure and assess cardiovascular risk factors. A detailed history, including alcohol and illicit drug use, alternative therapies, family history, and any history of chemotherapy, should be obtained. Features that increase the likelihood of heart failure include the presence of paroxysmal nocturnal dyspnea (>2-fold likelihood) and the presence of an S_3 (11 times greater likelihood). The likelihood of heart failure is decreased 50% by the absence of dyspnea on exertion and by the absence of crackles on pulmonary auscultation. Elevated jugular venous pressure and an S_3 are independently associated with adverse outcomes, including progression of heart failure.

Diagnosis

In patients who present with acute dyspnea of undetermined etiology, B-type natriuretic peptide (BNP) levels can be used to quickly differentiate between dyspnea secondary to heart failure (elevated BNP) and dyspnea related to pulmonary disease (low to normal BNP). The Breathing Not Properly study evaluated patients who presented to the emergency department with dyspnea. Patients who had heart failure had a mean BNP level greater than 600 pg/mL (600 ng/L), whereas those with noncardiac causes of dyspnea had levels of approximately 50 pg/mL (50 ng/L). Patients with a history of left ventricular dysfunction but not an acute exacerbation had a BNP level of approximately 200 pg/mL (200 ng/L). BNP levels increase with age and worsening kidney function and are reduced in patients with an elevated BMI.

BNP levels alone are not diagnostic for heart failure but should be used only as an initial test to guide the diagnostic evaluation in patients with dyspnea of uncertain etiology. BNP levels should not be used to follow a patient's clinical course. There is no benefit to following BNP levels during a hospitalization to determine if diuresis has been adequate. Additionally, routine use of BNP measurement in outpatients with heart failure is not helpful for determining if a patient is fluid overloaded.

A 12-lead electrocardiogram (ECG) should be obtained for all patients with heart failure. An ECG can be helpful to evaluate for possible myocardial infarction, tachyarrhythmia, or left ventricular hypertrophy. A chest radiograph should be obtained to evaluate for concomitant pulmonary disease. Chest radiography can also be helpful for identifying vascular congestion indicating volume overload or pleural effusions.

The initial laboratory assessment of heart failure should include electrolyte levels, urinalysis and kidney function, glucose and lipid levels, liver chemistry tests, and thyroid-stimulating hormone levels. Although thyroid disease is an uncommon cause of heart failure, hypothyroidism and hyperthyroidism are potentially reversible causes of heart failure with appropriate treatment. Coronary disease causes approximately two thirds of cases of heart failure, and an acute coronary syndrome should be suspected as a cause of new heart failure or an exacerbating factor in patients with preexisting heart failure. If an acute coronary syndrome is suspected as precipitating heart failure, measurement of troponin levels may be useful. However, troponin levels are occasionally mildly elevated in patients with an exacerbation of heart failure owing to wall stress and subendocardial ischemia or with acute myocarditis. An elevated troponin level does not guide therapy in this setting but can be used as a marker of more progressive heart failure and worse prognosis. Routine evaluation for unusual causes of heart failure, including hemochromatosis, Wilson disease, multiple myeloma, and myocarditis, should not be performed. An evaluation for other unusual causes of heart failure should not be performed routinely in all patients but should only be performed when there are suggestions of specific diseases by history or physical examination.

The most important diagnostic test in the evaluation of heart failure is transthoracic echocardiography. An echocardiogram will give an assessment of ejection fraction as well as information about possible causes. For example, identification of wall motion abnormalities increases suspicion for coronary artery disease and myocardial ischemia. Echocardiography also allows assessment for aortic and mitral valve disease, with the caveat that mitral regurgitation is often caused by the remodeling process of heart failure and is therefore secondary to the heart failure rather than the primary cause (functional mitral regurgitation). Additionally, the left ventricular end-diastolic dimension can be helpful for evaluating the chronicity of the disease process as well as prognosis. Patients with acute heart failure syndromes and a dilated left ventricle likely have a chronic disease process with delayed onset or recognition of symptoms. A small left ventricle (particularly without wall thinning) is associated with a greater chance of recovery of ejection fraction compared with a markedly dilated left ventricle. Also, a combination of findings on echocardiography may provide a clue to the cause of heart failure. For example, left ventricular hypertrophy and bi-atrial enlargement in a patient with reduced ejection fraction suggests a restrictive cardiomyopathy. The left ventricular hypertrophy of HFpEF is usually secondary to hypertension and should not be confused with the severe hypertrophy characteristic of hypertrophic cardiomyopathy (see Myocardial Disease). Patients with HFpEF often have mild to moderate left ventricular hypertrophy (<15 mm in any region).

Cardiac magnetic resonance (CMR) imaging is used increasingly in the evaluation of patients with heart failure. CMR imaging can be used to assess wall motion abnormalities, global wall function, and viability. Additionally, it can be used to assess tissue perfusion, tissue injury (inflammation or necrosis), fibrosis, infiltration (sarcoid or amyloid), or iron deposition.

Endomyocardial biopsy is rarely indicated for the evaluation of acute heart failure. Patients with progressive heart failure on medical therapy who have malignant arrhythmias should undergo biopsy to evaluate for giant cell myocarditis. Biopsy is also reasonable for patients with new-onset heart failure unresponsive to standard medical therapy. Endomyocardial biopsy can assist in the diagnosis of amyloidosis and hemochromatosis, which are diffuse processes amenable to diagnosis by biopsy techniques; sarcoidosis, on the other hand, can be quite patchy and is less likely to be discovered on endomyocardial biopsy.

There is no role for routine right heart catheterization for the diagnosis or management of patients with heart failure. In patients admitted to the hospital with heart failure, routine right heart catheterization has not been demonstrated to decrease either mortality or rehospitalization rates compared with usual care. Right heart monitoring can be helpful in patients with advanced heart failure who are refractory to medical therapy. Symptomatic hypotension and worsening kidney function may be suggestive of low cardiac output but could also be caused by infection or progression of disease. A right heart catheterization directly measuring cardiac output and filling pressures can guide therapy toward improving hemodynamics (higher stroke volume and lower filling pressures) with inotropic agents and/or more aggressive diuresis if the filling pressures are high. Right heart catheterization is also indicated in patients being evaluated for heart transplantation. Pulmonary hypertension is a risk factor for poor outcomes following heart transplantation because the right ventricle of the donor heart is not accustomed to pumping against high pulmonary pressures and may fail.

Evaluation for Ischemia

Although coronary artery disease is the most common cause of heart failure, owing to expense and radiation exposure, the routine investigation for coronary disease by stress testing or cardiac catheterization or other imaging modalities (such as CMR imaging, PET, or CT) is no longer considered part of the routine evaluation of all patients with newly diagnosed heart failure. Cardiac catheterization should be performed in patients presenting with angina or significant ischemia. Additionally, cardiac catheterization is recommended for patients presenting with chest pain that may or may not be of cardiac origin and those with previously diagnosed coronary artery disease without chest pain if they are eligible for revascularization. Noninvasive stress testing is reasonable in patients with a history of coronary artery disease to evaluate for reversible ischemia, as revascularization can dramatically improve left ventricular function. Additionally, patients with multiple risk factors for coronary disease should undergo noninvasive testing to evaluate for signs of ischemia. If stress testing identifies significant ischemic myocardium, coronary angiography should be considered. **H**

KEY POINTS

- B-type natriuretic peptide levels can be useful to distinguish cardiac from noncardiac causes of dyspnea in the urgent care setting.

HVC
- In patients with heart failure, with the exception of thyroid disease, an extensive evaluation of unusual causes of heart failure should not be performed unless there are suggestions of specific diseases by history or physical examination.

- The most important diagnostic test in the evaluation of heart failure is transthoracic echocardiography, which allows assessment of left ventricular ejection fraction as well as information regarding potential causes, clinical course, and prognosis.

Medical Therapy for Systolic Heart Failure

The treatment of patients with HFrEF (systolic heart failure) comprises treatment of the acute exacerbation followed by institution of long-term therapy to decrease morbidity and mortality and improve symptoms in patients with chronic heart failure. The initial therapy for patients presenting with acute heart failure and volume overload is a diuretic. An ACE inhibitor or angiotensin receptor blocker (ARB) should also be started unless the patient has symptomatic hypotension. Once the acute heart failure episode has stabilized, all patients should be treated with a β-blocker.

The long-term therapy of heart failure is based on the patient's functional status as measured by New York Heart Association (NYHA) functional class (**Table 15**) and signs and symptoms of volume overload. In addition to ACE inhibitors and β-blockers, other treatments for heart failure that have been shown to decrease mortality and future hospitalizations include aldosterone antagonists and, specifically for black patients, hydralazine-isosorbide dinitrate (**Table 16**). Several additional medications have been shown to improve symptoms but have no effect on mortality.

TABLE 15. New York Heart Association (NYHA) Functional Class

Class	Description
I	No limitations of physical activity
II	Slight limitation of physical activity
III	Marked limitation of physical activity
IIIA	Symptoms with less than ordinary activity
IIIB	Symptoms with minimal exertion
IV	Unable to carry on any physical activity without symptoms

TABLE 16. Medical Therapy for Heart Failure with Reduced Ejection Fraction

Therapies that Decrease Mortality
ACE inhibitors/angiotensin receptor blockers
β-Blockers
Aldosterone antagonists (if NYHA class II to IV)
Hydralazine/isosorbide dinitrate (black patients with NYHA class III/IV symptoms)

Therapies that Improve Symptoms
Digoxin
Diuretics
Inotropic agents
Vasodilators

NYHA = New York Heart Association.

ACE Inhibitors and Angiotensin Receptor Blockers

ACE inhibitors have been shown to decrease mortality, decrease symptoms of heart failure, improve functional capacity, and improve left ventricular ejection fraction. All patients with HFrEF should be started on an ACE inhibitor. The patient should be started on a low dose, which can be up-titrated as tolerated based on blood pressure and symptoms. Higher doses of ACE inhibitors compared with lower doses have been shown to decrease heart failure hospital admissions but not mortality. In patients with baseline hypotension, it is important to initiate ACE inhibitor therapy, but the dose should not be maximized prior to initiating β-blockade because the combination of both agents is superior to therapy with either one alone. Caution should be used when initiating ACE inhibitor therapy in patients with chronic kidney disease, and the patient's kidney function should be monitored closely. However, the presence of kidney dysfunction should not be considered a contraindication to the initiation of these agents; recent guidelines suggest initiating therapy in patients with a serum creatinine level below 3.0 mg/dL (265.2 µmol/L).

A common adverse effect of ACE inhibitors is a dry, nonproductive cough, which occurs in up to 20% of patients. For these patients, it is reasonable to switch to an ARB instead. Less information regarding mortality is available for ARBs, so they should not be used as first-line therapy. Other common adverse effects of both drugs include hyperkalemia and, occasionally, worsening kidney function. In patients with angioedema while taking ACE inhibitors, ARBs should not be used as an alternative because there are reports of angioedema also occurring with these agents.

β-Blockers

β-Blockers should be started in all patients with HFrEF after acute decompensation is treated and the patient is hemodynamically stable. These drugs block the adverse effects of chronic neurohormonal activation on cardiac function. Three β-blockers have been shown to decrease mortality, reduce heart failure symptoms, and improve left ventricular ejection fraction in patients with HFrEF: metoprolol succinate, carvedilol, and bisoprolol. It is important to use one of these three agents because they are the only ones that have a demonstrated benefit in patients with heart failure. Other β-blockers, including short-acting metoprolol (metoprolol tartrate), have not shown similar benefit. Some patients experience increased fatigue on β-blockade, but the vast majority experience an improvement in heart failure symptoms.

Initiating and Managing ACE Inhibitor and β-Blocker Therapy

Patients with acute heart failure and volume overload should initially be started on an ACE inhibitor. Typically, a short-acting agent such as captopril should be used in divided daily doses so that if the patient experiences symptomatic hypotension, the effect will be transient. ACE inhibitors should be titrated based on blood pressure and the presence or absence of adverse effects. For patients with new-onset heart failure and volume overload, a β-blocker should not be initiated until the patient is euvolemic or close to euvolemic.

In contrast to ACE inhibitors, in which the dose can be rapidly titrated upward, β-blockers should be started at a very low dose once patients are euvolemic because these agents have a negative inotropic effect. Instead of up-titrating the drug on a daily basis, titration of a β-blocker should be performed slowly at 1- to 2-week intervals, on an outpatient basis. A number of studies have demonstrated a dose-response effect with β-blockers. High doses compared with low doses of β-blockers have been shown to be more beneficial for both mortality reduction and the reduction of heart failure symptoms. Although patients are often discharged on low doses, these agents should be up-titrated to the maximal tolerated doses after the patient has been discharged (**Table 17**). Limitations to maximal up-titration include symptomatic hypotension and bradycardia. Once the heart rate is below 60/min, the current dose can be maintained. A history of COPD is not a contraindication to initiating β-blocker therapy, and there is no evidence that the nonselective β-blockers are not tolerated in these patients.

TABLE 17. Therapeutic Doses of β-Blockers for Treatment of Heart Failure with Reduced Ejection Fraction

Agent	Target Dosage
Carvedilol	25 mg BID (50 mg BID if >85 kg [187 lb])
Metoprolol succinate	200 mg daily
Bisoprolol	10 mg daily

BID = twice daily.

Diuretics

Diuretics are the mainstay of therapy for symptoms of heart failure associated with volume overload. To avoid hypovolemia, the lowest dose of diuretic necessary should be used. Loop diuretics are the most commonly used agents. In patients with refractory heart failure, the addition of a thiazide diuretic is occasionally used to augment the effects of the loop diuretic. There is no advantage to a continuous intravenous infusion versus bolus therapy in decompensated heart failure. Adverse effects of diuretics include hypokalemia, hypomagnesemia, and worsening kidney function. As electrolyte abnormalities can lead to malignant arrhythmias, electrolytes should be frequently measured in patients receiving high doses. Additionally, patients should be counseled to restrict their sodium and fluid intake.

Digoxin

Digoxin has been used for decades for the treatment of heart failure. Digoxin has not been shown to reduce mortality but does decrease hospitalizations for HFrEF in comparison with placebo. In short-term trials, digoxin has been shown to improve heart failure symptoms, quality of life, and exercise tolerance. The withdrawal of digoxin in patients is associated with increasing heart failure symptoms.

Therapy with digoxin should be closely followed. It is reasonable to check a serum digoxin level when a patient is stable. Patients with kidney impairment, low body mass, and older age have reduced metabolism of digoxin and can quickly develop a toxic level. It is important to check a digoxin level in patients with worsening kidney function. Retrospective analyses have shown that serum levels greater than 1 ng/mL (1.28 nmol/L) are associated with increased risk of mortality, most commonly related to arrhythmias.

Aldosterone Antagonists

Aldosterone antagonists (spironolactone, eplerenone) have been studied in patients with heart failure and NYHA functional class II to IV symptoms and have been shown to reduce mortality and morbidity. For patients with class II symptoms, the benefit has been shown only in those with a history of prior hospitalization or an elevated BNP level. The principal side effect of these agents is hyperkalemia. Spironolactone and eplerenone have not been compared with one another, but in clinical trials, gynecomastia occurs specifically with spironolactone. Because of the risk of kidney dysfunction and hyperkalemia, these drugs should be used only in patients with a serum creatinine level below 2.5 mg/dL (221 μmol/L) in men or below 2.0 mg/dL (176.8 μmol/L) in women, and with a serum potassium level below 5.0 mEq/L (5.0 mmol/L). Additionally, if the patient is on potassium supplementation, this should be discontinued when therapy is initiated. Electrolytes and kidney function should be checked 1 week after initiation of therapy and be closely monitored over time. Aldosterone antagonists should be used very cautiously in elderly patients. These drugs are not effective as diuretics at the doses used in heart failure therapy (12.5-25 mg/d for spironolactone, 25-50 mg/d for eplerenone).

Isosorbide Dinitrate and Hydralazine

The combination of isosorbide dinitrate and hydralazine is an alternative therapy for patients with heart failure who have kidney dysfunction that limits therapy with either ACE inhibitors or ARBs. In this setting, this combination is used for its vasodilating properties. More recently, based on retrospective data from earlier clinical trials, a clinical trial in black patients with heart failure and reduced ejection fraction and NYHA class III and IV symptoms was performed that demonstrated a reduction in mortality with a specific formulation of this combination compared with placebo. There was a high incidence of adverse effects (primarily peripheral edema, dizziness, gastrointestinal symptoms, and headaches) and drug withdrawal. For black patients, studies have demonstrated improvements in quality of life in addition to a mortality benefit. Note that this combination was studied as an additional therapy for patients already on an ACE inhibitor or an ARB and a β-blocker, not as a replacement therapy, and should only be instituted after these agents have been maximized.

Calcium Channel Blockers

Because of their vasodilating effects, calcium channel blockers have been closely studied for their potential role in the management of heart failure. Unfortunately, the non-dihydropyridine calcium channel blockers (for example, diltiazem or verapamil) also have myocardial depression activity and have been demonstrated to either have no benefit or worse outcomes in patients with heart failure. Patients who have been treated for hypertension with diltiazem or verapamil should have those agents discontinued once a diagnosis of heart failure has been made. The second-generation dihydropyridine calcium channel blockers, such as amlodipine and felodipine, have been shown to be safe in patients with heart failure, but do not reduce morbidity or mortality. For patients who are still hypertensive on high doses of ACE inhibitors and β-blockers, a peripherally acting dihydropyridine calcium channel blocker can be used as an antihypertensive agent. H

- Initial therapy for all patients with heart failure with reduced ejection fraction should include an ACE inhibitor; those with volume overload should be given a diuretic, and once the acute heart failure episode has stabilized, all patients should be placed on a β-blocker.

- β-Blockers in the treatment of heart failure should be started at a very low dose and up-titrated slowly, at 1- to 2-week intervals.

- Aldosterone antagonists should be started in patients with New York Heart Association class II to IV symptoms with appropriate kidney function and a potassium level below 5.0 mEq/L (5.0 mmol/L).

- The addition of isosorbide dinitrate and hydralazine to standard heart failure therapy is associated with improvements in quality of life and a mortality benefit in black patients.

Management of Heart Failure with Preserved Ejection Fraction

ACE inhibitors, ARBs, β-blockers, and aldosterone antagonists have been studied in patients with HFpEF. Unfortunately, none of these agents have demonstrated any clinical benefit compared with placebo. At this time, no medications have demonstrated a reduction in mortality in this patient population. Therapy for HFpEF should instead be based on treating the causes and symptoms of the heart failure. Hypertension is a common cause of HFpEF, and aggressive control of blood pressure is necessary. Additionally, controlling tachycardia can be helpful in patients with atrial arrhythmias.

Patients with HFpEF are often quite volume sensitive, with a small therapeutic window between hypovolemia and hypervolemia. Judicious use of diuretics to maintain euvolemia is important. These patients should be encouraged to monitor their weight closely, as small differences in volume can quickly cause volume overload and subsequent hospital admissions.

Device Therapy

Sudden cardiac death is the cause of death in approximately 50% of patients with heart failure. The only reliable predictor of an arrhythmic event is left ventricular ejection fraction. For this reason, implantable cardioverter-defibrillators (ICDs) are used for primary prevention of sudden cardiac death in patients with heart failure and low ejection fraction.

Implantable Cardioverter-Defibrillator for Prevention of Sudden Cardiac Death

In patients with mild to moderate heart failure symptoms and left ventricular ejection fraction less than or equal to 35%, placement of an ICD reduces mortality compared with medical therapy or placebo in patients with both ischemic and nonischemic etiologies (**Table 18**). ICDs are indicated for patients with NYHA functional class II and III symptoms, ejection fraction less than or equal to 35% on guideline-directed medical therapy, and a life expectancy of at least 1 year. As patients with class IV symptoms have a reduced life expectancy, ICDs are not indicated in this population except in patients who are awaiting transplantation or undergo placement of a mechanical circulatory device.

ICDs should only be placed after patients are on guideline-directed medical therapy. For patients with recent onset of heart failure who have a reasonable chance of recovery of function, one should wait upwards of 6 months with the patient on adequate medical therapy and then reassess ventricular function to determine if the ejection fraction is still less than 35% prior to implantation. Specifically, patients treated with revascularization for coronary artery disease may have improvement in ejection fraction, which should be re-measured after revascularization.

Cardiac Resynchronization Therapy

In approximately 30% of patients, heart failure progression is accompanied by dyssynchrony (dysfunctional ventricular electromechanical coordination) manifested by prolongation of the QRS duration or a left bundle branch block. Biventricular pacing, or cardiac resynchronization therapy (CRT), involves pacing the right and left ventricles simultaneously. In addition to the usual placement of a pacer lead in the apex of the right ventricle, an additional lead is placed through the coronary sinus down a coronary vein on the lateral wall of the left ventricle. This simultaneous pacing has been demonstrated to increase ejection fraction, decrease heart failure symptoms, and reduce mortality in patients with HFrEF and ECG evidence of dyssynchrony. The 2013 American College of Cardiology Foundation/American Heart Association heart failure management guideline makes a strong recommendation with strong supporting evidence for CRT therapy in patients with an ejection fraction less than or equal to 35%, NYHA functional class III to IV symptoms on guideline-directed medical therapy, and left bundle branch block with QRS duration greater than or equal to 150 msec (see Table 18). A strong recommendation with weaker evidence is provided for patients with NYHA functional class II symptoms.

Patients with NYHA class I symptoms caused by ischemia and a left bundle branch block with a QRS duration greater than 150 msec have shown some benefit with CRT therapy, but the risk-benefit ratio is high owing to adverse effects of the therapy, and it is currently a class IIb recommendation. Adverse effects include infection at the site of the device, inappropriate firings, and occasional tricuspid valve regurgitation. **H**

TABLE 18. Indications for Device Therapy in Heart Failure

Implantable Cardioverter-Defibrillator (for primary prevention)

NYHA class II or III while taking guideline-directed medical therapy[a] *and*

Expectation of survival >1 year *and*

Either of the following:

Ischemic cardiomyopathy ≥40 days post MI or nonischemic cardiomyopathy with ejection fraction ≤35% (primary prevention)

History of hemodynamically significant ventricular arrhythmia or cardiac arrest (secondary prevention)

Biventricular Pacemaker (cardiac resynchronization therapy)

All of the following:

NYHA class II to IV

Ejection fraction ≤35%

On guideline-directed medical therapy

Ventricular dyssynchrony (LBBB with a QRS duration ≥150 msec)

LBBB = left bundle branch block; MI = myocardial infarction; NYHA = New York Heart Association.

[a]Also NYHA class I in patients with ischemic cardiomyopathy and ejection fraction <30% (MADIT-II criteria: Moss AJ, Zareba W, Hall WJ, et al; Multicenter Automatic Defibrillator Implantation Trial II Investigators. Prophylactic implantation of a defibrillator in patients with myocardial infarction and reduced ejection fraction. N Engl J Med. 2002;346(12):877-883. [PMID: 11907286])

Recommendations from Yancy CW, Jessup M, Bozkurt B, et al; American College of Cardiology Foundation; American Heart Association Task Force on Practice Guidelines. 2013 ACCF/AHA guideline for the management of heart failure: a report of the American College of Cardiology Foundation/American Heart Association Task Force on Practice Guidelines. J Am Coll Cardiol. 2013 Oct 15;62(16):e147-239. [PMID: 23747642]

KEY POINTS

- An implantable cardioverter-defibrillator is recommended for patients with New York Heart Association class II or III heart failure, a left ventricular ejection fraction less than or equal to 35% after treatment with guideline-directed medical therapy, and a life expectancy of at least 1 year.

- Cardiac resynchronization therapy is recommended for patients with New York Heart Association class II to IV heart failure, a left ventricular ejection fraction less than or equal to 35% on guideline-directed medical therapy, and a left bundle branch block with QRS duration greater than or equal to 150 msec.

Assessment of Chronic Heart Failure

Patients with chronic heart failure should be serially assessed for progression of disease in the outpatient setting. At each visit, it is important to assess current symptoms and functional capacity, volume status, and the adequacy of the medical therapy (both appropriate doses and the appropriate medications as heart failure progresses). Of equal or greater importance is repeated patient education, including reminding patients to take their medications as prescribed, measure their weight daily, avoid dietary sodium, watch their fluid intake, and exercise regularly. Patients who appropriately take their medications and avoid sodium and excess fluid intake can greatly improve their functional status.

Despite multiple studies demonstrating the benefit of medical therapies in heart failure, fewer than 60% of patients are discharged from the hospital on ACE inhibitor and β-blocker therapy. It is important to review medications at every visit to ensure that patients are on the appropriate therapy.

Serial B-Type Natriuretic Peptide Assessment

Serial assessment of BNP levels in patients with chronic heart failure have been evaluated in a number of studies. Although higher BNP levels are associated with increased mortality, change in level in an individual patient does not predict progression of disease. Additionally, there is no evidence of benefit to using BNP for serially following patients to assess volume status or for dose adjustment of medications.

Echocardiography in Chronic Heart Failure

Echocardiography should be performed in patients with severe left ventricular dysfunction after optimization of medical therapy to determine if the left ventricular ejection fraction has improved to above 35% before consideration of ICD implantation. For patients with chronic heart failure who are clinically stable, echocardiography rarely provides diagnostic benefit, and obtaining annual echocardiograms is not likely to change therapy or outcome. For patients hospitalized with acute heart failure, obtaining a repeat echocardiogram to evaluate left ventricular function or for worsening valvular abnormalities is reasonable. If a patient has progressive heart failure symptoms as an outpatient, a repeat echocardiogram can be helpful to evaluate for progressive valvular abnormalities, new wall motion abnormalities, or an increase in left ventricular size that may alter treatment and affect prognosis.

Assessing Prognosis

Multiple retrospective studies have been performed looking at methods to evaluate prognosis in patients with heart failure. Current 1-year survival rates for patients undergoing heart transplantation or placement of a left ventricular assist device are between 85% and 90%. Patients with a higher risk of death should be considered for these therapies. Important risk factors for death include NYHA class IV symptoms, repeat hospitalizations, hyponatremia (serum sodium <133 mEq/L [133 mmol/L]), worsening kidney function, higher doses of diuretics, intolerance of ACE inhibitors or β-blockers, and arrhythmias resulting in ICD firings. Patients with multiple risk factors should be referred to a heart failure cardiologist for further evaluation. Additionally, occasional discussions with patients regarding end-of-life issues and their wishes for advanced heart failure therapy should be initiated while the patient is still stable. Patients' advanced care plans often change over time.

Cardiopulmonary exercise testing is routinely performed to assess prognosis in patients being evaluated for transplantation. Patients with a low oxygen consumption (peak O_2 consumption <14 mL/kg/min) or a high ratio of ventilation-to–carbon dioxide production ($\dot{V}E/\dot{V}CO_2$ >34) have a poor 1-year prognosis.

The Seattle Heart Failure model (www.SeattleHeart FailureModel.org) is an online program that uses clinical characteristics to predict outcomes in patients with heart failure. This model can be used to help assess prognosis based on clinical characteristics and can be used to guide patients as they ask questions about their prognosis.

KEY POINTS

- Patients with chronic heart failure should be seen regularly for assessment of clinical status as well as ongoing patient education regarding taking medications as prescribed, measuring their weight daily, reducing dietary sodium and avoiding excess fluid intake, and exercising regularly.

- In patients with chronic heart failure who are clinically stable, annual or more frequent follow-up echocardiography rarely provides therapeutic or diagnostic benefit and is not recommended.   **HVC**

Inpatient Management of Heart Failure

Acute Decompensated Heart Failure

Patients with heart failure admitted to the hospital usually have symptoms of volume overload as the primary concern. Reasons to admit patients include progressive heart failure symptoms with dyspnea at rest, an inability to respond to oral diuretics, recurrent ICD firings, symptoms of ischemia, worsening kidney function, and signs of poor perfusion (such as cool extremities, a low pulse pressure, or pulsus alternans). Therapy is primarily focused on diuresis. Additional evaluation should be performed to determine the reasons for the decompensation, including a review of medications and whether the patient was taking his or her medications properly, an echocardiogram to look for reversible causes of worsening function, and, if appropriate, an evaluation for ischemia. Generally, the initial dose of intravenous diuretic should be at least equivalent to the total daily oral dose. If the patient does not respond appropriately to that dose, rapid up-titration should be performed to assist in fluid removal. The patient's usual outpatient medications (for example, ACE inhibitor, β-blocker) should be continued unless the patient is hypotensive or demonstrates signs of poor perfusion, in which case dose reduction or discontinuation of both the ACE inhibitor and β-blocker should be considered. In patients with signs of low-output heart failure (hypotension, worsening kidney or liver function, cool extremities), the β-blocker should be discontinued.

Patients should be adequately diuresed during the hospitalization. Orthopnea and an elevated central venous pressure are suggestive of elevated filling pressures. Patients often have symptomatic improvement before they are euvolemic, and striving to achieve euvolemia may result in a reduction in readmission rates. Volume status can be difficult to assess and a

CONT.

careful physical examination is required. Patients should be assessed for signs of volume overload even if they have reached a goal or "dry" weight, as this is not a reliable measure of euvolemia. Findings supportive of euvolemia include an estimated central venous pressure below 10 cm H_2O, no orthopnea, absence of peripheral edema, and reduced dyspnea. Despite the use of high-dose intravenous diuretic therapy and improvement in volume status during hospitalization, many patients are discharged before achieving euvolemic or decongested status. Objective markers of decongestion include net urine output, weight loss, evidence of hemoconcentration (increase in hematocrit and hemoglobin levels), and reduction in BNP level. These markers have been associated with lower rates of rehospitalization for heart failure in short-term follow-up.

Ultrafiltration can occasionally be used in patients admitted with volume overload when routine diuresis fails or patients are unresponsive to diuretic therapy. A recent randomized trial of ultrafiltration versus intravenous diuretics in patients with decompensated heart failure and worsening kidney function showed no difference in weight loss but worsened kidney function in patients treated with ultrafiltration.

Worsening kidney function, typically defined as a serum creatinine increase of 0.3 mg/dL (26.52 µmol/L) or greater during hospitalization for heart failure, is a common complication, occurring in up to 25% of patients. This event often triggers changes in medical therapy, including reduction or cessation of diuretics, ACE inhibitors or ARBs, or aldosterone antagonists. Retrospective studies have found that this complication is associated with worse survival long-term, but no therapies have been shown to prevent or reduce worsening kidney function in patients with heart failure.

Vasopressin antagonists can be used for the treatment of patients with hypervolemic or euvolemic hyponatremia. They are beneficial for correcting hyponatremia but have not demonstrated any mortality benefits.

Cardiogenic Shock

Cardiogenic shock is defined by persistent, symptomatic hypotension and end-organ dysfunction. Patients have acute kidney failure, evidence of liver dysfunction with elevated aminotransferase levels, poor peripheral perfusion with cool extremities, and decreased mental status. Cardiogenic shock requires intensive therapy with intravenous vasopressors. Patients who remain in shock despite intravenous therapy and with worsening organ function should be considered for mechanical support.

It is important to quickly rule out reversible causes in patients with cardiogenic shock. Reversible causes include acute myocardial infarction; ventricular septal or free wall rupture; and acute valvular regurgitation, possibly related to papillary muscle rupture, infection, or ascending aortic arch aneurysm with dissection of the aortic valve. Bedside echocardiography can be helpful in identifying structural causes of cardiogenic shock.

The initial therapy for cardiogenic shock includes vasoactive medications to increase cardiac output and raise blood pressure through peripheral vasoconstriction (**Table 19**). Patients with cardiogenic shock secondary to progressive heart failure are generally given an inotropic agent, such as dobutamine or milrinone (cleared by the kidneys). Patients with peripheral vasoconstriction (increased systemic vascular resistance) often benefit from the addition of a pure vasodilator such as sodium nitroprusside. Placement of a right heart catheter can be helpful to assess filling pressures, cardiac output, and systemic vascular resistance to help choose the appropriate medical regimen. Although the routine placement of a right heart catheter for patients admitted with heart failure has not been shown to improve outcomes, it should be considered to assist in therapeutic decision-making in patients with cardiogenic shock.

For patients with symptomatic hypotension and end-organ dysfunction despite vasopressor therapy, mechanical therapy should be considered. Mechanical support options

TABLE 19. Intravenous Vasoactive Medications Used for Treatment of Cardiogenic Shock

Medication	Mechanism	Inotropy	Vasodilation
Milrinone	Phosphodiesterase inhibitor	++	+
Dobutamine	β_1, β_2 receptors	++	(+) (at low dose)
			– (vasoconstriction, at high dose)
Nesiritide	Natriuretic peptide receptors	0	++
Sodium nitroprusside	Nitric oxide	0	++
Nitroglycerin	Nitric oxide	0	++ (mainly venous)
Vasopressin	V receptor	–	– (vasoconstriction)
Dopamine	D receptor	+	– (vasoconstriction, at high dose)
	β_1 receptors at intermediate dose		
	α_1 receptor at high dose		
Norepinephrine	Affinity for α_1, α_2 receptors greater than for β_1 receptors	+	– (vasoconstriction)

Strength of effect: ++ indicates very strong; + indicates strong; (+) indicates weak; 0 indicates neutral; – indicates opposite effect.

CONT. include intra-aortic balloon pumps and percutaneous or surgically implanted short-term mechanical ventricular assist devices (VADs). These assist devices have catheters that are placed into the vascular system (left atrium or ventricle); they then pump the blood into the aorta, essentially assisting the failing left ventricle. These devices augment cardiac output and improve end-organ perfusion. Because all of these devices require large catheters, a common complication is vascular compromise at the point of insertion.

Strategies to Prevent Readmission

At many U.S. hospitals, heart failure is the most common discharge diagnosis. Currently, 30-day readmission rates are greater than 20%, and reducing these admissions is a major focus of study and resources. Studies evaluating diuresis have shown that greater fluid removal during the hospitalization is associated with a lengthening of the time to readmission. Additionally, it is important that patients are discharged on appropriate medical therapy, including an ACE inhibitor and a β-blocker. Early physician follow-up, ideally within 7 days of discharge, has also been associated with a reduction in readmissions.

Because it is often difficult to schedule patients for an office visit within 1 week of discharge, multidisciplinary heart failure clinics have been created by a number of hospitals. These programs often include telephone monitoring of signs and symptoms, evaluating whether patients are actually taking their medications, educating patients on salt and fluid restriction, and providing a mechanism for early follow-up after hospitalization. **H**

KEY POINTS

- In hospitalized patients with acute volume overload, the initial dose of intravenous diuretic should be at least equivalent to the total daily oral dose; rapid up-titration should be performed if needed to assist in fluid removal.

- Reversible causes of cardiogenic shock include acute myocardial infarction, ventricular septal or free wall rupture, and acute valvular regurgitation.

HVC
- In patients discharged with a diagnosis of heart failure, early physician follow-up, ideally within 7 days of discharge, has been associated with a reduction in hospital readmissions.

Advanced Refractory Heart Failure

Once patients have progressed to advanced heart failure, the therapeutic options are limited to inotropic therapy, heart transplantation, mechanical circulatory support, and palliative care. Heart transplantation is the best option for patients with end-stage heart failure, with 50% survival rates approaching 13 years, but is limited by donor availability such that only 2000 transplants are performed in the United States annually. Candidates for transplant are therefore thoroughly evaluated for comorbidities that may limit survival. The upper age limit for heart transplant is 65 to 70 years. Patients with kidney dysfunction, diabetes with end-organ manifestations, malignancy, chronic infection, or other comorbidities are often denied transplant. Options for patients who are not candidates for heart transplantation include mechanical circulatory support as destination therapy and inotropic therapy. However, inotropic therapy does not decrease mortality and may actually increase it. The survival of inotropic-dependent patients is less than 10% at 1 year.

Mechanical Circulatory Support

With the development of continuous-flow left ventricular assist devices (LVADs), the survival of patients with advanced heart failure after implantation of these devices has dramatically improved. The pumps are surgically inserted into the left ventricle, and the blood is pumped through the device from the left ventricle to the aorta. The patients have a line (driveline) coming through the skin through which the power is transmitted to the pump. Ninety percent of patients receiving an LVAD as a bridge to heart transplantation are alive at 1 year. For patients who are not candidates for transplant and have an LVAD placed as destination therapy, the survival at 2 years is more than 60% and improving. Complications related to these devices include ischemic and hemorrhagic stroke (>10% of patients), driveline-related infections (approximately 30%), and gastrointestinal bleeding related to arteriovenous malformations (20% in some reports). **H**

Management of Post-Transplant Patients

The prognosis of heart transplant recipients has improved greatly in recent years. Most patients have no functional limitations and return to a normal quality of life. Patients typically begin on a three-drug immunosuppression regimen early after transplantation that includes a calcineurin inhibitor (cyclosporine or tacrolimus), an antiproliferative agent (mycophenolate mofetil, sirolimus, or everolimus), and prednisone. Most centers try to wean patients off of prednisone by 1 year. Immunosuppressive medications are associated with a number of adverse effects, including hypertension (>90% of patients) and new-onset diabetes (20% of patients). During the first year post-transplant, while doses of immunosuppressants are high, patients have an increased risk for infection. Rejection occurs in approximately 20% of patients in the first year but is almost nonexistent after the first year unless a patient stops taking immunosuppressants. Signs of rejection include heart failure and atrial arrhythmias (typically atrial flutter). However, most patients with rejection manifest no clinical symptoms, necessitating routine surveillance with endomyocardial biopsy. The surveillance interval varies; however, most centers perform biopsies between 1 and 5 years after transplant.

The long-term complications of heart transplant include cardiac allograft vasculopathy and malignancy. Cardiac allograft vasculopathy occurs in more than 50% of the patients by the fifth year after transplant. It is characterized by diffuse intimal thickening of the coronary arteries that starts distally and progresses proximally. For this reason, the usual therapies for coronary disease, such as percutaneous coronary intervention and coronary artery bypass grafting, are usually not beneficial. Lymphoproliferative disorders and skin cancer are the most common malignancies.

Because the heart in transplant patients is denervated, they usually do not experience typical ischemic chest pain, leading to atypical presentations of coronary artery disease and acute coronary syndromes. Additionally, without vagal innervation, heart rates tend to run between 90/min and 110/min. Heart transplant patients have a marked response to adenosine but are not responsive to digoxin or atropine. For transplant patients presenting with atrial arrhythmias, caution should be used before giving adenosine to diagnose the arrhythmia because it may cause prolonged atrioventricular conduction block.

KEY POINTS

- Cardiac allograft vasculopathy occurs in more than 50% of heart transplant recipients by the fifth year after transplant; because of its diffuse nature, revascularization is usually not beneficial.

- Because the heart in transplant patients is denervated, they usually do not experience typical ischemic chest pain, leading to atypical presentations of coronary artery disease and acute coronary syndromes.

Specific Cardiomyopathies

The most common cause of heart failure is coronary artery disease. Other common causes include hypertension and idiopathic cardiomyopathy. Approximately 10% of patients with heart failure have heart failure related to a specific etiology. This includes medication-induced cardiomyopathies (primarily chemotherapeutic agents), myocarditis, amyloidosis, sarcoidosis, infectious etiologies such as HIV, peripartum cardiomyopathies, and alcohol or other drug-induced cardiomyopathies. Others will be discussed later. Restrictive cardiomyopathies with such causes as chemotherapeutic agents, amyloidosis, and sarcoidosis are discussed in Myocardial Disease. Peripartum cardiomyopathy is discussed in Pregnancy and Cardiovascular Disease.

Takotsubo Cardiomyopathy

Takotsubo, or stress-induced, cardiomyopathy is a syndrome of reversible ventricular systolic dysfunction usually precipitated by an acute emotional or physiologic stress. Although takotsubo cardiomyopathy was initially described in elderly women following intense emotional stress, the syndrome may occur in men and in some patients an antecedent stress may not be identifiable. It is believed to be caused by sympathetic-mediated myocyte injury, but the precise pathogenesis is unknown. It often mimics an acute myocardial infarction with elevated troponin levels and electrocardiographic changes, but it is usually associated with normal coronary arteries. The hallmark is wall motion abnormalities that extend beyond a single coronary territory, identified by echocardiography or other imaging study. For example, on left ventriculogram, the apex of the heart will be hypokinetic and the mid heart will contract normally.

Characteristic electrocardiographic changes include ST-segment elevation and diffuse deep T-wave inversions with some prolongation of the QTc interval. Takotsubo cardiomyopathy is usually associated with recovery of systolic function in the acute period. Nevertheless, these patients should be treated with ACE inhibitors and β-blockers acutely. There is no accepted length of time to continue this therapy in patients whose left ventricular function returns to normal. For the rare patient who does not recover, this therapy should be continued.

Acute Myocarditis

Myocarditis usually presents with heart failure symptoms over a few days to weeks. Occasionally, patients have symptoms for several months before heart failure is discovered. The classic presentation of viral myocarditis includes a viral prodrome with fever, myalgia, and upper respiratory symptoms, but a prodrome is not required for the diagnosis. Patients present with dyspnea, chest pain, and arrhythmias. ECG abnormalities are often present, along with evidence of myocardial damage with elevated troponin levels.

Various infectious pathogens can cause myocarditis. The most common causes are adenovirus, coxsackievirus, and enterovirus. The pathogenesis of myocarditis is unclear and may involve direct infection of the myocardium with the virus or an immune system response to the infection.

Endomyocardial biopsy can define myocarditis with evidence of myocardial necrosis, degeneration, or both, with an adjacent inflammatory infiltrate. Indications for endomyocardial biopsy include ventricular arrhythmia, high-grade conduction block (type II or III) or lack of response to usual heart failure therapy.

Therapy for acute myocarditis is supportive and consists of usual heart failure therapy. Placebo-controlled immunosuppressive trials have not demonstrated improvements in mortality or ejection fraction. Patients often take months (6-12) to recover left ventricular function. Approximately 50% of patients eventually recover cardiac function; therefore, it is important to wait and not place an ICD for the usual indications (ejection fraction <35% and NYHA class II or III symptoms) until at least 6 months of heart failure therapy.

Giant Cell Myocarditis

Giant cell myocarditis is an acute, rapidly progressive form of myocarditis associated with ventricular arrhythmias and progressive cardiac dysfunction despite medical therapy. For unclear reasons, this process usually occurs in persons younger than 40 years. The underlying mechanism is unknown but is thought to be autoimmune. On endomyocardial biopsy, the pathognomonic "giant cell" is seen. Unlike other forms of myocarditis, aggressive immunosuppressive therapy has been shown to improve survival but this process is still often fatal. These patients should be considered for cardiac transplantation but often need to be bridged with VADs. There are case reports of giant cell myocarditis recurring post-transplantation.

Tachycardia-Mediated Cardiomyopathy

Sustained tachyarrhythmia for weeks to months can produce cardiomyopathy. The most common arrhythmias implicated are atrial fibrillation, atrial flutter, and tachycardia. Patients with very frequent premature ventricular contractions (≥10,000/d) can develop cardiomyopathy. Controlling heart rate with medications or ablation often results in improvement and resolution of heart failure for these patients. Patients with tachycardia should be evaluated for hyperthyroidism.

Myocardial Disease
Hypertrophic Cardiomyopathy
Clinical Presentation and Evaluation

Hypertrophic cardiomyopathy (HCM) is an inheritable cardiac disorder with a prevalence of 1 in 500 persons. More than 1400 sarcomeric mutations involving at least 11 different genes have been identified. The mutations demonstrate an autosomal dominant pattern of inheritance with high disease penetrance. Sporadic cases may also occur.

The major pathophysiologic mechanisms contributing to signs and symptoms of HCM are diastolic dysfunction and dynamic left ventricular outflow tract (LVOT) obstruction. Diastolic dysfunction arises from abnormal relaxation and poor myocardial compliance, leading to an increase in left ventricular filling pressures. Dynamic LVOT obstruction, present in approximately two thirds of patients, results from septal hypertrophy and anterior displacement of the mitral valve apparatus; this displacement also is associated with decreased coaptation of the valve leaflets and resultant mitral regurgitation (**Figure 11**, **Figure 12**). Dynamic LVOT obstruction is exacerbated by any drug therapy that increases contractility, such as digoxin or other inotropic agents. Obstruction is also

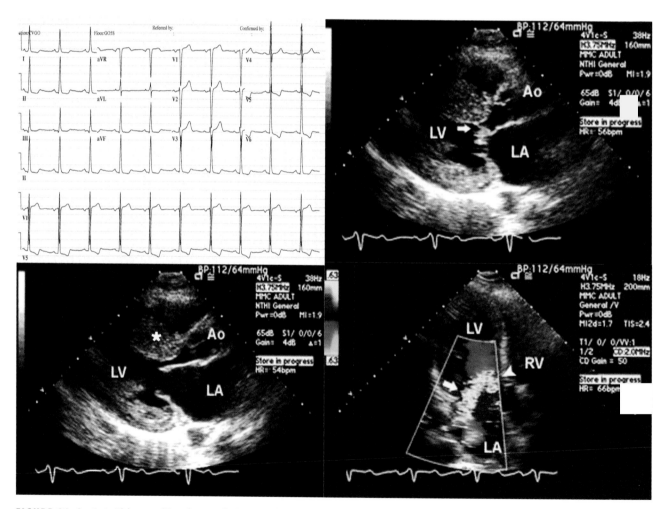

FIGURE 11. A patient with hypertrophic cardiomyopathy. Resting 12-lead electrocardiogram (*top left panel*) demonstrating findings of left ventricular hypertrophy and secondary ST-segment changes. Echocardiography (parasternal view) (*bottom left panel*) demonstrating severe myocardial hypertrophy of the ventricular septum (*asterisk*). Systolic anterior motion of the mitral valve is present (*arrow*) (*top right panel*). Apical long axis view of the left ventricle (*bottom right panel*). Systolic anterior motion of the mitral valve (*arrowhead*) leads to decreased coaptation of the mitral valve and secondary mitral regurgitation (*arrow*). Ao = ascending aorta; LA = left atrium; LV = left ventricle; RV = right ventricle.

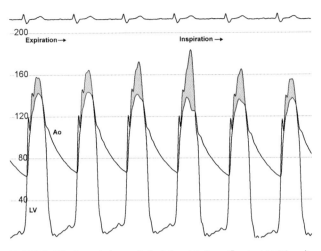

FIGURE 12. Dynamic changes in the left ventricular outflow tract (LVOT) gradient from obstructive hypertrophic cardiomyopathy during respiration. These hemodynamic tracings were taken during quiet respiration. Note that the LVOT gradient (*shaded*) increases significantly with expiration. These changes are mediated by respiratory-induced variation in ventricular afterload and have been described as *reversed pulsus paradoxus.* Ao = ascending aorta; LV = left ventricle.

worsened by reduced ventricular preload, such as from dehydration, or afterload, such as from vasodilator therapy.

Most patients with HCM have minimal or no symptoms. However, a subset develop exertional dyspnea, angina, presyncope, or syncope. Sudden cardiac arrest may be the initial manifestation of the disorder. HCM accounts for approximately 35% of sudden deaths among all persons younger than 35 years and is the leading cause of sudden death in this age group.

Several physical signs are helpful in diagnosing HCM in patients in whom it is suspected. The carotid upstroke typically is rapid and may be bifid (pulsus bisferiens—"twice beating") in those with LVOT obstruction. The jugular venous pulse may demonstrate a heightened *a* wave when there is significant infundibular hypertrophy. The apical impulse typically is sustained, localized, and may be bifid or trifid. An S_4 is frequently present, especially in younger patients. Paradoxical splitting of the S_2 also may occur with significant LVOT obstruction.

The murmur of dynamic LVOT obstruction is systolic with an ejection quality, frequently heard best at the left lower sternal border. Augmentation of the murmur occurs during maneuvers that decrease preload (squat-to-stand, Valsalva strain) and afterload (amyl nitrite inhalation). These maneuvers can help distinguish HCM from other causes of systolic murmurs, such as aortic stenosis and mitral regurgitation. Contrary to HCM, the murmurs of aortic stenosis and mitral regurgitation diminish with maneuvers that reduce preload.

The diagnosis of HCM typically is made by two-dimensional echocardiography and visualization of severe myocardial hypertrophy in the absence of a local or systemic etiology (**Figure 13**). The pattern of myocardial hypertrophy classically is described as asymmetric and involving principally the ventricular septum, but concentric, apical, and eccentric forms also are common. Cardiac magnetic resonance (CMR) imaging also may be used for diagnosis, particularly when there is eccentric or apical hypertrophy that may be difficult to visualize on echocardiography. Doppler echocardiography can accurately diagnose and quantify LVOT obstruction in most instances, with examinations performed at rest, with provocation (such as with amyl nitrite or dobutamine), or during exercise. LVOT obstruction is considered significant when the calculated pressure gradient is either 30 mm Hg or greater at rest, or 50 mm Hg or greater with provocation. In 80% to 90% of patients with HCM, electrocardiography (ECG) demonstrates findings of left ventricular hypertrophy.

Dynamic LVOT obstruction is present in approximately 25% of HCM patients at rest, with another 30% to 40% demonstrating obstruction only after provocative maneuvers. Patients can suffer from debilitating symptoms regardless of the presence of dynamic LVOT obstruction. However, because of the high prevalence of dynamic obstruction in patients with HCM and the availability of specific strategies that can reduce symptoms by alleviating it, clinicians should thoroughly evaluate for the presence and degree of obstruction.

HCM must be distinguished from other disorders that are associated with myocardial hypertrophy or increased wall thickness. These disorders include hypertensive heart disease, aortic stenosis, cardiac amyloidosis, Noonan syndrome, Fabry disease, and mitochondrial cardiomyopathy. Athlete's heart is a syndrome of myocardial hypertrophy that can be difficult to differentiate from HCM. Several clinical features are suggestive of athlete's heart, although a period of deconditioning (6 months or more) may be required to diagnose the presence of physiologic hypertrophy (**Table 20**, on page 45).

KEY POINT

- The systolic murmur of obstructive hypertrophic cardiomyopathy is augmented by maneuvers that decrease preload (squat-to-stand, Valsalva strain); in contrast, the systolic murmurs of aortic stenosis and mitral regurgitation diminish with maneuvers that reduce preload.

Clinical Course and Risk Stratification

Although symptoms of HCM can be debilitating and sudden cardiac death is a devastating complication, symptoms are minimal or absent and lifespan is normal in approximately 90% of patients with HCM. Atrial fibrillation occurs in 20% to 25% of patients with or without symptoms of obstruction. In some patients, owing to the underlying diastolic dysfunction, the loss of atrial systole from these arrhythmias can precipitate significant hemodynamic deterioration in addition to embolic risk. Contemporary investigations of unselected HCM populations demonstrate an incidence of sudden cardiac death of 0.5% to 0.8% per year. All patients with HCM should undergo

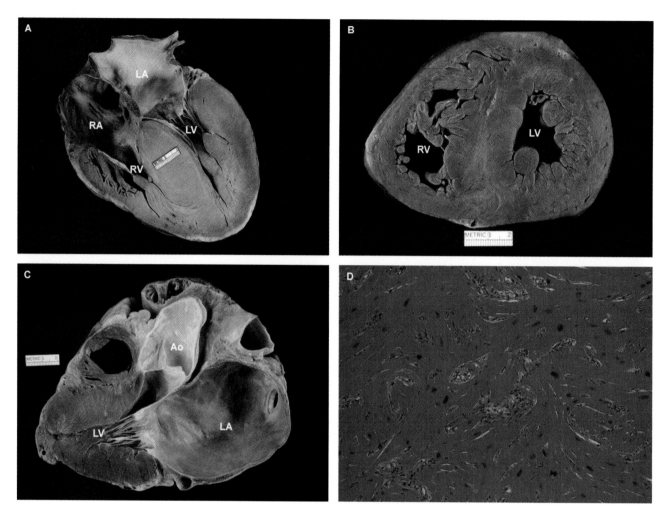

FIGURE 13. Pathology of hypertrophic cardiomyopathy. Gross specimens demonstrate severe myocardial hypertrophy due to hypertrophic cardiomyopathy with concentric hypertrophy (*A* and *B*) and apical hypertrophy (*C*). Microscopy demonstrates myocyte disarray, the histologic hallmark of hypertrophic cardiomyopathy (*D*). Ao = ascending aorta; LA = left atrium; LV = left ventricle; RA = right atrium; RV = right ventricle.

Images courtesy of Dr. William D. Edwards, Department of Pathology, Mayo Clinic.

risk stratification for sudden cardiac death (**Table 21**). Therapy with an implantable cardioverter-defibrillator (ICD) should be considered in patients with one or more risk factors. The clinical efficacy of ICDs for prevention of sudden cardiac death in HCM has been demonstrated in several large registries.

KEY POINT

- Placement of an implantable cardioverter-defibrillator should be considered in patients with hypertrophic cardiomyopathy with one or more major risk factors for sudden cardiac death: prior cardiac arrest, massive myocardial hypertrophy, family history of sudden cardiac death, ventricular tachycardia, blunted blood pressure response to exercise, unexplained syncope.

Management

The major management goals for patients with HCM are alleviation of symptoms, risk stratification for sudden cardiac death, ICD implantation for those at high risk, and family counseling.

Because a significant number of sudden deaths occur during or following exercise, abstention from competitive sports or strenuous aerobic activities is advised for all patients. Patients with HCM also should be counseled on the need to avoid dehydration and states of severe peripheral vasodilatation, such as from hot baths or saunas. Pregnancy generally is well tolerated, although precautions should be taken to minimize peripheral vasodilatation as for all patients with HCM.

Pharmacologic Treatment

Negative inotropic agents are the cornerstone of medical therapy for patients with symptomatic obstructive HCM. Negative inotropes (β-blockers, nondihydropyridine calcium channel blockers [verapamil], and disopyramide) depress contractility, thereby reducing the intraventricular flow velocities that predispose to LVOT obstruction. These agents also lengthen diastole, facilitating more time for ventricular filling. Appropriate drug therapy suffices for most patients with symptomatic obstructive HCM, although high doses may be required.

TABLE 20. Clinical Features Distinguishing Hypertrophic Cardiomyopathy from Athlete's Heart

Feature	Hypertrophic Cardiomyopathy	Athlete's Heart
Family history	Positive	Negative
Electrocardiography	Pathologic Q waves, T-wave inversions, conduction defects	Absence of these features
Doppler echocardiography	Diastolic filling abnormalities	Normal diastolic filling
Extent of hypertrophy	>15 mm	Often ≤12 mm
Pattern of hypertrophy	Asymmetric, concentric, or eccentric	Concentric
Left ventricular end-diastolic dimension	<45 mm	>55 mm
Gadolinium hyperenhancement on cardiac magnetic resonance imaging	Present	Absent
Objective exercise testing	% Predicted peak Vo_2 <100%	% Predicted peak Vo_2 >120% or >50 mL/kg/min
Genetic testing	Positive	Negative
Evaluation after period of deconditioning	No regression in hypertrophy	Regression >2 mm

Vo_2 = oxygen consumption.

TABLE 21. Risk Factors for Sudden Death in Patients with Hypertrophic Cardiomyopathy

Risk Factors	Comments
Major[a]	
Cardiac arrest (ventricular fibrillation)	Portends high rate of recurrence or death (11% per year)
Spontaneous sustained VT	
Family history of premature sudden death	Most predictive if occurs in a close relative or multiple relatives
Unexplained syncope	Most predictive if occurs in young patients, is exertional, or is recurrent
Left ventricular diastolic wall thickness ≥30 mm	
Blunted increase (<20 mm Hg) or decrease in systolic blood pressure on exercise	More predictive in patients <50 years of age
Nonsustained spontaneous VT	Less predictive if very brief (≤3 beats) and asymptomatic
Heart failure that has progressed to dilated cardiomyopathy with ejection fraction ≤35% and NYHA class II or III symptoms	Occurs in 5% to 10% of patients with hypertrophic cardiomyopathy
Possible Risk Factors in Individual Patients[a]	
Myocardial ischemia	May be a trigger for sustained ventricular arrhythmia in select patients
Left ventricular outflow obstruction	Gradient is modifiable with therapy
Delayed hyperenhancement with gadolinium on CMR imaging	Is common and is not an independent risk factor. However, severe extent is likely important and can be considered to be an arbitrating risk factor
Factors Not Predictive	
Ventricular arrhythmias inducible by electrophysiologic stimulation	Generally not considered to be of incremental value above noninvasive risk factors

CMR = cardiac magnetic resonance; NYHA = New York Heart Association; VT = ventricular tachycardia.

[a]Risk factors from Gersh BJ, Maron BJ, Bonow RO, et al; American College of Cardiology Foundation/American Heart Association Task Force on Practice Guidelines. 2011 ACCF/AHA Guideline for the Diagnosis and Treatment of Hypertrophic Cardiomyopathy: a report of the American College of Cardiology Foundation/American Heart Association Task Force on Practice Guidelines. Developed in collaboration with the American Association for Thoracic Surgery, American Society of Echocardiography, American Society of Nuclear Cardiology, Heart Failure Society of America, Heart Rhythm Society, Society for Cardiovascular Angiography and Interventions, and Society of Thoracic Surgeons. J Am Coll Cardiol. 2011 Dec 13;58(25):e212-60. [PMID: 22075469]

Positive inotropes (such as digoxin), vasodilators, and high-dose diuretics should be avoided, as these drugs exacerbate LVOT obstruction. Patients with atrial fibrillation and HCM should receive anticoagulation therapy with warfarin for stroke prevention, independent of cardiovascular risk factors. Although β-blockers are commonly prescribed in these patients, their use in the absence of symptoms or for prevention of sudden cardiac death is generally not recommended.

Septal Reduction Therapy

For patients with persistent, severe, drug-refractory symptoms caused by obstructive HCM, septal reduction therapy with surgical septal myectomy or percutaneous alcohol septal ablation should be considered.

Surgical myectomy is the gold standard therapy for relief of LVOT obstruction. In this procedure, a transaortic approach is typically used to resect the ventricular septum, often extending the resection to the base of the papillary muscles (**Figure 14**). In experienced centers, symptom relief with surgical myectomy occurs in more than 90% of patients with a low perioperative mortality rate (<1%). Long-term survival following myectomy has been found to be comparable to the expected survival of the general population.

Percutaneous alcohol septal ablation is an alternative therapy for septal reduction and may be particularly considered as an option for patients with high surgical risk. In this technique, a slightly oversized angioplasty balloon is placed in a septal perforating artery. The perfusion bed is delineated with contrast, followed by injection of desiccated alcohol. The alcohol results in a controlled infarction, which decreases ventricular systole and thereby ameliorates LVOT obstruction. A major limitation of alcohol ablation is the risk of pacemaker dependency. Pacemaker dependency occurs more frequently in patients with preexistent conduction disease. Incidence is 10% to 15% in patients with a normal ECG but up to 50% in patients with preprocedural left bundle branch block or a wide QRS interval. The decision to implant a pacemaker or ICD in the event of heart block with septal reduction therapy is based primarily on risk factors for sudden death.

In comparison to surgical myectomy, alcohol septal ablation has been associated with similar rates of clinical improvement, as measured by symptoms of heart failure and objective measures of peak myocardial oxygen consumption on treadmill testing. Few data on long-term follow-up after alcohol septal ablation are available, leading to recommendations that this procedure be restricted to relatively older patients as the long-term consequences of the therapeutic infarction of septal ablation are relatively unknown. Current national guidelines recommend that surgical myectomy and alcohol septal ablation should only be performed in centers of expertise, in the context of a longitudinal, comprehensive care program dedicated to patients with HCM.

Role of Genetic Testing and Screening

All first-degree relatives of patients with HCM should undergo screening for the disease. This recommendation is

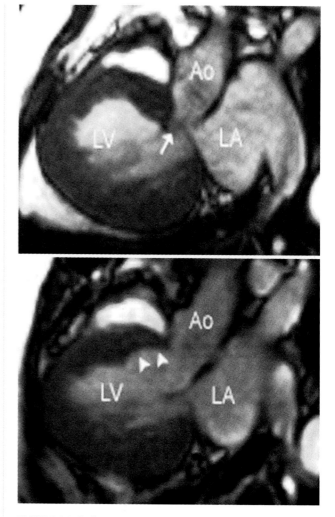

FIGURE 14. Cardiac magnetic resonance (CMR) imaging of hypertrophic cardiomyopathy before and after surgical myectomy. Prior to surgery, there is systolic anterior motion of the mitral valve owing to ventricular septal hypertrophy (*arrow*) (*top panel*). Surgery facilitates direct resection of the basal ventricular septum (*arrowheads*), leading to reconstruction of the left ventricular outflow tract and relief of obstruction (*bottom panel*). Ao = ascending aorta; LA = left atrium; LV = left ventricle.

based on the inheritable nature of HCM, the potential for sudden cardiac death, and the demonstrated efficacy of ICDs. Screening consists of physical examination, ECG, and two-dimensional echocardiography (or CMR imaging), with screening intervals recommended according to age, symptoms, and family history (**Table 22**). Ongoing screening of first-degree relatives who are initially free of the disease is recommended throughout adulthood because of the possibility of disease expression at any age.

Genetic testing of patients with HCM can identify pathologic mutations, which can then be used to screen family members for HCM. Genetic counseling is an important facet of the care of patients with HCM, regardless of whether genetic testing is performed. Counseling enables informed decision-making about the risks and benefits of testing and facilitates

TABLE 22. Recommended Screening Intervals for Evaluation of First-Degree Relatives of Patients with Hypertrophic Cardiomyopathy

Age Group	Recommendation
<12 years	Screening optional unless: Presence of symptoms Family history of malignant ventricular tachyarrhythmias Patient is competitive athlete in an intense training program Other clinical suspicion of early LV hypertrophy
12 to 18-21 years	Every 12 to 18 months
>18-21 years	At symptom onset or at least every 5 years (more frequently in families with malignant tachyarrhythmias or late onset)

LV = left ventricular.

NOTE: These recommendations are for relatives of patients with hypertrophic cardiomyopathy in whom genetic testing is negative, inconclusive, or not performed.

Recommendations from Gersh BJ, Maron BJ, Bonow RO, et al; American College of Cardiology Foundation/American Heart Association Task Force on Practice Guidelines. 2011 ACCF/AHA Guideline for the Diagnosis and Treatment of Hypertrophic Cardiomyopathy: a report of the American College of Cardiology Foundation/American Heart Association Task Force on Practice Guidelines. Developed in collaboration with the American Association for Thoracic Surgery, American Society of Echocardiography, American Society of Nuclear Cardiology, Heart Failure Society of America, Heart Rhythm Society, Society for Cardiovascular Angiography and Interventions, and Society of Thoracic Surgeons. J Am Coll Cardiol. 2011 Dec 13;58(25):e212-60. [PMID: 22075469]

the interpretation of the results, which can include known pathologic mutations and likely pathogenic mutations, as well as variants of unknown significance.

Genetic testing is performed as a panel, with the mutations associated with the greatest likelihood of pathologic consequences being β-myosin heavy chain, myosin-binding protein C, troponin T, troponin I, α-tropomyosin, actin, regulatory light chain, and essential light chain. A negative genetic test result does not rule out HCM in patients with phenotypic evidence of disease, so their immediate family members still should undergo interval screening. Whereas all patients with HCM can be considered for genetic testing to facilitate diagnosis in family members, the decision to pursue testing is individualized based on likelihood of detecting mutations, patient and family desire, and reimbursement concerns. The likelihood of detecting mutations is increased with a positive family history and a reversed curvature morphology of the ventricular septum. In reversed curvature, the hypertrophy of the septum is maximal in the mid-portion, with relatively less hypertrophy in the apical and basal segments. To date, genetic test results have not been strongly linked to risk of sudden cardiac death, so they should not be used for risk stratification.

KEY POINT

- All first-degree relatives of patients with hypertrophic cardiomyopathy should undergo screening for the disease, with screening intervals recommended according to age, symptoms, and family history.

Restrictive Cardiomyopathy

Clinical Presentation and Evaluation

Primary restrictive cardiomyopathy is an idiopathic disorder characterized by nondilated, poorly compliant ventricles, leading to severe diastolic dysfunction, elevated filling pressures,

and heart failure. In rare cases, restrictive cardiomyopathy is familial, with an autosomal dominant pattern of inheritance. Restrictive cardiomyopathy is a diagnosis of exclusion and must be distinguished from constrictive pericarditis (see later), eosinophilic syndromes, radiation-induced disease, storage diseases (such as Fabry disease, hemochromatosis), as well as infiltrative cardiomyopathies, such as amyloidosis and sarcoidosis. Patients with other forms of heart failure can also have restrictive patterns of diastolic ventricular filling but are not defined as having a primary restrictive cardiomyopathy.

Patients with restrictive cardiomyopathy may present at any age, with symptoms and signs of pulmonary and systemic congestion. The diagnosis can be considered when there is severe diastolic dysfunction and dilated atria in the absence of ventricular hypertrophy or cavity dilatation. Systolic function is preserved in most patients or, at least, is disproportionately high given the degree of diastolic dysfunction. Pulmonary hypertension, secondary to diastolic dysfunction, is common.

Endomyocardial biopsy can be performed for patients with suspected restrictive cardiomyopathy to evaluate for infiltrative disease, such as storage diseases or amyloidosis, when clinical assessment or less invasive testing (such as protein electrophoresis or fat biopsy) is inconclusive. The yield of biopsy is low in disorders with patchy myocardial involvement such as sarcoidosis.

Differentiating Restrictive Cardiomyopathy from Constrictive Pericarditis

Both restrictive cardiomyopathy and constrictive pericarditis present with elevation of diastolic pressures and heart failure that is disproportionate to the degree of systolic dysfunction. Distinction of the two disorders is important, as pericardiectomy will result in symptom relief and improvement in longevity in patients with constriction. Imaging and hemodynamic evaluation are most useful for differentiating these entities.

Distinguishing constrictive pericarditis and restrictive cardiomyopathy with physical examination can be challenging, as these conditions have similar signs. In both conditions, peripheral edema with elevation of the jugular venous pulse can be evident. The contour of the jugular venous pulse demonstrates prominent y descents owing to accentuation of early ventricular filling, and may rise (or fail to fall) with inspiration because of poor effective operative compliance (Kussmaul sign). In both disorders, if systolic function is preserved, the apical impulse characteristically is not displaced nor diffusely enlarged. In constriction, the apical impulse may be diminished. An early diastolic filling sound may be present in both disorders, attributable to either a "knock" in constrictive pericarditis or an S_3 (right- or left-sided) in restrictive cardiomyopathy. Because of severe diastolic abnormalities, physical findings of pulmonary hypertension are relatively more common in restrictive cardiomyopathy.

Measurement of B-type natriuretic peptide may be useful, as this biomarker is released at high levels in response to wall tension with restrictive cardiomyopathy ($\geq$400 pg/mL [400 ng/L]) but is usually normal or only mildly elevated in constriction (<100 pg/mL [100 ng/L]). CT imaging may demonstrate pericardial thickening and possibly calcification in constrictive pericarditis, although the pericardium can also be normal in thickness in a small subset of patients.

A hemodynamic evaluation is frequently required to distinguish restrictive cardiomyopathy from constriction. As a myocardial disease, restrictive cardiomyopathy may predominantly affect left ventricular filling, resulting in elevated left ventricular end-diastolic pressure and resultant pulmonary hypertension. In patients with constriction, the total cardiac volume is fixed by the rigid pericardium. As a result, there is enhancement of ventricular interdependence and resultant equalization of right and left ventricular diastolic pressures and reciprocal changes in the filling and stroke volume of the right and left ventricles during inspiration (see Pericardial Disease). These reciprocal changes during inspiration can be detected by either echocardiography or cardiac catheterization and are not present in patients with restrictive cardiomyopathy. **H**

Management

The primary goals in the management of restrictive cardiomyopathy are optimization of diastolic filling and relief of pulmonary and systemic congestion. Negative chronotropic agents, such as calcium channel blockers and β-blockers, are beneficial, as they lengthen the diastolic filling period and improve myocardial relaxation. Loop diuretics may be utilized; however, these agents should be used judiciously owing to the underlying poor ventricular compliance, which leads to the need for a relatively high ventricular filling pressure to maintain forward cardiac output. ACE inhibitors (or angiotensin receptor blockers) may improve diastolic function, but the benefit of these drugs in patients with heart failure due to restrictive cardiomyopathy is less certain than in patients with systolic dysfunction. Digoxin, which increases intracellular calcium, should

not be used in patients with restrictive cardiomyopathy. Atrial fibrillation, with loss of atrial contractile function, may lead to decompensated heart failure in patients with restrictive cardiomyopathy, but rhythm control may be challenging because of chronic left atrial pressure elevation and dilation.

The overall prognosis is generally poor in patients with idiopathic restrictive cardiomyopathy, with a 5-year survival of approximately 64%. Prognosis is affected by functional status, and cardiac transplantation should be considered in patients with severe refractory symptoms.

KEY POINTS

- Restrictive cardiomyopathy is characterized by severe diastolic dysfunction and, frequently, pulmonary hypertension.
- Restrictive cardiomyopathy is a diagnosis of exclusion and must be distinguished from constrictive pericarditis, eosinophilic syndromes, and infiltrative diseases.

Cardiac Tumors

Tumor Types

Cardiac tumors are usually metastatic, arising from carcinoma of the lung, breast, kidney, esophagus, or liver, or from blood dyscrasias, such as leukemia or lymphoma. Malignant melanoma is commonly associated with cardiac metastases. In autopsy series, cardiac involvement occurs in 10% to 15% of all patients with metastatic malignancy.

Primary cardiac tumors are exceedingly rare (0.02% to 0.06%) and are mostly benign. The most common primary cardiac tumors in adults are myxomas, followed by lipomas and papillary fibroelastomas. Myxomas are connective tissue tumors with cells encompassed within mucopolysaccharide stroma, with an appearance that may be villous, smooth, or friable. Myxomas may arise as part of the Carney complex, an autosomal dominant disorder associated with pigmentation abnormalities (blue nevi), cardiac and extracardiac myxomas, schwannomas, and endocrine tumors. Lipomas are fatty cell tumors that typically arise in the subendocardial layer. Papillary fibroelastomas are pedunculated tumors with frond-like arms, usually present on the left-sided valves of the heart. Malignant sarcomas of various types (angiosarcoma, fibroma, rhabdomyosarcoma, leiomyosarcoma) also have been described with cardiac involvement, accounting for approximately 15% of primary cardiac tumors.

Clinical Presentation and Evaluation

Manifestations of cardiac tumors depend on their location and size. Cardiac tumors that arise near or involve valves may obstruct blood flow or cause regurgitation, leading to pulmonary or systemic congestion. The auscultatory findings associated with left atrial myxoma are classically described as resembling those of a mitral stenosis murmur with an accompanying sound of a "tumor plop"; this finding, however, occurs in the minority of patients (10% to 15%). Patients with a myxoma may report constitutional symptoms, such as fever, anorexia, and weight loss, which are likely related to tumor cytokine production. Embolization, from either tumor fragments or associated thrombi, may cause neurologic symptoms or other systemic sequelae. Such embolization is relatively more common with villous or friable myxomas and papillary fibroelastomas. In a series of 74 patients with left atrial myxoma, systemic embolization occurred in 12%. Cardiac tumors, particularly lipomas and malignant sarcomas, may either directly invade or be located within myocardium, causing heart block or impairment of contractility. Pericardial effusion with or without tamponade also is a common manifestation.

Imaging (echocardiography, CT, or CMR imaging) is needed for the detection and evaluation of cardiac tumors. Myxomas characteristically are pedunculated and gelatinous, arising most commonly in the left atrium with the stalk adherent to the fossa ovalis (85% of cases) (**Figure 15**). Papillary fibroelastomas, whose origin may be related to trauma, typically involve left-sided cardiac valves or the left ventricular outflow tract. Papillary fibroelastomas have a central core stalk with fronds and often are mobile, with an appearance resembling a sea anemone (**Figure 16**). Lipomas typically are found within the subendocardium, although involvement of valves has been reported. Sarcomas frequently infiltrate the myocardium. Although sarcomas may occur in the right atrium, myxomas predominate as the cause of primary cardiac tumors in both atria.

Management

The need for surgical resection is dependent on the size, location, and malignant nature of the cardiac tumor, in addition

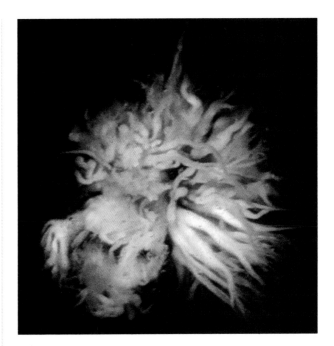

FIGURE 16. Gross pathologic specimen of a papillary fibroelastoma.

Image courtesy of Dr. William D. Edwards, Department of Pathology, Mayo Clinic.

to symptoms and risk of embolization. Myxomas should be resected after diagnosis owing to the risk of embolization and cardiovascular complications, including the potential for sudden death. Survival for patients after surgical resection of myxoma is comparable to that of healthy individuals. Myxomas may recur, with a reported incidence varying between 5% and 13%, with recurrence being more common in younger patients and those with Carney complex or a positive family history. Routine surveillance with imaging is indicated to monitor for recurrence, which usually occurs at the original site of the tumor.

Surgical resection is often considered for papillary fibroelastoma, particularly if the lesion is large (>10 mm), highly mobile, or associated with systemic embolization.

Treatment of tumors with myocardial involvement is challenging. In particular, sarcomas are difficult to treat owing to their widespread, invasive nature and the high recurrence rates despite surgical resection. Survival is improved when there is complete resection and no metastatic involvement (median survival, 15 to 18 months versus 2 to 5 months). Cardiac transplantation using an allograft or autograft may be a therapeutic option in selected patients. In the autograft procedure, the tumor is resected from an excised heart, followed by reconstruction and auto-implantation of the heart into the patient.

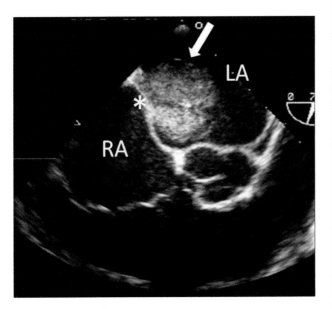

FIGURE 15. Transesophageal echocardiography across the right atrium (RA) and left atrium (LA) demonstrates a large mass (*arrow*) attached to the atrial septum in proximity of the fossa ovalis (*asterisk*); the mass was surgically removed and proved to be a left atrial myxoma.

KEY POINT

- Myxomas should be resected after diagnosis owing to the risk of embolization and cardiovascular complications, including the potential for sudden death.

Arrhythmias

Antiarrhythmic Medications

Antiarrhythmic medications are used to prevent recurrent arrhythmias and maintain sinus rhythm. Although antiarrhythmic medications have historically been organized according to their predominant mechanism of action using the Vaughan-Williams classification system (**Table 23**), it is increasingly recognized that this nomenclature system has limitations because most antiarrhythmic drugs have several mechanistic actions.

The membrane-active antiarrhythmic agents (class I and class III) principally affect ion channels. Class I agents decrease impulse formation and speed of depolarization and are often used in patients with atrial arrhythmias and no structural heart disease. Several class IA agents are used less frequently,

although they are helpful in specific situations (see Table 23), including the use of procainamide in patients with preexcited atrial fibrillation. Class IC agents are avoided in patients with coronary artery disease and structural heart disease as they have been shown to cause proarrhythmic activity (ventricular arrhythmias) and increase mortality. Class II agents (β-blockers) and class IV agents (nondihydropyridine calcium channel blockers) are frequently used to slow heart rates in patients with supraventricular or atrial arrhythmias; however, they should be avoided in patients who have atrial fibrillation with preexcitation. Class III agents are used to treat atrial and ventricular arrhythmias. These agents are cleared by the kidneys and should be avoided in patients with significant chronic kidney disease owing to increased toxicity and proarrhythmia. Because class III agents lead to QTc-interval prolongation, initiation of this therapy is usually done on an inpatient basis

TABLE 23. Antiarrhythmic Medications				
Classification	**Mechanism of Action**	**Individual Agents/ Examples**	**Effects**	**Use**
Class IA	Sodium channel blockade with some potassium channel blockade	Quinidine, procainamide, disopyramide	Decreases speed of depolarization and prolongs repolarization	Pre-excited atrial fibrillation (procainamide), Brugada syndrome (quinidine), SVT, atrial fibrillation, and ventricular arrhythmias
Class IB	Sodium channel blockade	Lidocaine, mexiletine, phenytoin	Decreases speed of depolarization	Ventricular arrhythmias
Class IC	Sodium channel blockade	Flecainide, propafenone	Decreases speed of depolarization and shortens repolarization	Atrial fibrillation, SVT, ventricular arrhythmias; avoid with CAD or structural heart disease.
Class II	β-adrenergic blockade	Metoprolol, propranolol, carvedilol, atenolol, bisoprolol	Decreases sympathetic tone; suppresses automaticity, sinoatrial conduction, and AV conduction	Rate control of atrial arrhythmias, SVT, ventricular arrhythmias; avoid if pre-excitation is present.
Class III	Potassium channel blockade	Sotalol, dofetilide	Prolongs action potential duration	Atrial fibrillation, atrial flutter, ventricular arrhythmias; avoid in CKD.
Class IV	Calcium channel blockade (nondihydropyridines)	Verapamil, diltiazem	Suppresses sinoatrial and AV conduction	SVT, rate control of atrial arrhythmias, triggered arrhythmias (e.g., outflow tract VT); avoid if pre-excitation is present.
Multichannel blockers	Several, including potassium, sodium, and calcium channel blockade	Amiodarone, dronedarone	Multiple mechanisms, although they act principally by extending repolarization	Atrial arrhythmias, ventricular arrhythmias
Adenosine receptor agonists	A_1-receptor agonist	Adenosine	Slows or blocks sinoatrial and AV nodal conduction	Termination of SVT
Cardiac glycoside	Increasing vagal activity	Digoxin	Slows AV nodal conduction	Rate control of atrial fibrillation

AV = atrioventricular; CAD = coronary artery disease; CKD = chronic kidney disease; SVT = supraventricular tachycardia; VT = ventricular tachycardia.

with regular assessment of the QTc interval. Patients taking class III agents should avoid other QT-prolonging medications, and serum potassium and magnesium levels should be checked regularly.

Amiodarone, a multichannel blocker, is among the most commonly used antiarrhythmic medications. It is frequently used to treat atrial fibrillation in older persons and to prevent recurrent ventricular tachycardia. Amiodarone is the preferred antiarrhythmic agent in patients with structural heart disease and heart failure. Although highly effective, amiodarone has multiple toxicities. Amiodarone therapy is associated with risks for thyroid toxicity, hepatotoxicity, lung toxicity, photosensitivity, corneal and lenticular deposits, optic neuropathy, and other neurologic adverse effects. Patients on amiodarone require routine monitoring of thyroid and liver function, pulmonary function testing at baseline and with symptoms, and periodic ophthalmologic evaluation. Amiodarone interacts with several medications. Patients on amiodarone require lower doses of warfarin, statins, and digoxin. Dronedarone is a multichannel blocker used to treat atrial fibrillation. Owing to increased mortality in patients with heart failure or permanent atrial fibrillation, its use should be restricted to patients with intermittent atrial fibrillation and no overt heart failure.

Digoxin is an oral positive inotropic agent that acts on the sodium–potassium exchanger and has vagal properties that lead to decreased atrioventricular (AV) nodal conduction. As a result of its vagal mechanism, it primarily controls the heart rate at rest and is less effective during activity. Adenosine is an A_1-receptor blocker that can inhibit AV conduction. Adenosine is frequently used as a therapeutic agent to terminate supraventricular tachycardia.

KEY POINT

- Calcium channel blockers and β-blockers are often used to treat supraventricular and atrial arrhythmias; however, these agents should be avoided in patients who have atrial fibrillation with preexcitation.

Approach to the Patient with Bradycardia

Clinical Presentation

Symptoms of bradycardia (heart rate less than 60/min) include fatigue, exertional intolerance, dyspnea, lightheadedness, and syncope. Bradycardia can result from pathology in the sinus node, the AV node, or the His-Purkinje system. Physicians should maintain a high suspicion for reversible causes of bradycardia, including elevated intracranial pressure, hypothyroidism, hyperkalemia, Lyme disease, and medication effects (most commonly AV nodal blockers, especially β-blockers and digoxin).

The diagnostic evaluation of bradycardia includes (1) establishing a correlation between the rhythm (bradycardia) and symptoms and (2) excluding severe conduction abnor-malities that require urgent intervention. Evaluation includes a careful history, a focused laboratory evaluation (including an assessment of thyroid function), resting 12-lead electrocardiogram (ECG), exercise treadmill testing to assess the heart rate response to exercise (chronotropic competence), and ambulatory ECG monitoring based on the nature and frequency of the patient's episodes or symptoms (see Diagnostic Testing in Cardiology). Rarely, electrophysiologic testing can be used to help ascertain if sinus node dysfunction is present. $\blacksquare$

Sinus Bradycardia

Sinus bradycardia (sinus rhythm with a heart rate <60/min) may be appropriate in several situations, including in trained athletes or during sleep, when the heart rate may fall as low as 30/min. The most common intrinsic cause of inappropriate or pathologic sinus bradycardia (sinus node dysfunction) is age-related myocardial fibrosis in the vicinity of the sinus node. The most common extrinsic cause of sinus bradycardia is medication effect. Sinus node dysfunction can also present with chronotropic incompetence, and this is frequently overlooked. Other, less common, causes of sinus node dysfunction include right coronary ischemia, intracranial hypertension, postsurgical scarring after cardiothoracic surgery, and infiltrative or inflammatory disorders (such as sarcoidosis).

Atrioventricular Block

AV block is classified as first degree, second degree, or third degree. First-degree AV block is characterized by prolonged AV conduction, which manifests on the ECG as a PR interval greater than 200 msec. First-degree AV block is not a true block because all P waves conduct to the ventricles. It has been associated with an increased risk of atrial fibrillation, pacemaker implantation, and all-cause mortality in long-term follow-up.

In second-degree AV block, some P waves conduct to the ventricle and some do not. There are two forms of second-degree AV block. When progressive PR prolongation is observed prior to a blocked beat, second-degree Mobitz type 1 (Wenckebach block) is present. Second-degree Mobitz type 1 block is characterized by grouped beating and progressive shortening of the R-R intervals. Mobitz type 1 block is almost always localized to the AV node. It generally carries a benign prognosis and frequently improves with exercise or increased sympathetic tone.

When the PR interval is constant prior to nonconducted P waves, the second-degree block is termed Mobitz type 2 block. When 2:1 block is present, Mobitz type 1 versus type 2 block cannot be differentiated. Mobitz type 2 block usually represents block lower in the conduction system and has a higher risk of progression to complete heart block.

Third-degree AV block, or complete heart block, is defined as the failure of any P waves to conduct to the ventricles, and it is characterized by AV dissociation on the ECG.

Pacemakers

Pacemakers are indicated in patients with symptomatic brady-cardia in the absence of a reversible cause, hence the importance of establishing symptoms when evaluating patients with bradycardia. In patients with minimal symptoms, a persistent resting heart rate below 40/min is also considered an indication for permanent pacing. Pacemakers also are indicated in patients with evidence of AV conduction disturbances that have a high likelihood of progressing to complete heart block or life-threatening sudden asystole. Indications for permanent pacemaker implantation are shown in **Table 24**.

TABLE 24. Selected Indications for Permanent Pacing
Symptomatic bradycardia without reversible cause
Asymptomatic bradycardia with significant pauses (>3 seconds in sinus rhythm) or persistent heart rate <40/min
Atrial fibrillation with 5-second pauses
Asymptomatic complete heart block or Mobitz type 2 second-degree atrioventricular block
Alternating bundle branch block

Patients with intraventricular conduction delays have a low risk of progression to complete heart block (1%-3% annually) and do not require permanent pacing. When a patient develops new-onset conduction disease in the setting of an acute coronary syndrome, temporary pacing may be required, but decisions on permanent pacing should be delayed until a patient has been revascularized and stabilized to determine whether the arrhythmia persists.

Patients with pacemakers who require surgery should have a preoperative device evaluation to determine whether preoperative reprogramming of the device is necessary. Although "MRI conditional" pacemakers are now available, the presence of a pacemaker remains a contraindication to MRI scanning for most patients.

There are several types of implanted cardiac devices, with various capabilities. Implanted cardiac electronic devices include implanted loop monitors, pacemakers, implantable cardioverter-defibrillators (ICDs), and cardiac resynchronization devices. With the exception of subcutaneous ICDs, which do not utilize intracardiac leads, all ICDs also have pacemaker functions. **Table 25** reviews the various types of implanted

TABLE 25. Cardiac Implantable Electronic Devices for Treatment of Cardiac Rhythm Disorders			Functions		
Device	Components	Indications	Pacemaker Function	Antitachycardia Pacing	Defibrillation
Pacemaker	Pulse generator and intravascular leads (single- or dual-chamber)	Sinus node dysfunction, atrioventricular block, or other causes of non-reversible symptomatic bradycardia	Yes	No	No
Implantable cardioverter-defibrillator	Defibrillator and intravascular leads (single- or dual-chamber)	To provide continuous monitoring and treatment of ventricular arrhythmias	Yes	Yes	Yes
Subcutaneous implantable cardioverter-defibrillator	Defibrillator and a single lead that are entirely under the skin (extravascular); no transvenous leads	To provide continuous monitoring and treatment of ventricular arrhythmias	No	No	Yes
Cardiac resynchronization therapy-pacing (CRT-P)	Pulse generator and intravascular leads, including a pacing lead in the coronary sinus to pace the left ventricle	To restore electrical synchrony between the ventricles in patients with heart failure	Yes	No	No
Cardiac resynchronization therapy-defibrillator (CRT-D)	Defibrillator and intravascular leads, including a pacing lead in the coronary sinus to pace the left ventricle	To restore electrical synchrony between the ventricles in patients with heart failure and to monitor and treat ventricular arrhythmias	Yes	Yes	Yes

CONT.

cardiac electronic devices, their functions, and their general indications. **H**

> **KEY POINT**
>
> - A pacemaker is indicated for symptomatic bradycardia without a reversible cause as well as for atrioventricular conduction abnormalities that are likely to progress to complete heart block.

Approach to the Patient with Tachycardia

Patients with symptomatic tachycardia often report palpitations, lightheadedness or dizziness, chest discomfort, dyspnea, exertional intolerance, or syncope. Some patients are asymptomatic and are found to have arrhythmias incidentally during monitoring in the setting of hospitalization or other medical care. The most important part of the evaluation is the documentation of tachycardia and correlation with symptoms (see Diagnostic Testing in Cardiology). In addition to a history and physical examination, all patients with tachycardia should have a resting 12-lead ECG. Most patients with tachycardia should undergo echocardiography to exclude the presence of structural heart disease and thyroid function evaluation.

In both hospital and ambulatory settings, sinus tachycardia (sinus rhythm with heart rate >100/min) is the most commonly encountered tachycardia. Sinus tachycardia is usually caused by physiologic distress, including pain, fever, anemia, or anxiety. The evaluation and treatment of sinus tachycardia are directed at the underlying etiology. Significant sinus tachycardia in a critically ill patient is a worrisome finding as it usually indicates advanced physiologic compromise, including respiratory failure, insufficient cardiac output, or severe infection.

Older patients with palpitations are more likely to have atrial fibrillation, atrial flutter, or ventricular tachycardia (VT). Although VT is often associated with hemodynamic compromise, VT is often well tolerated, whereas many patients have hemodynamically significant supraventricular tachycardia or atrial arrhythmias. Therefore, vital signs are not helpful in determining the nature of an arrhythmia.

In younger persons with tachycardic symptoms, supraventricular tachycardias are more common, including AV nodal reentrant tachycardia (AVNRT) and accessory pathway–mediated tachycardia. Patients with an accessory pathway often have evidence of anterograde conduction and a delta wave on ECG.

Atrial and ventricular ectopy are present in many—if not most—persons. The frequency of ectopy and symptoms usually dictate both the work-up and subsequent management. **H**

> **KEY POINT**
>
> - In addition to a resting electrocardiogram, diagnostic testing for most patients with tachycardia should include an echocardiogram and evaluation of thyroid function.

Supraventricular Tachycardias

Clinical Presentation

Supraventricular tachycardias (SVTs) are a group of arrhythmias that arise in atrial tissue or the AV node. Because conduction of supraventricular impulses below the AV node is conducted normally, the ECG in SVT usually reveals a narrow-complex tachycardia, although the QRS complexes can be wide (>120 msec) in the presence of bundle branch block, aberrancy, pacing, or anterograde accessory pathway conduction (antidromic tachycardia).

SVTs include abnormal electrical activity arising in the atrium (premature atrial contractions, tachycardia, atrial fibrillation and flutter, multifocal atrial tachycardia) or AV node (junctional tachycardia, AVNRT, atrioventricular reciprocating tachycardia [AVRT]). Because they are so common and for the purpose of this review, atrial fibrillation and atrial flutter are discussed separately; the rest of this section will focus exclusively on the other SVTs.

SVT can occur in all age groups but is frequently encountered in younger patients. SVT is more common in women than men and usually occurs without structural heart disease, although this should be evaluated with an echocardiogram. Patients with SVT often have repeated episodes of tachycardia. Patients may have palpitations, a sensation of pounding in the neck, fatigue, lightheadedness, chest discomfort, dyspnea, presyncope, and, less commonly, syncope.

The ECG classification of SVT is usually based on the relationship of the P wave and the QRS complex. In short-RP tachycardias (RP interval < PR interval), the P wave closely follows the QRS complex. In long-RP tachycardias (RP interval > PR interval), the P wave is more than half the distance between the QRS complexes. Short-RP tachycardias include typical AVNRT, AVRT, and junctional tachycardia. Junctional tachycardias are less common in adults, but they can occur in patients with digoxin intoxication and other conditions. Long-RP tachycardias include atypical AVNRT, sinus tachycardia, atrial tachycardia, and the permanent form of junctional reciprocating tachycardia.

Episodes of SVT can often be terminated with Valsalva maneuvers (bearing down), carotid sinus massage, or facial immersion in cold water. Adenosine can be used to terminate SVT and to help diagnose the etiology. Termination with adenosine often suggests AV node dependence (AVNRT and AVRT), whereas continued atrial activity (P waves) during AV block can help identify atrial flutter and atrial tachycardia. **H**

Premature Atrial Contractions and Atrial Tachycardia

Atrial ectopy can be isolated (premature atrial contractions [PACs]), occur in salvos, or be sustained (atrial tachycardia). PACs are extremely common, and the frequency increases with age. Only 1% of persons in the general population have no PACs during ambulatory ECG monitoring. However, PAC burden is associated with increased risk of atrial fibrillation.

Symptomatic PACs are typically treated with β-blockers or calcium channel blockers.

Atrial tachycardia can occur in patients with or without structural heart disease; when symptomatic, first-line treatment is a β-blocker or nondihydropyridine calcium channel blocker (diltiazem or verapamil). Second-line treatment includes catheter ablation or antiarrhythmic drug therapy. In general, success rates for ablation of atrial tachycardia are lower than those for other SVTs.

Multifocal atrial tachycardia, characterized by multiple (≥3) P-wave morphologies and a heart rate greater than 100/min, is frequently seen in patients with end-stage COPD. Treatment is usually directed at the underlying etiology and electrolyte disturbances, although β-blockers and calcium nondihydropyridine calcium channel blockers can be used cautiously.

Atrioventricular Nodal Reentrant Tachycardia

AVNRT is the most common type of SVT, accounting for two thirds of all patients with SVT (excluding atrial fibrillation and atrial flutter). AVNRT is caused by reentrant conduction within the AV node, utilizing both the fast and slow pathways (**Figure 17**). In *typical* AVNRT, the electrical conduction goes down the slow pathway and conducts back up toward the

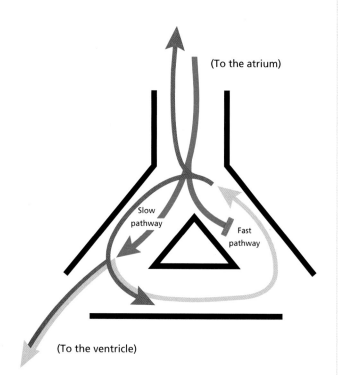

(To the atrium)

Slow pathway

Fast pathway

(To the ventricle)

FIGURE 17. Mechanism of typical atrioventricular nodal reentrant tachycardia. The slow pathway has a short refractory period, and the fast pathway has a long refractory period. The *blue line* represents anterograde conduction down the slow pathway; conduction does not occur down the fast pathway because it is refractory. The *yellow line* represents impulse conduction into the ventricle and retrograde up the fast pathway, which is no longer refractory. The *red line* represents completion of the circuit with activation of the atria and ventricles.

atrium over the fast pathway (slow-fast). This leads to a short RP interval with a retrograde P wave inscribed very close to the QRS complex. The closely coupled retrograde P waves may be buried in the QRS complexes and may not be visible, or they may appear as a pseudo R′ wave in lead V$_1$ and a pseudo S wave in the inferior leads. In *atypical* AVNRT, conduction goes down the fast pathway and returns to the atrium via the slow pathway (fast-slow); this leads to a long RP interval. Rarely, AVNRT can involve conduction over more than one slow pathway (slow-slow AVNRT).

Beyond acute termination with physical maneuvers or adenosine, treatment to prevent recurrent AVNRT includes AV nodal blocking therapy with β-blockers or nondihydropyridine calcium channel blockers. Patients who have recurrent AVNRT or do not tolerate or prefer to avoid long-term medical therapy are usually referred for catheter ablation, which has a high success rate. The major risk of ablation is a 1% risk of injury to the AV node requiring pacemaker implantation.

Atrioventricular Reciprocating Tachycardia

AVRT is an accessory pathway (bypass tract)–mediated tachycardia. Accessory pathway conduction is often observed as preexcitation on ECG. Because of early ventricular activation over the accessory pathway, the PR interval is shortened and the initial part of the QRS complex is slurred (delta wave) because of ventricular depolarization adjacent to the pathway. In AVRT, conduction is anterograde over the AV node (orthodromic AVRT) or anterograde over the accessory pathway (antidromic AVRT). Orthodromic AVNRT, the most common type of AVRT (more than 90% to 95% of cases) is characterized by a narrow QRS complex resulting from conduction over the AV node and the His-Purkinje system. Antidromic AVRT is characterized by a wide, slurred QRS complex resulting from conduction over the bypass tract and activation of the ventricle without use of the specialized conduction system. Adenosine can be given to terminate orthodromic AVRT; however, adenosine or other AV nodal blockers are contraindicated in preexcited atrial fibrillation and antidromic AVRT. AV nodal blockade in patients with these rhythms can promote rapid conduction down the bypass tract and induction of ventricular fibrillation (VF).

Patients with evidence of preexcitation on their resting ECG (delta wave) and symptomatic SVT have Wolff-Parkinson-White (WPW) syndrome. Up to one third of patients with WPW syndrome have or will develop atrial fibrillation. Rapid conduction over an accessory pathway in atrial fibrillation can lead to VF and sudden cardiac death (SCD), although this is a relatively rare event. Risk factors for VF in WPW syndrome include documented AVRT, multiple bypass tracts, Ebstein anomaly (right heart enlargement and severe tricuspid valve regurgitation), and a rapidly conducting accessory pathway. WPW syndrome is often seen in patients with Ebstein anomaly.

In general, evaluation of a patient with preexcitation includes a 12-lead ECG, echocardiogram, ambulatory ECG monitoring, and an exercise stress test. Stress testing is an effective means of noninvasive risk stratification for patients with preexcitation. Loss of preexcitation during exercise generally indicates low risk. Electrophysiology (EP) testing can help determine rapidity of conduction and risk for sudden death; it also can help localize the pathway and facilitate catheter ablation, which has a high success rate (although success depends on the location of the bypass tract). In general, catheter ablation is first-line therapy for patients with preexcitation and symptoms. Antiarrhythmic agents are reserved for second-line therapy, particularly in patients with accessory pathways in close vicinity to the AV node.

Management of asymptomatic preexcitation on ECG is controversial. In the absence of symptoms, however, invasive testing is generally not required, unless the patient has a high-risk occupation, such as an airline pilot or bus driver. **H**

KEY POINTS

- Therapeutic options for prevention of recurrence of atrioventricular nodal reentrant tachycardia include atrioventricular nodal blocking drugs and catheter ablation.
- First-line therapy for Wolff-Parkinson-White syndrome (preexcitation with symptoms) is catheter ablation.

Atrial Fibrillation

Atrial fibrillation is the most common sustained cardiac arrhythmia. The diagnosis of atrial fibrillation is based upon the demonstration of disorganized atrial activity, seen as an irregularly irregular ventricular response on ECG. Fibrillation of the atrial myocardium can lead to stasis and intracardiac thrombus formation. In patients older than 40 years, the lifetime risk of atrial fibrillation is 1 in 4. The incidence of atrial fibrillation is age-related, and more than 10% of persons aged 80 years and older have atrial fibrillation. Atrial fibrillation is associated with a fivefold increased risk of stroke as well as an increased risk of heart failure and dementia. Atrial fibrillation can occur secondary to reversible or acute physiologic insults, including hyperthyroidism, cardiac surgery, and pulmonary embolism. More commonly, atrial fibrillation is the result of long-standing disease affecting the heart, particularly hypertension, structural heart disease, and obstructive sleep apnea.

Clinical Presentation

As with most arrhythmias, patients with atrial fibrillation can experience a wide range of symptoms, including palpitations, lightheadedness or dizziness, dyspnea, exercise intolerance, chest pain, and syncope. Some patients are asymptomatic and are found to have atrial fibrillation as an incidental finding on ECG. In its most severe forms, particularly in patients with advanced diastolic dysfunction or restrictive cardiomyopathy, atrial fibrillation can result in hemodynamic compromise. Some patients initially present with heart failure caused by tachycardia-induced cardiomyopathy.

Atrial fibrillation is classified as first-detected, paroxysmal, persistent, or long-standing persistent atrial fibrillation. Paroxysmal atrial fibrillation starts and stops spontaneously. Persistent atrial fibrillation lasts for 7 days or more and requires electrical or pharmacologic cardioversion. Long-standing persistent atrial fibrillation is persistent atrial fibrillation that is more than 1 year in duration.

Acute Management

Both acute and chronic management of atrial fibrillation are based on three therapeutic goals: (1) preventing stroke, (2) controlling the heart rate (preventing tachycardia/rapid ventricular rates), and (3) symptom relief. Once a diagnosis of atrial fibrillation is made, a search for reversible causes should be completed, including an evaluation of thyroid function. Patients with atrial fibrillation should undergo screening for sleep apnea with more extensive testing if the clinical history is suggestive. An echocardiogram should be obtained to investigate potential valvular or other structural heart disease.

Acute Anticoagulation

In patients with newly discovered atrial fibrillation in whom cardioversion will not be performed, institution of intravenous anticoagulation is usually not necessary. In these patients, oral anticoagulation can be started based on risk factors (see Long-Term Management). If cardioversion is planned, anticoagulation therapy is based on the duration of atrial fibrillation. For patients who are known to have been in atrial fibrillation for less than 48 hours, preprocedural anticoagulation is not necessary as the risk of thrombus formation is low. Patients with atrial fibrillation of unclear duration or those with atrial fibrillation for more than 48 hours require preprocedural anticoagulation. These patients should receive 3 weeks of therapeutic anticoagulation prior to cardioversion. Alternatively, transesophageal echocardiography (TEE) can be performed to look for an intracardiac thrombus. If TEE is negative for thrombus, acute cardioversion can be performed immediately. All patients (regardless of the duration of atrial fibrillation) must be anticoagulated at the time of cardioversion and after cardioversion for a minimum of 4 weeks owing to an increased risk of thromboembolic events after restoration of sinus rhythm.

Cardioversion and Acute Rate Control

Many patients who present with an initial episode of atrial fibrillation convert spontaneously, often within hours. However, the presence of hypotension, myocardial ischemia, or heart failure is an indication for immediate cardioversion regardless of the duration of atrial fibrillation. Acute cardioversion of atrial fibrillation should be synchronized to the R wave so as to avoid an "R-on-T" event and provocation of VF.

Patients with rapid ventricular conduction require heart rate control in order to improve cardiac function and symptoms. Target heart rates should be between 60/min and 110/min in the acute setting. Acute rate control is most often achieved with β-blockers or nondihydropyridine calcium channel blockers. Intravenous medications, including metoprolol, esmolol, diltiazem, and verapamil, can be used, with subsequent transition to oral formulations. In patients with mild symptoms, oral agents can be considered without initial intravenous therapy. Calcium channel blockers should be avoided in patients with left ventricular dysfunction. Digoxin can be added to improve rate control, especially in patients with heart failure. Patients with evidence of preexcitation should not be treated with β-blockers or calcium channel blockers. In patients with preexcited atrial fibrillation, procainamide is the treatment of choice.

If cardioversion is favored because of significant symptoms despite rate control, pharmacologic or electrical cardioversion can be pursued. Class IC agents (flecainide, propafenone) or ibutilide (an intravenous class III medication) can be considered for pharmacologic cardioversion in patients without structural heart disease. **H**

Long-Term Management
Anticoagulation

Stroke is the most concerning consequence of atrial fibrillation. The absolute risk of stroke is 4% per year among patients with nonvalvular atrial fibrillation, but comorbidities can increase the risk 15 to 20 times. Hypertension is an important risk factor for both atrial fibrillation and stroke; therefore, aggressive blood pressure control is paramount in the management of atrial fibrillation.

Stroke prevention with antithrombotic therapies is predicated on a patient's aggregate risk profile. Several risk stratification scores are available to clinicians. In patients with nonvalvular atrial fibrillation, the $CHADS_2$ score was, until recently, the basis for most guideline and consensus documents. Owing to the limited ability of the $CHADS_2$ score to discern between low and intermediate risk, the CHA_2DS_2-VASc risk score was developed and now is the recommended score to assess risk of stroke in patients with nonvalvular atrial fibrillation (**Table 26**). The CHA_2DS_2-VASc score is particularly

TABLE 26. Risk Stratification Scores, Adjusted Stroke Rates, and Antithrombotic Therapy Recommendations

Score	Incidence of Ischemic Stroke (per 100 patient-years)[a]	Antithrombotic Therapy[b]
$CHADS_2$ Score[c]		
0	0.6	Aspirin or no therapy
1	3.0	Aspirin or OAC
2	4.2	OAC
3	7.1	OAC
4	11.1	OAC
5	12.5	OAC
6	13.0	OAC
CHA_2DS_2-VASc Score[d]		
0	0.2	None
1	0.6	None or aspirin or OAC
2	2.2	OAC
3	3.2	OAC
4	4.8	OAC
5	7.2	OAC
6+	10.3	OAC

OAC = oral anticoagulation.

[a]Data from Friberg L, Rosenqvist M, Lip GY. Evaluation of risk stratification schemes for ischaemic stroke and bleeding in 182 678 patients with atrial Fibrillation cohort study. Eur Heart J. 2012 Jun;33(12):1500-10. [PMID: 22246443]

[b]$CHADS_2$ recommendations from Fuster V, Rydén LE, Cannom DS, et al; American College of Cardiology; American Heart Association Task Force; European Society of Cardiology Committee for Practice Guidelines; European Heart Rhythm Association; Heart Rhythm Society. ACC/AHA/ESC 2006 guidelines for the management of patients with atrial fibrillation: full text: a report of the American College of Cardiology/American Heart Association Task Force on practice guidelines and the European Society of Cardiology Committee for Practice Guidelines (Writing Committee to Revise the 2001 guidelines for the management of patients with atrial fibrillation) developed in collaboration with the European Heart Rhythm Association and the Heart Rhythm Society. Europace. 2006 Sep;8(9):651-745. Erratum in: Europace. 2007 Sep;9(9):856. [PMID: 16987906]. CHA_2DS_2-VASc recommendations from January CT, Wann LS, Alpert JS, et al; ACC/AHA Task Force Members. 2014 AHA/ACC/HRS guideline for the management of patients with atrial fibrillation: a report of the American College of Cardiology/American Heart Association Task Force on practice guidelines and the Heart Rhythm Society. Circulation. 2014 Dec 2;130(23):e199-267. [PMID: 24682347]

[c]$CHADS_2$ scoring (maximum 6 points): One point each is given for heart failure, hypertension, age ≥75 years, and diabetes mellitus. Two points are given for previous stroke/transient ischemic attack.

[d]CHA_2DS_2-VASc scoring (maximum 9 points): One point each is given for heart failure, hypertension, diabetes mellitus, vascular disease (prior myocardial infarction, peripheral arterial disease, aortic plaque), female sex, and age 65 to 74 years. Two points each are given for previous stroke/transient ischemic attack/thromboembolic disease and age ≥75 years.

helpful in patients with 0 or 1 CHADS$_2$ risk factors. In addition to the CHADS$_2$ points, this score gives an additional point for age 65 to 74 years, female sex, and the presence of atherosclerotic disease, and gives 2 points for age 75 or older. Patients with a CHADS$_2$ score of 0 or 1 who have a CHA$_2$DS$_2$-VASc score of 2 or more may benefit from oral anticoagulation. Certain high-risk features, such as mitral stenosis or rheumatic heart disease, prior systemic embolism, a prosthetic heart valve, left atrial appendage thrombus, and hypertrophic cardiomyopathy require oral anticoagulation regardless of risk score.

For patients who are treated with aspirin, the recommended dose is 81 to 325 mg daily. For patients who require oral anticoagulation, several agents are now available. Dose-adjusted warfarin (a vitamin K antagonist) remains an effective low-cost alternative for stroke prevention in patients with a higher risk of stroke. The efficacy and safety of warfarin therapy are closely associated with the amount of time in the therapeutic range (INR 2-3). The chief limitations of warfarin are its need for frequent INR monitoring and adjustment and its numerous food and drug interactions. Recently, several new oral anticoagulants have been approved by the FDA for the prevention of stroke in patients with nonvalvular atrial fibrillation, including dabigatran, rivaroxaban, and apixaban (**Table 27**). Warfarin remains the agent of choice in patients with valvular atrial fibrillation, generally defined as atrial fibrillation with mitral stenosis or mitral valve replacement.

Dabigatran is superior to warfarin for the prevention of stroke and is associated with less intracranial bleeding, but carries a higher risk of gastrointestinal bleeding. Rivaroxaban is noninferior to warfarin for the prevention of stroke or systemic embolism and is associated with less intracranial and fatal bleeding. Similar to patients receiving dabigatran, patients on rivaroxaban have a higher risk of gastrointestinal

bleeding compared with warfarin. Apixaban also is superior to warfarin for the prevention of stroke and is associated with less bleeding overall, including intracranial bleeding, but similar rates of gastrointestinal bleeding. All of the novel oral anticoagulants are cleared by the kidneys. Thus, dose adjustment is required based on estimated glomerular filtration rate (eGFR), and these agents are contraindicated in patients with end-stage kidney disease. For this reason, annual measurement of serum creatinine level is recommended for patients treated with these drugs. All of the novel oral anticoagulants have shorter half-lives relative to warfarin; however, there are no quick, readily available serum assays to accurately determine anticoagulant activity. Furthermore, currently there is no antidote for these agents in patients with severe hemorrhage.

In patients with concomitant coronary artery disease and atrial fibrillation, antithrombotic therapy presents significant challenges. For most patients with stable coronary artery disease, single-agent therapy with an oral anticoagulant is sufficient for prevention of both acute coronary syndromes and stroke events. Combination antiplatelet and oral anticoagulant therapy increases the risk of bleeding, including intracranial hemorrhage. However, patients with an acute coronary syndrome or revascularization in the previous 12 months are thought to benefit from combination therapy with low-dose aspirin (<100 mg/d) and oral anticoagulation. In patients who receive a coronary stent, triple therapy with low-dose aspirin (<100 mg/d), a thienopyridine (such as clopidogrel), and warfarin is indicated for as short a period as possible. In patients with a drug-eluting stent, this period may extend to 6 months or a year. Ongoing clinical trials are evaluating the combination of anticoagulant therapy for atrial fibrillation and antiplatelet agents for coronary artery disease.

TABLE 27.	Anticoagulants FDA-Approved for Stroke Prevention in Atrial Fibrillation			
Medication	**Reversibility**	**Frequency**	**Type of AF**	**Cautions**
Warfarin (vitamin K antagonist)	Yes	Dosing adjusted to INR	Valvular or nonvalvular	Avoid in pregnancy. Caution with idiopathic thrombocytopenic purpura, HIT, hepatic disease, protein C or S deficiency. Many drug interactions.
Dabigatran (direct thrombin inhibitor)	No	Twice daily	Nonvalvular	Decrease dose if CrCl 15-30. Caution with P-glycoprotein inhibition.
Rivaroxaban (factor Xa inhibitor)	No[a]	Once daily	Nonvalvular	Avoid with CrCl <30, moderate hepatic disease. Caution with mild hepatic disease
Apixaban (factor Xa inhibitor)	No[a]	Twice daily	Nonvalvular	Avoid with severe hepatic disease, strong dual inhibitors or inducers of CYP3A4 and P-glycoprotein. Caution with moderate hepatic disease.

AF = atrial fibrillation; CrCl = creatinine clearance (mL/min/1.73 m^2); HIT = heparin-induced thrombocytopenia.

[a]Early data suggest that factor Xa inhibitors may be able to be reversed with prothrombin complex concentrates. Additionally, several "antidotes" are in development for the factor Xa inhibitors.

Rate Versus Rhythm Control

There is no evidence of a survival advantage or reduction in stroke with restoration and maintenance of sinus rhythm in patients with atrial fibrillation, including those with heart failure. Therefore, the decision to institute a rate or rhythm control strategy largely depends on symptoms and patient preference. Patients who are asymptomatic can be managed with rate control only, with a resting heart rate goal of less than 110/min. Patients with tachycardia-induced cardiomyopathy, heart failure, or left ventricular ejection fraction of less than 40% may require more stringent rate control (heart rate 60-80/min at rest). AV nodal blockers, including β-blockers and nondihydropyridine calcium channel blockers, can be used to control the heart rate. Combination therapy is often required to adequately control the heart rate. In addition to assessing the resting heart rate, assessment of the heart rate with activity should be considered, either with ambulatory ECG monitoring, a stress test, or a 6-minute walk test.

In patients who continue to have symptoms despite adequate rate control, a rhythm control strategy should be considered to improve quality of life. Rhythm control may require cardioversion followed by antiarrhythmic therapy. Antiarrhythmic drug selection is based on patient comorbidities and the safety profile of the antiarrhythmic drugs. Some patients with infrequent symptomatic atrial fibrillation may not require daily therapy. Patients with infrequent atrial fibrillation and neither structural heart disease nor conduction disease may benefit from a "pill-in-the pocket" approach, whereby patients take a class IC drug (flecainide or propafenone) only when they develop an episode of atrial fibrillation. Patients who follow this approach should be taking an AV nodal blocker or should take one before taking their "pill in the pocket." The first time this approach is used, it should take place in a monitored setting to ensure that the patient can safely tolerate the therapy without development of proarrhythmia or conduction disturbance (for example, post-termination pause). Regardless of the rate or rhythm control strategy used, stroke prevention should be guided by patient risk (CHA_2DS_2-VASc score).

Nonpharmacologic Strategies

In patients who have refractory symptomatic atrial fibrillation despite antiarrhythmic drug therapy, catheter ablation with pulmonary vein isolation is an effective rhythm control therapy. Atrial fibrillation ablation is best reserved for patients with early atrial fibrillation without evidence of significant left atrial enlargement and those without multiple comorbidities. The success rates for atrial fibrillation ablation are variable, but in patients with paroxysmal atrial fibrillation, between 70% and 90% are symptom-free at 1 year. Complications can include intraprocedural or late tamponade, vascular complications, and a 0.5% to 1% risk of stroke. Patients who develop dyspnea months to years after an atrial fibrillation ablation may have pulmonary vein stenosis. Anticoagulation is mandatory for the first 2 to 3 months after ablation, and thereafter is guided by risk factors. In patients with symptomatic atrial fibrillation who are undergoing cardiac surgery for other reasons, the maze procedure can be performed as a means of maintaining sinus rhythm.

Patients with refractory symptomatic tachycardia despite attempts at rate and rhythm control may be candidates for AV node ablation. In this approach, patients receive a pacemaker and undergo therapeutic ablation of the AV node, rendering them pacemaker-dependent but no longer tachycardic. These patients remain in atrial fibrillation and still require stroke prevention therapy.

KEY POINTS

- All patients with atrial fibrillation who undergo cardioversion require anticoagulation therapy for a minimum for 4 weeks following the procedure.

- The CHA_2DS_2-VASc score for estimating stroke risk in atrial fibrillation is similar to the $CHADS_2$ score but better differentiates low- and intermediate-risk patients; in addition to heart failure, hypertension, age, diabetes mellitus, and previous stroke, the CHA_2DS_2-VASc score incorporates lower age (65-74 years), sex, and the presence of atherosclerotic disease.

- Options for long-term anticoagulation in patients with atrial fibrillation include warfarin, dabigatran, rivaroxaban, and apixaban; the latter three agents do not require blood monitoring and lack the food and drug interactions of warfarin, but they are substantially more expensive.

Atrial Flutter

Unlike atrial fibrillation, atrial flutter is an organized macro-reentrant rhythm with discrete and organized atrial activity on the ECG, usually with an atrial rate of 250/min to 300/min. Although they are distinct rhythms, atrial fibrillation and atrial flutter are often found in the same patients because of similar risk factors and pathophysiology. Episodes of atrial flutter can induce atrial fibrillation and vice-versa.

Typical atrial flutter has a sawtooth appearance on ECG, with negative flutter waves in the inferior leads and positive flutter waves in lead V_1 (**Figure 18**). Typical atrial flutter is caused by counterclockwise reentry around the tricuspid annulus. Atypical flutter can be clockwise or can occur in other locations in the atria, including the left atrium after atrial fibrillation ablation.

In many respects, atrial flutter is managed similar to atrial fibrillation, including stroke prevention. However, owing to the atrial rate and the ratio of conduction through the AV node (for example, 2:1 or 4:1), rate control of atrial flutter can be difficult and often requires large doses of AV nodal blockers. Therefore, atrial flutter is usually managed with a rhythm control strategy. Catheter ablation of typical atrial flutter is often preferred owing

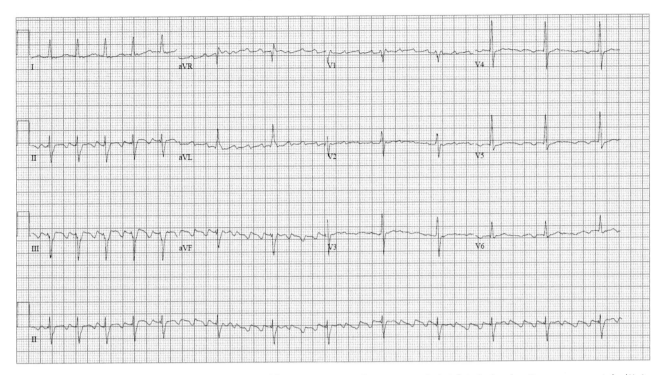

FIGURE 18. In this electrocardiogram demonstrating typical atrial flutter, negative sawtooth waves are seen in the inferior leads and positive waves are seen in lead V_1. In the bottom rhythm strip, 2:1 and 4:1 conduction patterns are seen.

to a high success rate and lower complication rate relative to other ablation procedures. In asymptomatic patients in whom rate control can be achieved, a medical rate control strategy is acceptable.

Wide-Complex Tachycardias

A wide-complex tachycardia is any tachycardia (heart rate ≥100/min) with a QRS complex of 120 msec or greater. The differential diagnosis includes supraventricular rhythms with aberrant conduction (such as underlying bundle branch block), preexcitation, paced rhythms, and ventricular tachycardia.

Often, patients present with a wide-complex tachycardia of unknown etiology. In adults with structural heart disease, 95% of wide-complex tachycardias are VT. Wide-complex tachycardias that are positive in lead aVR, have a QRS morphology that is concordant in the precordial leads (monophasic with the same polarity), have a QRS morphology other than typical right or left bundle branch block, and exhibit extreme axis deviation (-90° to ±180°, sometimes called a northwest axis), are usually VT. The presence of AV dissociation, fusion beats (QRS complex created by fusion between a sinus capture beat and a VT beat), and capture beats (sinus beat that captures the myocardium in between VT beats) are all highly suggestive of VT.

When the origin of a wide-complex tachycardia cannot be determined, VT should be assumed until expert consultation can be obtained.

Ventricular Arrhythmias
Premature Ventricular Contractions

Premature ventricular contractions (PVCs) are common and can occur in up to 75% of healthy persons. Patients with PVCs generally report palpitations and a sensation of skipped beats. Forceful palpitations with PVCs are usually caused by exaggerated cardiac filling during the pause after the PVC. PVCs are more common in patients with hypertension, left ventricular hypertrophy, prior myocardial infarction, and other forms of structural heart disease. For patients with bothersome palpitations, the first diagnostic test is an ECG. If the diagnosis is not established, 24- to 48-hour ambulatory monitoring is used to diagnose and quantify the frequency of PVCs and determine if they are monomorphic or polymorphic. Frequent PVCs (>10% of all beats or ≥10,000 PVCs in a 24-hour period) can lead to tachycardia-induced myopathy. Patients with frequent PVCs or polymorphic PVCs should undergo echocardiography or other cardiovascular imaging (such as cardiac magnetic resonance [CMR] imaging) to evaluate for the presence of structural heart disease.

In patients without high-risk features (such as syncope, a family history of premature SCD, coronary artery disease, or structural heart disease), PVCs (including ventricular bigeminy and trigeminy) are generally benign and do not require additional testing or treatment. Treatment should be limited to those with symptoms or a high burden of PVCs (≥10,000 in a 24-hour period). Treatment for PVCs usually begins with β-blocker or nondihydropyridine calcium channel blocker therapy. Antiarrhythmic drug therapy can also be used when PVCs persist despite β-blockade or calcium channel blockade. EP study and catheter ablation can be considered in patients who cannot tolerate medical therapy or if medical therapy fails to suppress the PVCs.

Ventricular Tachycardia with Structural Heart Disease

In structural heart disease, including both ischemic and nonischemic cardiomyopathy, the presence of myocardial scar tissue facilitates reentry and the development of VT. VT can present as nonsustained or sustained VT (>30 seconds). In patients with ventricular scarring, VT is usually regular and monomorphic. **Figure 19** shows ECG findings of monomorphic VT in a patient with cardiac sarcoidosis. In patients with structural heart disease, VT may lead to hypotension, syncope, degeneration into VF, and cardiac arrest. Alternatively, short runs of VT or slow sustained VT may be well tolerated or asymptomatic.

All patients with VT should undergo resting ECG, exercise treadmill testing to provoke the arrhythmia, and cardiac imaging to evaluate for structural heart disease. Patients with ischemic cardiomyopathy who present with VT should undergo an ischemia evaluation and revascularization if indicated. Patients with cardiomyopathy and heart failure should receive optimal medical therapy in order to reduce their risk of ventricular arrhythmia. Patients with structural heart disease or cardiomyopathy and sustained VT/VF should undergo ICD implantation for secondary prevention. In patients with an ICD, if VT recurs despite β-blocker therapy, antiarrhythmic drug therapy should be considered. In most patients with structural heart disease, amiodarone is first-line antiarrhythmic drug therapy. Patients with recurrent VT despite medical therapy should be considered for EP study and catheter ablation, which has been shown to reduce ICD shocks and thus improve quality of life.

Idiopathic Ventricular Tachycardia

VT in patients without structural heart disease is considered idiopathic. Patients often present with palpitations in early adulthood (20-40 years of age). Episodes are often provoked by stress, emotion, or exercise. Syncope is uncommon. Idiopathic VT usually arises from the outflow tracts, the fascicles, or the papillary muscles. Outflow tract tachycardias, the most common type, are triggered arrhythmias that can arise from the right or left ventricular outflow tracts. They are adenosine-sensitive and often exhibit repetitive salvos. Right ventricular outflow tract tachycardia has a left bundle branch block appearance with tall R waves in the inferior leads. Pharmacologic therapy for idiopathic VT includes calcium channel blockers (especially verapamil) or β-blockers. When symptoms continue despite these measures, catheter ablation can be considered. ICDs are rarely indicated in patients with idiopathic VT owing to the benign prognosis and efficacy of other therapies.

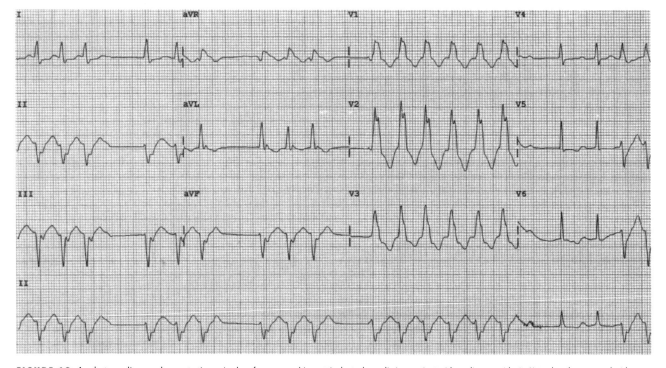

FIGURE 19. An electrocardiogram demonstrating episodes of monomorphic ventricular tachycardia in a patient with cardiac sarcoidosis. Note that the repeated wide-complex beats do not resemble a typical bundle branch block pattern. There are several sinus beats (narrow complexes) that help ascertain the etiology of the wide beats as ventricular tachycardia.

- In patients with premature ventricular contractions without high-risk features, reassurance is usually sufficient; treatment should be limited to those with symptoms or frequent episodes.

Inherited Arrhythmia Syndromes

The diagnosis and management of inherited arrhythmia syndromes are complicated by the variable penetrance and variable expressivity often observed. Characteristics and treatment of the most important inherited syndromes are reviewed in **Table 28**. The presence of unexplained premature (younger than 35 years) death or sudden death in a first-degree family member should raise suspicion for the possible presence of an inherited arrhythmia syndrome and referral to a cardiovascular specialist. Genetic testing has facilitated the diagnostic evaluation of these disorders, particularly when an affected family member has a known pathogenic mutation. Patients with a family history of SCD and unexplained syncope are particularly at high risk and merit aggressive evaluation.

Long QT syndrome is one of the most common inherited arrhythmias and is defined by the presence of a prolonged QTc interval (>440 msec in men and >460 msec in women) accompanied by unexplained syncope or ventricular arrhythmia. The presence of a prolonged QTc interval alone is not sufficient for a diagnosis of long QT syndrome. The diagnostic criteria include ECG findings, symptoms, and in some cases, results of genetic testing. There are many causes of a prolonged QTc interval, most of them are acquired, including medications such as antiarrhythmic agents, antibiotics (macrolides and fluoroquinolones), antipsychotic drugs, and antidepressants (a list can be accessed at http://crediblemeds.org/); structural

heart disease; and electrolyte abnormalities. Patients with a QTc interval greater than 500 msec are at greatest risk for SCD. First-line therapy for long QT syndrome is β-blocker therapy. Patients with cardiac arrest or those who have recurrent events (syncope or VT) despite β-blocker therapy should undergo ICD implantation. Patients with documented long QT syndrome should avoid participation in competitive athletics.

Short QT syndrome is a rare and genetically heterogeneous disorder characterized by a short QT interval, usually less than 340 msec (or QTc <350 msec). It is inherited in an autosomal dominant pattern. Patients can present with atrial and ventricular arrhythmias and syncope. Short QT syndrome carries a high risk for SCD, and ICD placement is recommended for all patients.

Brugada syndrome, an autosomal dominant disorder associated with mutations in the sodium channel gene, is characterized by right precordial ECG abnormalities, including ST-segment coving (ST-segment elevation that descends into an inverted T wave) in leads V_1 through V_3 with or without right bundle branch block (**Figure 20**), VF, and cardiac arrest. Brugada syndrome is more common in men and in persons of Asian descent. Arrhythmic events often occur at night during sleep. The ECG abnormalities can be variable and may be unmasked by fever or pharmacologic challenge with sodium channel blockade (for example, procainamide infusion). Risk stratification in patients with Brugada syndrome is principally based upon the presence or absence of syncope; those with syncope or ventricular arrhythmia should undergo ICD placement. Patients with recurrent ventricular arrhythmias and/or ICD shocks often benefit from quinidine antiarrhythmic drug therapy.

Catecholaminergic polymorphic VT is a rare disorder characterized by polymorphic ventricular arrhythmias and

TABLE 28. Inherited Arrhythmia Syndromes		
Disorder	**Characteristic Findings**	**Treatment[a]**
Long QT syndrome	Syncope, QTc interval usually >460 msec, torsades de pointes	β-Blockers, ICD, exercise restriction
Short QT syndrome	Syncope, QT interval <340 msec, atrial fibrillation, VT, VF	ICD in all patients
Brugada syndrome	Syncope, VF, coved ST-segment elevation in early precordial leads (V_1-V_3)	ICD
Catecholaminergic polymorphic VT	Syncope, polymorphic or bidirectional VT during exercise or emotional distress	β-Blockers, ICD, exercise abstinence
Early repolarization syndrome	Syncope, inferior and lateral early repolarization on ECG, VF	ICD
ARVC/D	Syncope, T-wave inversions in leads V_1 to at least V_3, monomorphic VT, abnormal signal-averaged ECG, frequent PVCs, and abnormal right ventricular size and function on echocardiography or CMR imaging	ICD, β-blockers, antiarrhythmic medications, exercise abstinence

ARVC/D = arrhythmogenic right ventricular cardiomyopathy/dysplasia; CMR = cardiac magnetic resonance; ECG = electrocardiography; ICD = implantable cardioverter-defibrillator; PVCs = premature ventricular contractions; QTc = corrected QT interval; VF = ventricular fibrillation; VT = ventricular tachycardia.

[a]Treatment recommendations for ICDs in inherited arrhythmia syndromes are guided by risk stratification with criteria that are often disease specific. Additionally, antiarrhythmic drugs are often required in several syndromes for recurrent ventricular arrhythmias.

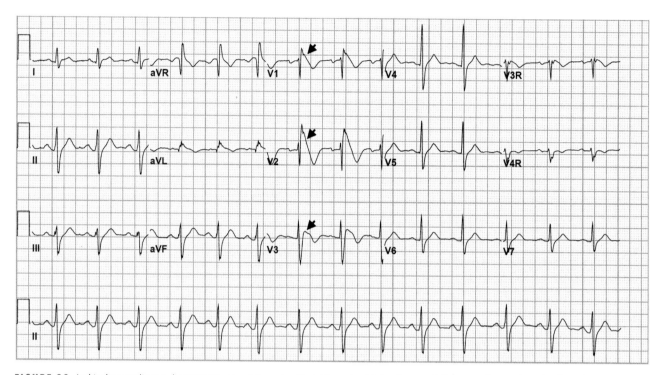

FIGURE 20. In this electrocardiogram demonstrating a type 1 Brugada pattern, ≥2 mm J-point elevation, coved ST-segment elevation (*arrowheads*), and T-wave inversions are seen in leads V₁ to V₃.

cardiac arrest usually provoked by high-adrenergic states, including strong emotion and exercise. Patients with this disorder usually have provocable arrhythmias with exercise or epinephrine infusion. Treatment includes β-blocker therapy and often ICD placement. Patients with the disorder should abstain from exercise.

In patients with unexplained VF arrest, particularly when provoked during exercise, early repolarization syndrome should be considered. Whereas early repolarization (J-point elevation) is a common and benign finding on ECG, the presence of inferior and lateral early repolarization more than 1 mm in a patient with VF or cardiac arrest should be considered early repolarization syndrome. In patients with VF or cardiac arrest, ICD implantation is indicated.

Hereditary structural heart disease, such as hypertrophic cardiomyopathy (see Myocardial Disease) or arrhythmogenic right ventricular cardiomyopathy/dysplasia (ARVC/D), often manifests as sudden cardiac arrest in a young person. ARVC/D is characterized by fibrous and fibro-fatty changes of the right ventricle and subsequent ventricular arrhythmias. Penetrance is variable and age-related, with many patients presenting between puberty and young adulthood. Patients with ARVC/D usually have ventricular ectopy or monomorphic VT, although patients with severe disease may have heart failure. The diagnosis of ARVC/D is guided by diagnostic criteria that include ECG abnormalities, family history, the presence of arrhythmias, and structural abnormalities of the right ventricle as seen on cardiac imaging. ARVC/D is usually progressive, and those with ARVC/D should abstain from exercise, as it may

accelerate disease progression and arrhythmogenesis. Patients with ARVC/D and cardiac arrest or risk factors (nonsustained VT, inducible VT) are offered ICD placement. β-Blockers are first-line therapy for ventricular arrhythmia; however, antiarrhythmic therapy with sotalol or amiodarone or catheter ablation is often required for recurrent VT.

Sudden Cardiac Arrest
Epidemiology and Risk Factors

SCD is defined as instantaneous death or sudden collapse within 1 hour of symptoms. Unwitnessed death is considered SCD if the patient was known to be well within 24 hours of the event. Most episodes of SCD are caused by ventricular arrhythmias (VT/VF arrest). In the general population, the risk of SCD is 1/1000 per year. The incidence is greatest in patients with preexisting structural heart disease; however, most episodes of SCD occur in patients with normal left ventricular function. Risk factors for SCD include (but are not limited to) heart failure, diminished left ventricular function, prior myocardial infarction, unexplained syncope, left ventricular hypertrophy, nonsustained ventricular arrhythmia, chronic kidney disease, and obstructive sleep apnea.

Acute Management

Patients with cardiac arrest require immediate cardiopulmonary resuscitation (CPR) and advanced cardiac life support. The two most important interventions for patients in cardiac arrest are high-quality CPR chest compressions and rapid

H CONT. defibrillation in patients with VT/VF arrest. Basic life support guidelines now emphasize the acronym CAB (Chest compressions, Airway, Breathing) to highlight the importance of immediate, rapid, and sustained chest compressions and de-emphasizing assisted breathing. Once a code has been called or the emergency medical system has been activated and an automated external defibrillator has been requested, the patient's pulse should be checked immediately. If no definite pulse is detected within 10 seconds, chest compressions should begin without delay. In patients with VT/VF, time to defibrillation is an important determinant of the likelihood of survival to hospital discharge. Therefore, when a shockable rhythm is present, defibrillation should be performed as rapidly as possible.

Once CPR has been started, the 2010 American Heart Association guidelines on CPR and emergency cardiovascular care dictate management based upon the presence or absence of a shockable rhythm. In patients with asystole or pulseless electrical activity (PEA), CPR is continued with reassessment of rhythm status for a shockable rhythm every 2 minutes. Epinephrine (1 mg intravenously) should be given every 3 to 5 minutes, although vasopressin (40 units intravenously) can replace the first or second dose of epinephrine. Atropine is not recommended for the treatment of asystole or PEA arrest. Further management of PEA arrest should include ascertainment and treatment of any correctable etiology (for example, tamponade). In patients with VT/VF, a shock is advised with immediate resumption of CPR and reassessment of the rhythm in 2 minutes. Epinephrine should be given after the second shock and every 3 to 5 minutes thereafter. If VT/VF continues despite three shocks and epinephrine, amiodarone should be given as a bolus.

Patients with symptomatic bradycardia and hemodynamic distress should first be treated with atropine. If atropine is ineffective, dopamine or epinephrine infusions can be attempted until transcutaneous pacing or a temporary pacing wire (preferred) can be implemented.

Post-resuscitation care includes therapeutic hypothermia in patients who remain comatose. Complications of therapeutic hypothermia include ventricular arrhythmias during rewarming and infectious complications, including sepsis. Hemodynamics and oxygenation should be optimized in the post-arrest setting. Moderate glycemic control is also recommended. Patients with evidence of acute coronary syndrome should undergo immediate catheterization and revascularization provided there are no contraindications.

Device Therapy for Prevention of Sudden Cardiac Death

Patients with sustained ventricular arrhythmias or cardiac arrest without a reversible etiology have a class I recommendation for secondary prevention ICD placement. In patients with structural heart disease who meet specific criteria, ICDs are indicated for primary prevention (see Heart Failure). ICD battery life is approximately 7 to 10 years but is variable. Although ICD malfunction is rare, when it occurs, it is often due to a problem with the intracardiac leads.

Patients with modern ICDs have few limitations. In general, light to moderate exercise, including sexual intercourse, is permissible and is associated with improvement in cardiovascular health and quality of life. However, some disorders carry specific restrictions (see Table 28). Patients with ICDs should avoid strenuous upper extremity exercises, including weight lifting, because these activities can damage the leads coursing through the chest. Electromagnetic interference can lead to inappropriate detection of VT/VF and shocks; therefore, patients should avoid large sources of electromagnetic interference, including arc welding and high-voltage machinery. During surgery, ICDs may need to be reprogrammed or have a magnet applied to avoid false detection of VT/VF due to electrocautery. For this reason, patients with ICDs should have an evaluation or device programming recommendation from their electrophysiologist before undergoing invasive procedures or surgery.

Patients who experience shocks need to contact their ICD physician. Patients who experience more than one shock in 24 hours or any shock accompanied by dyspnea, chest pain, syncope, or heart failure symptoms require emergency medical care. **H**

KEY POINT

- Implantable cardioverter-defibrillator placement is indicated for secondary prevention in patients with sustained ventricular arrhythmias (>30 sec) or cardiac arrest without a reversible etiology.

Device Infection **H**

Between 1993 and 2008, the use of cardiac implanted electronic devices increased by 96%. As a result, the number of patients susceptible to device infection seen in clinical practice has increased dramatically. Device infections range from infections involving the site of device placement (pocket infection) to infective endocarditis. Most device infections are due to staphylococcal infections, particularly *Staphylococcus epidermidis* and *S. aureus*. When caring for patients with cardiac implanted electronic devices who present with symptoms of infection, clinicians must have a high suspicion for device infection.

Patients with cardiac device infection can present with fever, chills, and malaise. The physical examination may reveal erythema, pocket swelling, and drainage from the pocket. Laboratory findings frequently include anemia, leukocytosis, and an elevated erythrocyte sedimentation rate. In patients with suspected device infection, multiple blood cultures should be drawn. Echocardiography (most often with transesophageal echocardiography) should be performed to identify intracardiac or lead vegetations. The device pocket should never be aspirated for diagnostic purposes because puncturing the pocket can damage the leads or introduce infection.

Once a cardiac device infection is diagnosed, treatment includes complete removal of all hardware, debridement of the pocket, sustained antibiotic therapy, and reimplantation at a new site (if and when appropriate). Suppressive antibiotic therapy without complete removal of the device is not curative and is associated with a high fatality rate. **H**

- In a patient with suspected implanted cardiac device infection, the device pocket should never be aspirated for diagnostic purposes because puncturing the pocket can damage the leads or introduce infection.

- Treatment of implanted cardiac device infection comprises complete hardware removal and pocket debridement, sustained antibiotic therapy, and reimplantation at a new site if appropriate.

Pericardial Disease

Acute Pericarditis

Clinical Presentation

Acute pericarditis may occur as part of a systemic disorder or in isolation. Although there are many potential causes of acute pericarditis, most cases are idiopathic or presumed to be viral or autoimmune in origin. In developing countries and susceptible individuals, tuberculosis and HIV infection are common causes of acute pericarditis. Other causes include neoplasm, trauma, uremia, thoracic irradiation, and certain medications (hydralazine, penicillin, chemotherapeutic agents).

Acute pericarditis may be diagnosed on the basis of typical symptoms of chest pain, a pericardial friction rub, distinctive electrocardiographic (ECG) abnormalities, and supportive data from noninvasive testing. Chest pain characterizes the clinical presentation in 90% to 95% of patients, with additional symptoms related to the underlying cause. Chest pain due to acute pericarditis typically is sharp, anterior, and positional, and it is aggravated by maneuvers that increase pericardial pressure (cough, inspiration) and orthostasis (decreased pain in the upright position). These characteristics may be useful in distinguishing pericarditis from acute myocardial ischemia; however, these features also are frequently present in other chest pain syndromes, such as aortic dissection, costochondritis, and pulmonary embolism. Fever may also be present with acute pericarditis.

A pericardial friction rub is considered to be a hallmark of acute pericarditis. A pericardial rub occurs in 35% to 80% of patients, with or without a pericardial effusion. Three components may be auscultated, attributable to atrial systole, ventricular systole, and early rapid ventricular diastolic filling. Pericardial rub intensity and location can vary, but it is characteristically heard at the left lower sternal border. It is best heard during a held end-expiration with the patient leaning forward. This maneuver allows distinction from a pleuropericardial or pleural rub, which are present only during respiration.

Evaluation

ECG changes frequently occur in patients with acute pericarditis owing to inflammation of the visceral pericardium (or epicardium). Typical ECG changes are concave upward ST-segment elevation and PR-segment abnormalities, with elevation in lead aVR and depression in all other leads. PR-segment abnormalities are due to atrial involvement (**Figure 21**). Although the ECG abnormalities typically are diffuse, certain causes (such as cardiac perforation, trauma, or

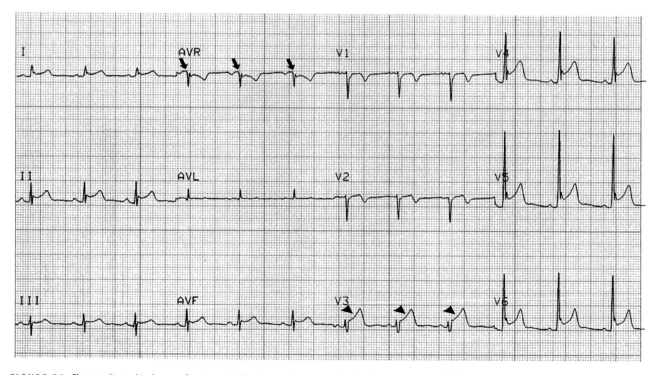

FIGURE 21. Electrocardiographic changes of acute pericarditis. Concave ST-segment elevation is present in most of the leads (*arrowheads*). The PR segment is depressed in all leads except aVR (*arrows*).

segmental myocardial infarction) may result in localized changes. Sinus tachycardia and electrical alternans also are frequently seen. Several ECG features should be routinely considered to help to distinguish the changes of acute pericarditis from myocardial ischemia and early repolarization (**Table 29**).

Other noninvasive tests can be used to support the diagnosis of acute pericarditis but are limited in their sensitivity and specificity. Inflammatory markers, such as erythrocyte sedimentation rate, leukocyte count, and C-reactive protein level, may be elevated. Increases in biomarkers of cardiac injury (cardiac troponin T or troponin I) indicate concomitant myocarditis (that is, myopericarditis). Cardiomegaly may be seen on chest radiographs if a large pericardial effusion in present.

Echocardiography should be performed in all patients with suspected acute pericarditis to evaluate for the presence of a hemodynamically significant pericardial effusion. Although a pericardial effusion occurs in 50% to 60% of patients, its absence does not rule out the diagnosis of acute pericarditis.

Although evaluation for a cause is usually warranted in patients with acute pericarditis, the diagnostic yield of standard testing is low, with an etiology identified in fewer than 20% of cases. Important causes to consider for further evaluation are those that require specific therapy, such as neoplastic disorders, autoimmune disease, trauma (for example, postsurgical pericarditis), and infection (such as tuberculosis). Evaluation for specific causes of acute pericarditis should be considered according to the degree of clinical suspicion for disorders that would require therapy beyond treatment of the acute episode of pericarditis (for example, malignancy or autoimmune disease). Most cases of acute pericarditis are viral or idiopathic and responsive to anti-inflammatory drugs.

Pericardiocentesis can assist in diagnosis when other testing is inconclusive and is also indicated for obtaining a tissue sample if tuberculosis is suspected.

Management

Management goals for a patient with acute pericarditis are the identification and treatment of potential underlying causes, symptom relief with anti-inflammatory agents, and the recognition and treatment of pericardial effusions that are hemodynamically significant. Most patients with acute pericarditis can be managed as outpatients. Patients with acute pericarditis are at increased risk for developing atrial fibrillation and flutter, which may require treatment for symptom management and reversion to sinus rhythm. Life-threatening complications due to effusion are rare but may develop rapidly. Clinical features indicative of increased risk and a potential need for hospitalization are the presence of fever, leukocytosis, acute trauma, abnormal cardiac biomarkers, immunocompromise, oral anticoagulant use (which may increase the risk of bleeding and tamponade), and large or hemodynamically significant pericardial effusions.

For analgesia and treatment of pericardial inflammation, NSAIDs provide effective relief in 70% to 80% of patients. The efficacy of medical therapy varies according to the underlying cause, with response rates greatest among those with idiopathic or presumed viral causes. Relatively high doses of these medications are required (aspirin, 650-1000 mg every 6 to 8 hours; ibuprofen, 400-800 mg every 8 hours; indomethacin, 50 mg every 8 hours). Slow tapering over a period of 2 to 4 weeks is recommended to reduce the risk of recurrent inflammation. In patients with pericarditis associated with myocardial infarction, NSAIDs other than aspirin should not be used. These agents can impair myocardial healing and increase the risk of mechanical complications in these patients.

Colchicine (0.5 to 1.2 mg/d for 3 months), in addition to NSAIDs, is an effective adjunctive therapy for acute pericarditis. The efficacy of colchicine has been demonstrated in several randomized and retrospective studies, which have shown significantly lower rates of treatment failure and recurrent pericarditis when used in conjunction with standard NSAID therapy. Colchicine is generally well tolerated; side effects include gastrointestinal distress and, less commonly, bone marrow suppression, myositis, and liver toxicity.

Glucocorticoids are not considered first-line therapy for acute pericarditis and are reserved for patients with contraindications to NSAIDs and those with refractory pericarditis. Glucocorticoids also may be considered in specific disease

TABLE 29.	Electrocardiographic Features for Differentiating Acute Pericarditis from Myocardial Ischemia	
Feature	**Acute Pericarditis**	**Myocardial Ischemia**
ST-segment contour	Concave upwards	Convex upwards
ST-segment lead involvement	Diffuse	Localized
Reciprocal ST-T wave changes	No	Yes
PR-segment abnormalities	Yes	No
Hyperacute T waves	No	Yes
Pathologic Q waves	No	Yes
Evolution	ST-segment change initially, then T-wave change	T-wave change initially, then ST-segment change
QT prolongation	No	Yes

CONT.

states that are potentially amenable to such therapy (for example, autoimmune disorders, uremic pericarditis). A 3-month course of prednisone (0.25 to 0.50 mg/kg daily starting dose) may be used in these circumstances, with a slow taper beginning at 2 to 4 weeks. Recurrent pericarditis has been reported to be more common among patients prescribed glucocorticoids, but these reports have been hampered by the tendency to use these agents in patients whose pericarditis has been refractory to other therapies. Thus, glucocorticoids are still considered to be an effective alternative therapy for these patients.

After an episode of acute pericarditis, as many as 30% of patients develop recurrent pericarditis. There is a low (<1%) risk of developing constrictive pericarditis. Recurrent pericarditis can be treated with anti-inflammatory agents with a slower, longer taper (for example, 4 months), the addition of colchicine, or the use of glucocorticoids. Etiologies of acute pericarditis other than viral or idiopathic causes should be suspected. **H**

KEY POINTS

- Echocardiography should be performed in patients with suspected acute pericarditis to evaluate for the presence of a hemodynamically significant pericardial effusion; however, the absence of an effusion does not rule out the diagnosis.

- First-line therapy for acute pericarditis is high-dose NSAIDs; colchicine can be used in conjunction with standard NSAID therapy.

- Glucocorticoids in the treatment of acute pericarditis are reserved for patients with contraindications to NSAIDs and those with refractory pericarditis.

H Constrictive Pericarditis

Clinical Presentation and Evaluation

Constrictive pericarditis is a chronic disorder that results from pericardial inflammation, fibrosis, and possibly calcification, leading to a loss of elasticity. Although many cases are idiopathic, causes of constrictive pericarditis include chest radiation therapy, cardiac surgery, trauma, post–myocardial infarction syndromes, and systemic diseases that affect the pericardium, such as connective tissue disease, malignancy, tuberculosis, and other infections.

The pericardium in constrictive pericarditis is rigid and noncompliant, resulting in a total cardiac volume that is largely fixed. Ventricular filling occurs rapidly in early diastole and terminates abruptly near mid-diastole owing to the pericardial restraint. With disease progression, the impairment in diastolic filling and increased intracardiac filling pressures leads to reduced end-diastolic ventricular volume and stroke volume. As a result, symptoms and signs of diminished cardiac output (such as fatigue) and evidence of volume overload characterize the clinical presentation of constrictive pericarditis.

The jugular venous pressure is elevated in nearly all patients, with prominent *x* and *y* descents. Physical findings that also may be present include a Kussmaul sign (jugular vein engorgement with inspiration), pericardial knock, pulsus paradoxus, pleural effusion, congestive hepatomegaly, and peripheral edema or ascites. In patients with long-standing constrictive pericarditis, hepatic failure and cirrhosis may be present.

The diagnosis of constrictive pericarditis can be made with a detailed hemodynamic evaluation using either Doppler echocardiography or cardiac catheterization. The basis for the diagnostic hemodynamic findings in constrictive pericarditis is the concept of enhanced ventricular interdependence, which classically results in equalization of diastolic pressures in all heart chambers. The noncompliant pericardium also prevents the complete transmission of respiratory changes in thoracic pressure to the cardiac chambers. Filling of the right and left ventricles varies significantly with respiration owing to marked changes in the early diastolic gradient emptying into these chambers (that is, dissociation of thoracic-cavitary pressures). During inspiration, the decrease in thoracic pressure leads to relatively less left ventricular filling, while the increase in caval blood flow augments right ventricular preload. Reciprocal changes in ventricular loading occur during expiration (**Figure 22**). Because

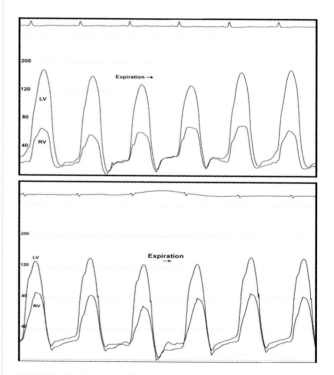

FIGURE 22. Comparison of hemodynamics of constrictive pericarditis versus restrictive cardiomyopathy. In constrictive pericarditis (*top panel*), there is significant enhancement of ventricular interdependence leading to discordance of the left ventricular and right ventricular pressures during respiration. Arrows indicate onset of expiration and subsequent respective changes in left ventricular and right ventricular systolic pressures. In restrictive cardiomyopathy (*bottom panel*), there is evidence of early rapid ventricular filling, but the ventricular pressures concordantly rise and fall during respiration. LV = left ventricle; RV = right ventricle.

CONT.

constrictive pericarditis does not involve the ventricular septum, bulging of the septum towards the left occurs during inspiration and returns towards the right during expiration, leading to marked enhancement of ventricular interdependence. The dissociation of thoracic and intracavitary pressures and the enhanced ventricular interdependence lead to reciprocal changes in filling and emptying of the right and left ventricles, which manifest as alterations in right- and left-sided forward stroke volumes during respiration (see Figure 22). These findings are distinct from restrictive cardiomyopathy, in which there is not significant enhancement of ventricular interdependence or dissociation of intracavitary-intrathoracic pressures (**Table 30**). Restrictive cardiomyopathy is characterized by severe left ventricular diastolic dysfunction due to myocardial abnormalities or infiltration.

Differentiation of constrictive pericarditis from restrictive cardiomyopathy is clinically important because surgical treatment of constrictive pericarditis may be curative of the condition, but there are no therapies that significantly improve the natural history of restrictive cardiomyopathy.

Other echocardiographic findings supportive of the diagnosis of constrictive pericarditis are increased pericardial thickness and plethora of the inferior vena cava. Pericardial thickening, with or without calcification, can also be detected with cardiac CT or cardiac magnetic resonance (CMR) imaging (**Figure 23**).

A subset of patients with chronic constrictive pericarditis develop effusive constrictive pericarditis. There typically is minimal pericardial fluid present in constrictive pericarditis; in some patients, however, pericardial inflammation

TABLE 30. Characteristics of Constrictive Pericarditis, Restrictive Cardiomyopathy, and Cardiac Tamponade

Characteristic	Constrictive Pericarditis	Restrictive Cardiomyopathy	Cardiac Tamponade
Mechanism	Rigid, inelastic pericardium resulting in fixed cardiac volume	Myocardial disease with severe diastolic dysfunction	Increased intrapericardial pressure compromises ventricular filling
Hemodynamic implications	Rapid and limited diastolic filling due to pericardial restraint; increased intracardiac filling pressures, diminished cardiac output, and volume overload	Diastolic abnormalities lead to elevated ventricular filling pressures and pulmonary hypertension	Ventricular filling is impaired with a reduction in cardiac output; jugular venous and pulmonary venous pressures increased
Physical examination	↑ JVP, Kussmaul sign, pericardial knock, diminished apical impulse, congestion (peripheral edema, pleural effusion, congestive hepatopathy)	↑ JVP, Kussmaul sign, pericardial knock, diminished apical impulse, congestion (peripheral edema, pleural effusion, congestive hepatopathy)	↑ JVP, pulsus paradoxus, hypotension, reflex tachycardia
Electrocardiography	No characteristic findings	No characteristic findings	Decreased voltage, sinus tachycardia, electrical alternans
Chest radiography	Pericardial calcification	Atrial enlargement	Enlarged cardiac silhouette ("water-bottle" heart)
Echocardiography	Pericardial thickening/calcification; respiratory variation in filling of right and left ventricles; ventricular septal shift during respiration; plethora of inferior vena cava	Markedly dilated atria with preserved systolic function; severe impairment of myocardial relaxation	Pericardial effusion, diastolic collapse of right atrium and ventricle, enlargement of inferior vena cava, ventricular septal shifting during respiration, respiratory changes in mitral inflow
CMR imaging/CT	Pericardial thickening/calcification	Normal pericardium	Pericardial effusion
Hemodynamic right and left heart catheterization	Prominent x and y descents; elevated atrial pressures; elevated and equalized diastolic LV and RV pressures (within 5 mm Hg); decreased transmission of intrathoracic pressure causes discordance of LV and RV pressures and stroke volume during respiration (enhanced ventricular interdependence)	Prominent x and y descents; elevated atrial pressures; concordance of LV and RV pressures during respiration	Prominent x descents and blunted y descents; elevated atrial pressures; blunting/loss of early ventricular diastolic filling wave
BNP	Normal or minimally elevated	Elevated	Normal or low

BNP = B-type natriuretic peptide; CMR = cardiac magnetic resonance; JVP = jugular venous pressure; LV = left ventricular; RV = right ventricular.

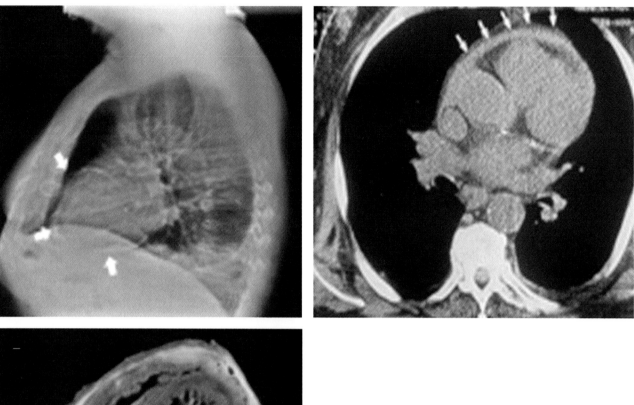

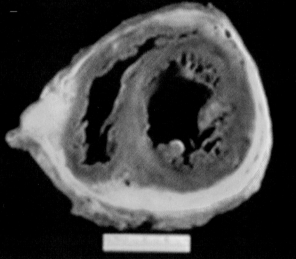

FIGURE 23. Constrictive pericarditis. Chest radiograph (*top left panel*) showing pericardial calcification (*arrows*). CT scan (*top right panel*) demonstrating pericardial thickening (*arrows*). Gross pathology (*bottom left panel*) demonstrating severe pericardial calcification.

Pathology image courtesy of Dr. William D. Edwards, Department of Pathology, Mayo Clinic.

results in an effusion that is placed under pressure by the inelastic pericardium. Although this does not typically cause the hemodynamic changes seen with cardiac tamponade, it may change the clinical presentation. Symptoms of low cardiac output, systemic congestion, and an elevated jugular venous pulse occur, as in constrictive pericarditis; however, a pericardial knock may be absent and the y descent of the jugular venous pulse may be less prominent. The etiology is similar to that of chronic constriction, although tuberculous pericarditis is particularly prone to this clinical presentation. Effusive constrictive pericarditis should be suspected in a patient with residual symptoms and signs of persistent atrial pressure elevation after successful pericardiocentesis. The diagnosis can be made with either echocardiography or cardiac catheterization.

Management

Some patients with constrictive pericarditis can have reversible or transient inflammation, such as post-pericardiotomy syndrome after cardiac surgery, that responds to anti-inflammatory agents. Thus, it may be reasonable to perform a trial of medical therapy (such as NSAIDs) before pericardiectomy surgery in some patients presenting with constrictive pericarditis, particularly those with mild symptoms, a potentially reversible cause of acute inflammation, and no evidence of chronic constriction. Diuretic therapy may reduce volume overload and improve symptoms transiently.

Cardiac surgery with pericardiectomy is the definitive treatment for relief of heart failure in patients with constrictive pericarditis. Because of the complexity of the procedure, this surgery is best performed in experienced centers where a total pericardiectomy, with removal of as much of the pericardium as is technically possible, may be achieved. Patients treated with total pericardiectomy have been shown to have improved outcomes relative to those who undergo more limited procedures. Predictors of poor outcome after surgical pericardiectomy include advanced age, severe symptoms, chronic kidney disease, pulmonary hypertension, left ventricular dysfunction, and radiation therapy as the underlying cause of constrictive pericarditis. In one study, the 7-year survival after pericardiectomy was 27%, 66%, and 88%, respectively, for patients with constrictive pericarditis due to radiation, prior cardiac surgery, and an idiopathic cause. Medical therapy with diuretics can improve symptoms or be palliative in patients who are not surgical candidates, but the chronic nature of the disorder can prove to be drug-refractory.

KEY POINTS

- In some patients with constrictive pericarditis, particularly those with mild symptoms, a potentially reversible cause of acute inflammation, and no evidence of chronic constriction, it may be reasonable to perform a trial of medical therapy before surgery.
- Cardiac surgery with pericardiectomy is the definitive treatment for relief of heart failure in patients with constrictive pericarditis.

Cardiac Tamponade

Clinical Presentation and Evaluation

The normal pericardium contains 15 to 50 mL of plasma ultrafiltrate. The rate of accumulation and the absolute amount of pericardial fluid surrounding the heart above the normal baseline level determine the hemodynamic effects of an effusion. Cardiac tamponade occurs when intrapericardial pressure exceeds intracardiac pressure, leading to impairment of ventricular filling throughout the entire diastolic period.

Virtually any disorder that causes a pericardial effusion can result in cardiac tamponade. Malignancy is the most common atraumatic etiology, with breast and lung cancer being the most frequent. Other important causes are idiopathic or viral pericarditis, complications of invasive cardiac procedures, aortic dissection with disruption of the aortic valve annulus, tuberculosis, uremia, and pericarditis or ventricular rupture from a myocardial infarction.

During cardiac tamponade, venous return and ventricular filling become impaired owing to excess intrapericardial pressure. This impairment precipitates elevation and equalization of diastolic pressures in the heart, including increased pulmonary venous and right atrial pressures, and ultimately, a reduction in cardiac output. With inspiration, filling pressure to the left ventricle falls, leading to a reduction in the stroke volume. The fall in left ventricular stroke volume during inspiration manifests as a relative decrease in pulse pressure or peak systolic pressure and is the hallmark finding of

pulsus paradoxus (a decrease in the systolic pressure of >10 mm Hg with inspiration) in these patients. As compensation for the reduced stroke volume and hypotension, tachycardia is usually present.

Less common presentations of cardiac tamponade also need to be considered in some patients. A loculated pericardial effusion may occur after cardiac surgery or in other postoperative settings. It may occur in the posterior pericardial space adjacent to the atria, posing challenges for detection by echocardiography. Posterior loculated effusions should be suspected in postoperative patients with hemodynamic instability. Low-pressure cardiac tamponade occurs without elevated jugular venous pressure because the intracardiac filling pressures are low. Examples include patients with malignancy or tuberculosis complicated by severe dehydration. Pneumopericardium with cardiac tamponade may result from gas-forming bacterial pericarditis after penetrating chest trauma.

Cardiac tamponade should be suspected when there is a compatible history, hypotension, and an elevated jugular venous pressure and pulsus paradoxus. An enlarged cardiac silhouette may be seen on chest radiograph ("water-bottle heart"). The ECG typically demonstrates sinus tachycardia and electrical alternans. Echocardiography readily detects pericardial effusions and is the primary modality for diagnosing cardiac tamponade (**Figure 24**). Signs of cardiac tamponade include diastolic collapse of the right atrium and right ventricle, ventricular septal shifting with respiration, and enlargement of the inferior vena cava. With Doppler echocardiography, respiratory variation in mitral inflow can be detected early in the evolution of tamponade. Moreover, the changes in mitral inflow are highly sensitive, and may precede changes in cardiac output, blood pressure, and other echocardiographic evidence of tamponade. Respiratory changes in mitral inflow resolve after pericardiocentesis unless an effusive-constrictive physiology is present.

The signs of cardiac tamponade also can be evident with invasive hemodynamic catheterization. Characteristic findings include prominent x descents and blunted y descents on the atrial tracings (**Figure 25**) and elevated ventricular diastolic pressures with blunting or loss of the early rapid ventricular filling wave, which is the hallmark of cardiac tamponade that distinguishes it from other diastolic disorders. Other hemodynamic findings include equalization of left- and right-sided end-diastolic pressures, reduced cardiac output, and alterations in the systolic ejection period or pulse pressure that result from decreased stroke volume (analogous to pulsus paradoxus).

Management

Intravenous normal saline and, if needed, vasopressors should be administered to stabilize the hemodynamics in a patient with cardiac tamponade. Although the presentation includes symptoms and signs of heart failure, reduction of intravascular volume by diuresis may exacerbate the hemodynamic abnormalities of tamponade.

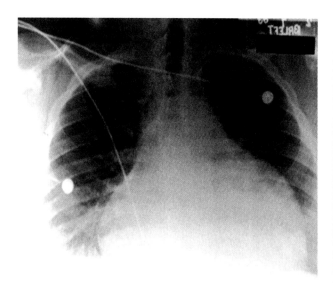

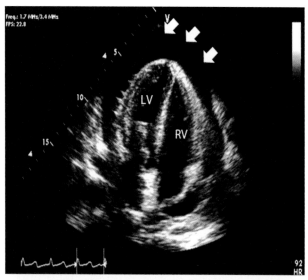

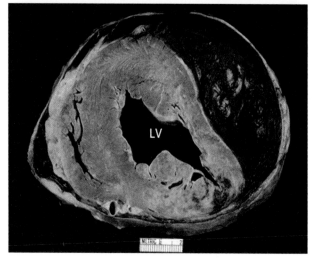

FIGURE 24. Cardiac tamponade. Chest radiograph (*top panel*) showing "water-bottle heart." Transthoracic echocardiogram (*middle panel*) showing a large pericardial effusion (*arrows*). Gross pathology (*bottom panel*) of cardiac tamponade. LV = left ventricle; RV = right ventricle.

Pathology image courtesy of Dr. William D. Edwards, Department of Pathology, Mayo Clinic.

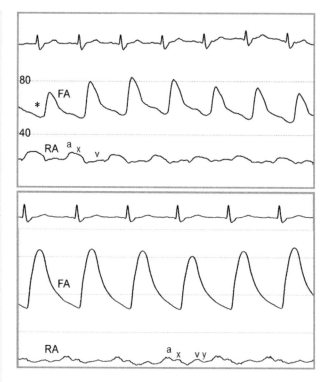

FIGURE 25. Invasive hemodynamic features of cardiac tamponade. Y-axis indicates pressure (mm Hg). Hypotension and pulsus paradoxus (*asterisk*) in the femoral artery (FA) pressure tracing and loss of the *y* descent in the right atrial (RA) pressure tracing are evident (*top panel*). Following pericardiocentesis, there is a rise in arterial pressure and return of the *y* descent in the RA pressure tracing (*bottom panel*).

Pericardiocentesis with echocardiographic guidance is the most expeditious treatment for cardiac tamponade, with a lower complication rate than blind or ECG-guided pericardiocentesis. Pericardiocentesis should be avoided when treating tamponade associated with aortic dissection. In these patients, abrupt return of ventricular ejection may exacerbate the dissection and precipitate acute decompensation. During attempts at needle passage with pericardiocentesis, the tense pericardium may discharge fluid from the pericardial effusion into the pleural space. This effect can be immediately recognized on echocardiography and may obviate further attempts at pericardiocentesis, as acute relief of tamponade may occur.

Although the vast majority of pericardial effusions can be treated percutaneously, some still require surgical drainage. A surgical approach also may be required for viscous or loculated effusions, those resulting from bacterial infections, posterior effusions that can be difficult to approach from any thoracic approach, and malignant effusions with a high likelihood of recurrence. In addition, recent hemorrhage into the pericardium may result in pericardial clot formation that can be difficult to remove with a catheter. Pericardiocentesis in the setting of aortic dissection may exacerbate the intimal tear owing to the abrupt increase in stroke volume that occurs with relief of cardiac tamponade. Surgical therapy most commonly consists of a pericardial window to allow drainage of fluid; some

CONT.

CONT.

patients require an open pericardiectomy. Open pericardiectomy can be beneficial when there is a diagnostic need for pericardial tissue. **H**

> **KEY POINT**
>
> - Pericardiocentesis with echocardiographic guidance is the most expeditious treatment for cardiac tamponade.

Valvular Heart Disease

Pathophysiology of Valvular Heart Disease

Valvular heart disease (VHD) comprises cardiac dysfunction due to structural or functional abnormalities of the cardiac valves. Dysfunction results from either failure of the valves to competently close (regurgitation) or to effectively open (stenosis). Causes of VHD have changed markedly in developed countries over the past 50 years, with a shift away from rheumatic disease and toward calcific, degenerative, and congenital causes. Rheumatic heart disease continues to be the primary cause of VHD in the developing world.

The effect of VHD on the heart and on the patient varies based on the affected valve and the mechanism of dysfunction:

- Aortic stenosis causes chronic pressure overload that typically leads to concentric left ventricular (LV) hypertrophy with increased wall thickness and normal chamber size to compensate for increased LV afterload.

- Chronic aortic regurgitation causes increased LV preload and afterload, leading to increased LV volume and mass.

- Mitral stenosis causes increased pressure within the left atrium (LA), leading to increased pulmonary venous pressure, pulmonary hypertension, and atrial dilation.

- Chronic mitral regurgitation causes volume overload (increased preload) of the LV and LA, leading to increased LA size and pressure and LV dilation.

Many of these changes in cardiac structure occur gradually because of physiologic mechanisms that compensate for the increased loading conditions. For this reason, patients remain asymptomatic for some time even in the setting of significant valve disease. The exception to this is acute valve lesions, in which the compensatory changes do not have sufficient time to develop.

Diagnostic Evaluation of Valvular Heart Disease

History and Physical Examination

The initial evaluation of the patient with possible VHD serves to diagnose, quantify, and assess mechanisms of valve dysfunction. The evaluation should focus on disease severity, symptoms, quality of life, expected benefits of intervention compared with medical therapy or expectant management, patient desires, and local resources for surgery or intervention.

In many patients with chronic VHD, the development of symptoms is insidious and their onset may go unnoticed. Typical symptoms include exertional dyspnea, edema, and orthopnea. A thorough history provides the opportunity to assess daily activity and lifestyle changes that may effectively "mask" symptoms. This is important as the presence or absence of symptoms may play a pivotal role in deciding timing of intervention.

The physical examination, including cardiac auscultation, is the key first step in identifying the presence of VHD and the likely valve or valves involved and in helping to guide an appropriate diagnostic and therapeutic approach (**Figure 26**). A thorough cardiac examination entails determining the intensity of the murmur as well as specific characteristics that help define whether it is a clinically significant murmur. Not all murmurs require further evaluation (specifically echocardiography).

The clinical grading of both systolic and diastolic murmurs is based on a scale of 1 to 6 (**Table 31**). Diastolic murmurs are always considered abnormal and require further evaluation. Systolic murmurs may be either innocent or indicative of significant valve disease. Some murmurs are associated with normal valves but abnormal systemic processes (for example, anemia and other high-output states, such as hyperthyroidism) or increased flow (for example, a systolic murmur in the setting of aortic regurgitation). Innocent murmurs are characteristically brief and are associated with normal heart sounds and no hemodynamic abnormalities. Patients with grade 1 or 2 midsystolic murmurs who are asymptomatic with no associated findings and those with continuous murmurs suggestive of a venous hum or mammary souffle (a continuous murmur heard over the breast in lactating women) do not warrant echocardiographic evaluation.

The character of a murmur in response to clinical maneuvers is helpful in localizing the flow disturbance to a specific valve. For example, in general, right-sided murmurs increase with inspiration and left-sided murmurs increase with expiration. A Valsalva maneuver decreases the length and intensity of most murmurs, except for systolic murmurs associated with hypertrophic obstructive cardiomyopathy and mitral valve prolapse. Exercise causes the murmur of mitral stenosis to get louder, whereas isometric maneuvers, such as handgrip, increase the intensity of regurgitant murmurs such as aortic and mitral regurgitation. Postural maneuvers are ideal for differentiating hypertrophic obstructive cardiomyopathy and mitral valve prolapse from other murmurs as they are louder with standing and softer with squatting. Physical examination findings, such as an enlarged or displaced apical impulse, abnormal peripheral pulses, and timing and intensity of heart sounds (including extra heart

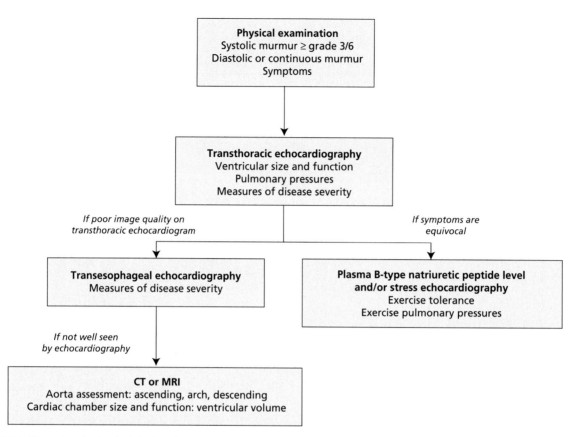

FIGURE 26. Diagnostic evaluation of valvular heart disease.

Grade	Description
1	Faintest murmur that can be heard (with difficulty)
2	Faint murmur but can be identified immediately
3	Moderately loud murmur
4	Loud murmur associated with a palpable thrill
5	Very loud murmur but cannot be heard without the stethoscope
6	Loudest murmur; can be heard without a stethoscope

TABLE 31. Clinical Grading of Murmurs

sounds such as an S_3 or S_4 or a systolic ejection click) may help identify specific valve lesions as well. Common valve lesions and heart murmurs are further described in **Table 32**.

Laboratory and Imaging Tests

Electrocardiography (ECG) and chest radiography are often performed during the initial evaluation. ECG provides valuable insight into rhythm (such as the presence of atrial fibrillation) and cardiac chamber enlargement. Chest radiography is essential when interpreting dyspnea or clinical signs of heart failure with evidence of cardiac enlargement and pulmonary vascular redistribution. Chest radiography may also provide secondary

clues (such as a dilated left ventricle in the setting of chronic aortic regurgitation), but its utility in the evaluation of VHD is less than other modalities, especially echocardiography.

Transthoracic echocardiography (TTE) with color flow and spectral Doppler imaging is the primary noninvasive means of evaluating cardiac murmurs as well as the primary means for following the course of VHD. TTE is indicated for patients with the following (see Figure 26):

- Systolic murmurs ≥grade 3/6 or late or holosystolic murmurs

- Diastolic or continuous murmurs

- Murmurs with accompanying symptoms

TTE permits assessment of LV size and function (systolic and diastolic), estimation of pulmonary artery pressure (an indirect estimate based on the tricuspid regurgitant jet velocity), and determination of disease severity. Echocardiography also helps establish a reference point for future comparisons if significant abnormalities are detected. Transesophageal echocardiography (TEE) provides improved image quality over TTE as the probe has only the thin tissue of the esophagus through which to image. TEE is indicated for patients with severe disease who need further quantification, better identification of leaflet involvement (particularly for patients with mitral regurgitation), or when poor image quality on TTE limits

TABLE 32. Valvular and Other Cardiac Lesions and Their Associated Examination Findings

Cardiac Condition	Characteristic Murmur	Location	Radiation	Associated Findings	Severity and Pitfalls
Aortic stenosis	Mid-systolic; crescendo-decrescendo	RUSB	Right clavicle, carotid, apex	Enlarged, nondisplaced apical impulse; S_4; bicuspid valve without calcification will have systolic ejection click followed by murmur	Severe aortic stenosis may include decreased A_2; high-pitched, late peaking murmur; diminished and delayed carotid upstroke Radiation of murmur down the descending thoracic aorta may mimic mitral regurgitation
Aortic regurgitation	Diastolic; decrescendo	LLSB (valvular) or RLSB (dilated aorta)	None	Enlarged, displaced apical impulse; S_3 or S_4; increased pulse pressure; bounding carotid and peripheral pulse	Acute, severe regurgitation murmur may be masked by tachycardia, short duration of murmur Severity in chronic regurgitation is difficult to assess by auscultation
Mitral stenosis	Diastolic; low pitched, decrescendo	Apex (heard best in left lateral decubitus position)	None	Opening snap after S_2 if leaflets mobile; irregular pulse if atrial fibrillation present	Interval between S_2 and opening snap is short in severe mitral stenosis Intensity of murmur correlates with transvalvular gradient P_2 may be loud if pulmonary hypertension present
Mitral regurgitation	Systolic; holo- or late systolic	Apex	To axilla or back; occasionally anteriorly to precordium	Systolic click in mitral valve prolapse; S_3; apical impulse hyperdynamic and may be displaced if dilated left ventricle; in mitral valve prolapse, Valsalva maneuver moves onset of clicks and murmur closer to S_1; handgrip increases murmur intensity	Acute, severe regurgitation may have soft or no holosystolic murmur, mitral inflow rumble, S_3
Tricuspid stenosis	Diastolic; low pitched, decrescendo; increased intensity during inspiration	LLSB	Nonradiating	Elevated central venous pressure with prominent *a* wave, signs of venous congestion (hepatomegaly, ascites, edema)	Low-pitched frequency may be difficult to auscultate, especially at higher heart rate

(Continued on the next page)

TABLE 32. Valvular and Other Cardiac Lesions and Their Associated Examination Findings *(Continued)*

Cardiac Condition	Characteristic Murmur	Location	Radiation	Associated Findings	Severity and Pitfalls
Tricuspid regurgitation	Holosystolic	LLSB	LUSB	Merged and prominent *c* and *v* waves in jugular venous pulse; murmur increases during inspiration	Right ventricular impulse below sternum Pulsatile, enlarged liver with possible ascites May be higher pitched if associated with severe pulmonary hypertension
Pulmonary stenosis	Systolic; crescendo-decrescendo	LUSB	Left clavicle	Pulmonic ejection click after S_1 (diminishes with inspiration)	Increased intensity of murmur with late peaking
Pulmonary regurgitation	Diastolic; decrescendo	LLSB	None	Loud P_2 if pulmonary hypertension present	Murmur may be minimal or absent if severe due to minimal difference in pulmonary artery and right ventricular diastolic pressures
Innocent flow murmur	Midsystolic; grade 1/6 or 2/6 in intensity	RUSB	None	Normal intensity of A_2; normal splitting of S_2; no radiation	May be present in conditions with increased flow (e.g., pregnancy, fever, anemia, hyperthyroidism)
Hypertrophic obstructive cardiomyopathy	Systolic; crescendo-decrescendo	LLSB	None	Enlarged, hyperdynamic apical impulse; bifid carotid impulse with delay; increased intensity during Valsalva maneuver or with squatting to standing	Murmur may not be present in nonobstructive hypertrophic cardiomyopathy
Atrial septal defect	Systolic; crescendo-decrescendo	RUSB	None	Fixed, split S_2; right ventricular heave; rarely, tricuspid inflow murmur	May be associated with pulmonary hypertension, including increased intensity of P_2, pulmonary valve regurgitation
Ventricular septal defect	Holosystolic	LLSB	None	Palpable thrill; murmur increases with hand-grip, decreases with amyl nitrite	Murmur intensity and duration decrease as pulmonary hypertension develops (Eisenmenger syndrome) Cyanosis if Eisenmenger syndrome develops

A_2 = aortic valve component of S_2; LLSB = left lower sternal border; LUSB = left upper sternal border; P_2 = pulmonary valve component of S_2; RLSB = right lower sternal border; RUSB = right upper sternal border.

image interpretation. The disadvantage compared with TTE is that it is invasive, requiring sedation and technical expertise distinct from TTE.

For stenotic lesions, Doppler-derived velocities across the affected valve allow calculation of pressure gradients and valve area. Based on the conservation of mass principle, the measured flow through one heart chamber region and measured velocity of blood across the region (stenotic valve) of interest can be used to calculate the area of the stenotic valve.

Assessment of severity for regurgitant valves includes color Doppler jet size and the width of the narrowest segment of the regurgitant jet (vena contracta). Additional quantitative measures for regurgitant lesions, such as effective regurgitant orifice area, regurgitant volume, and proximal isovolumic surface area, although technically more demanding to acquire, are strongly associated with prognosis and should be measured routinely in patients with moderate or severe regurgitation by color Doppler jet size. Three-dimensional echocardiography, both transthoracic and transesophageal, provides additional information such as feasibility of repair (rather than replacement) and location of paravalvular leaks. Additional imaging, such as cardiac magnetic resonance (CMR) imaging or multidetector CT (MDCT), may provide information on LV function, aortic dimensions, chamber sizes and volumes, and coronary anatomy. Consistency of quantitative evaluation is important. Simple measurements, such as LV outflow tract diameter, may vary greatly in the same patient when obtained at different times and by different operators. These differences may affect valve area calculations and influence timing of surgery.

Cardiac catheterization can provide important hemodynamic information, especially when the severity of the valve disease as measured by noninvasive testing is not consistent with symptoms or physical examination severity, or when accurate assessment of pulmonary pressures or detection of intracardiac shunts is needed. Coronary angiography is recommended before valve surgery in patients with severe VHD and a history of coronary artery disease, suspected myocardial ischemia, or LV systolic dysfunction; in men older than 40 years and postmenopausal women; in patients with one or more cardiovascular risk factors; and in patients in whom mitral regurgitation is thought to be caused by LV dysfunction. These patients may require concomitant revascularization at the time of surgery.

For patients in whom symptoms are equivocal, adjunctive evaluation (such as B-type natriuretic peptide measurement, exercise evaluation for tolerance/symptoms, and blood pressure response to exercise), assessment of pulmonary artery pressures, and LV outflow tract gradient (by TTE or cardiac catheterization) may be helpful.

KEY POINTS

- Patients with grade 1 or 2 midsystolic murmurs who are asymptomatic with no associated findings and those with continuous murmurs suggestive of a venous hum or mammary souffle do not warrant echocardiographic evaluation. **HVC**

- Transthoracic echocardiography is indicated for the evaluation of valve disease in patients with systolic murmurs grade 3/6 intensity or greater; late or holosystolic murmurs; diastolic or continuous murmurs; or any murmur with accompanying symptoms.

General Principles of Management of Valvular Heart Disease

Treatment is guided by valve lesion severity, which can be classified into four stages (A to D) in a system similar to that used for patients with heart failure (**Table 33**). The mainstay of treatment for VHD, both stenosis and regurgitation, is centered on interventions to treat the mechanical problem. The goals of treatment are both to improve symptoms and reduce the risk of complications such as irreversible ventricular dysfunction, pulmonary hypertension, and death. The most

TABLE 33.	Stages of Progression of Valvular Heart Disease	
Stage	**Definition**	**Description**
A	At risk	Patients with risk factors for development of VHD
B	Progressive	Patients with progressive VHD (mild-to-moderate severity and asymptomatic)
C	Asymptomatic severe	Asymptomatic patients who meet criteria for severe VHD:
		C1: Asymptomatic patients with severe VHD in whom the left or right ventricle remains compensated
		C2: Asymptomatic patients with severe VHD, with decompensation of the left or right ventricle
D	Symptomatic severe	Patients who have developed symptoms as a result of VHD

VHD = valvular heart disease.

Reprinted with permission of Elsevier Science and Technology Journals, from Nishimura RA, Otto CM, Bonow RO, et al. 2014 AHA/ACC guideline for the management of patients with valvular heart disease: executive summary: a report of the American College of Cardiology/American Heart Association Task Force on Practice Guidelines. J Am Coll Cardiol. 2014 Jun 10;63(22):2438-88. [PMID: 24603192]; permission conveyed through Copyright Clearance Center, Inc.

common indication for treatment is symptoms (**Table 34**) but other factors, including chamber dysfunction, chamber enlargement, and pulmonary hypertension may be indications for treatment. In general, for both stenotic and regurgitant lesions, symptoms occur before the development of ventricular dysfunction; however, some patients may have asymptomatic ventricular dysfunction. Medical therapy does not stall the progression of disease but is indicated for patients with symptoms and LV dysfunction who are awaiting valve repair or replacement, as well as for those who are not operative candidates. Preventive measures, such as statins for preventing progression of aortic stenosis, have not been shown to be useful.

The primary therapy for patients with severe VHD is valve repair or valve replacement with either bioprosthetic or mechanical valves. For patients with high surgical risks, percutaneous techniques for aortic valve replacement and mitral valve repair are now available.

Follow-up is essential in asymptomatic patients, as disease progression may occur over time (**Table 35**). After valve repair or replacement, patients should ideally be followed in conjunction with a cardiovascular specialist. **H**

TABLE 34.	Indications for Interventions for Valvular Heart Conditions	
Valve Lesion	**Indications to Intervene[a]**	**Interventions**
Aortic stenosis	Symptoms (class I)	Aortic valve replacement
	LVEF <50% (class I)	
	Moderate (class IIa) or severe (class I) aortic stenosis at time of other cardiac surgery	
	Abnormal blood pressure response (decrease in systolic blood pressure) during exercise (class IIa)	
	Asymptomatic patients with very severe aortic stenosis (class IIa)	
Aortic regurgitation	Symptoms (class I)	Aortic valve replacement
	LVEF <50% (class I)	
	Moderate (class IIa) or severe (class I) aortic regurgitation at time of other cardiac surgery	
	LV dilatation (end-systolic dimension >50 mm) (class IIa)	
Mitral stenosis	Symptoms (class I)	Percutaneous balloon valvotomy (if anatomy favorable by echocardiography with less than moderate mitral regurgitation and no left atrial thrombus)[b]
	Very severe mitral stenosis (MVA <1.0 cm^2) and no symptoms if valve morphology favorable for balloon valvotomy (class IIa)	
	Severe mitral stenosis at time of other cardiac surgery (class I)	Mitral valve replacement
Mitral regurgitation	Symptoms (class I)	Mitral valve repair if anatomy favorable (presence of annular dilation, mitral leaflet prolapse, or myxomatous changes without calcification or stenosis)
	LVEF 30%-60% (class I)	
	LV end-systolic diameter ≥40 mm (class I)	
	Moderate (class IIa) or severe (class I) mitral regurgitation at time of other cardiac surgery	Mitral valve replacement
	Pulmonary hypertension (PA systolic pressure ≥50 mm Hg) (class IIa)	
	New-onset atrial fibrillation (class IIa)	
Tricuspid regurgitation	Severe tricuspid regurgitation at time of surgery for left-sided valve (class I)	Tricuspid valve repair if anatomy favorable
	Symptoms due to severe, primary tricuspid regurgitation not responsive to medical therapy (class IIa)	Tricuspid valve replacement (bioprosthetic)

LV = left ventricle; LVEF = left ventricular ejection fraction; MVA = mitral valve area; PA = pulmonary artery.

[a]Strength of recommendation: class I: procedure should be performed; class IIa: procedure is reasonable.

[b]All patients considered for percutaneous balloon mitral valvotomy should undergo transesophageal echocardiography to assess for left atrial appendage clot and mitral regurgitation severity regardless of whether patient has sinus rhythm or atrial fibrillation.

Recommendations from Nishimura RA, Otto CM, Bonow RO, et al; American College of Cardiology/American Heart Association Task Force on Practice Guidelines. 2014 AHA/ACC guideline for the management of patients with valvular heart disease: executive summary: a report of the American College of Cardiology/American Heart Association Task Force on Practice Guidelines. J Am Coll Cardiol. 2014 Jun 10;63(22):2438-88. Erratum in: J Am Coll Cardiol. 2014 Jun 10;63(22):2489. [PMID: 24603192]

TABLE 35. Serial Evaluation of Asymptomatic Patients with Left-Sided Valvular Conditions

Factors Considered	Lesion Severity	Frequency
Aortic Stenosis		
Stenosis severity; rate of progression; LV systolic function; ascending aorta dilation if bicuspid aortic valve	At risk (V_{max} <2 m/s)	
	Mild (V_{max} 2.0-2.9 m/s or mean gradient <20 mm Hg)	Clinical eval yearly; echo every 3-5 y
	Moderate (V_{max} 3.0-3.9 m/s or mean gradient 20-39 mm Hg)	Clinical eval yearly; echo every 1-2 y
	Severe (V_{max} ≥4 m/s or mean gradient ≥40 mm Hg, AVA ≤1.0 cm^2)	Clinical eval yearly; echo every 6-12 mo
	Very severe (V_{max} ≥5 m/s or mean gradient ≥60 mm Hg)	Clinical eval yearly; echo every 6-12 mo
Mitral Stenosis		
Stenosis severity	Mild and moderate (MVA >1.5 cm^2, diastolic pressure half-time <150 msec)	Clinical eval yearly; echo every 3-5 y
	Severe (MVA ≤1.5 cm^2, diastolic pressure half-time ≥150 msec or ≥220 msec with very severe stenosis, PASP >30 mm Hg)	Clinical eval yearly; echo every 1-2 y for MVA 1.0-1.5 cm^2, every year for MVA <1.0 cm^2
Aortic Regurgitation		
Regurgitation severity; rate of progression; LV ejection fraction; LV chamber size; ascending aorta dilation if bicuspid aortic valve	Mild (VC <0.3 cm, ERO <0.10 cm^2, RV <30 mL/beat, RF <30%); normal EF	Clinical eval yearly; echo every 3-5 y
	Moderate (VC 0.3-0.6 cm, ERO 0.10-0.29 cm^2, RV 30-59 mL/beat, RF 30%-49%)	Clinical eval yearly; echo every 1-2 y
	Severe (VC >0.6 cm, ERO >0.3 cm^2, RV ≥60 mL/beat, RF ≥50%)	
	EF ≥50%; LVESD ≤50 mm	Clinical eval every 6-12 mo; echo every 6-12 mo, more frequently for dilating LV
	EF <50%; LVESD >50 mm	Clinical eval every 6-12 mo; echo every 6-12 mo, more frequently for dilating LV
Mitral Regurgitation		
Regurgitation severity; rate of progression; EF; LV chamber size	At risk (VC <0.3 cm)	Clinical eval yearly; echo only if symptomatic
	Mild and moderate (VC <0.7 cm, ERO <0.40 cm^2, RV <60 mL/beat, RF <50%)	Clinical eval yearly; echo every 3-5 y for mild severity, every 1-2 y for moderate severity
	Severe (VC ≥0.7 cm, ERO ≥0.4 cm^2, RV ≥60 mL/beat, RF ≥50%)	Clinical eval every 6-12 mo; echo every 6-12 mo, more frequently for dilating LV

AVA = aortic valve area; echo = echocardiography; EF = ejection fraction; ERO = effective regurgitant orifice; eval = evaluation; LV = left ventricle; LVESD = left ventricular end-systolic dimension; MVA = mitral valve area; PASP = pulmonary artery systolic pressure; RF = regurgitant fraction; RV = regurgitant volume; VC = vena contracta width; V_{max} = maximum aortic jet velocity.

Recommendations based on Nishimura RA, Otto CM, Bonow RO, et al; American College of Cardiology/American Heart Association Task Force on Practice Guidelines. 2014 AHA/ACC guideline for the management of patients with valvular heart disease: executive summary: a report of the American College of Cardiology/American Heart Association Task Force on Practice Guidelines. J Am Coll Cardiol. 2014 Jun 10;63(22):2438-88. Erratum in: J Am Coll Cardiol. 2014 Jun 10;63(22):2489. [PMID: 24603192]

KEY POINTS

- Medical therapy does not stall the progression of valvular heart disease but is indicated for patients with symptoms and left ventricular dysfunction who are awaiting valve repair or replacement, as well as for those who are not operative candidates.
- The mainstay of therapy for patients with severe valvular heart disease is either valve repair or valve replacement with bioprosthetic or mechanical valves.

Aortic Stenosis

Clinical Presentation and Evaluation

Aortic stenosis is the most common type of valvular heart disease in the United States and is typically caused by calcific degeneration of an otherwise normal aortic valve. Other causes include bicuspid aortic valve and rheumatic valve disease, the latter of which remains common worldwide and is almost always accompanied by mitral valve disease.

Calcific aortic stenosis is a disease of the elderly, and coronary artery disease and hypertension are common in these patients. Patients may present with heart failure symptoms, usually associated with preserved ejection fraction. Some patients present with decompensated heart failure associated with reduced cardiac output. The chronic increase in LV systolic pressure results in a compensatory increase in myocardial cell mass; interstitial fibrosis may follow, leading first to diastolic dysfunction and then to systolic dysfunction. Increased LV end-diastolic pressure results in pulmonary congestion. These and other adaptive and pathologic processes contribute to the three cardinal symptoms of aortic stenosis: angina, dyspnea, and syncope. Identification of the symptomatic patient is crucial; in the absence of symptoms, patients with aortic stenosis—even severe aortic stenosis—have a low risk of mortality, with a risk of sudden death estimated to be less than 1%. The rate of progression is approximately 0.1 cm² annually. Although variable, symptoms of heart failure, angina, or syncope generally begin once the valve area is below 1.0 cm². Once symptoms develop, prognosis is poor without valve replacement, with an average survival of less than 10% over the next 2 to 3 years.

TTE is essential in the initial diagnosis and follow-up of aortic stenosis, permitting quantification of valve area and gradients (see Table 35), chamber size, wall thickness, ventricular function, and coexistent valve disease. Echocardiographic findings for severe aortic stenosis include a heavily calcified aortic valve with restrictive leaflets, possibly a bicuspid aortic valve, and associated aortic regurgitation. TEE can provide additional information regarding leaflet anatomy (bicuspid, unicuspid) when TTE images are inadequate as well as information about concomitant aortic root abnormalities. If echocardiographic data conflict with clinical data or echocardiographic images are suboptimal, CMR imaging may be useful. It can assess leaflet anatomy, measure gradients, and, in patients with a bicuspid aortic valve, assess aorta and aortic root anatomy. Cardiac CT can be used to measure valve area when echocardiographic images are inadequate and to quantify calcification, a marker for risk of disease progression.

Some patients with calcific aortic stenosis have severe aortic stenosis based on valve area but a gradient that is less than 30 mm Hg. Whether symptoms in this "low-flow/low-gradient aortic stenosis" are caused primarily by aortic valve disease with resultant LV dysfunction or the effective valve is reduced owing to poor leaflet excursion ("pseudosevere aortic stenosis") can be best determined with dobutamine stress echocardiography. Key to this evaluation is the understanding of contractile reserve. Contractile reserve is defined as an increase in transaortic stroke volume of greater than 20% with dobutamine infusion. In patients with severe aortic stenosis and resultant LV dysfunction but with contractile reserve, the mean gradient will increase with dobutamine stress and the aortic valve area will remain below 1.0 cm²; these patients will benefit from aortic valve replacement. Those with an increase in aortic valve area to greater than 1.0 cm² or with a maximum

aortic jet velocity (V$_{max}$) below 4 m/s have moderate aortic stenosis and medical therapy is appropriate. Some patients with true aortic stenosis do not have contractile reserve and no change in LV function or aortic valve gradients is seen with dobutamine stress. These patients have a worse prognosis. A lack of contractile reserve is an indicator of higher surgical mortality but is not in itself a contraindication to surgery.

Paradoxic low-gradient aortic stenosis is a more recently described entity in which the measured aortic valve area is reduced in a setting of preserved ejection fraction (>50%) but reduced stroke volume (<35 mL/m²). Typically encountered in the elderly, it is associated with factors related to reduced stroke volume, such as small LV size and marked LV hypertrophy. This may cause the severity of aortic stenosis to be underestimated by echocardiography owing to the low gradient. Identifying these patients—who are usually symptomatic—is important, as these are patients who may benefit from aortic valve replacement.

Management

In asymptomatic patients with aortic stenosis, identifying those who are in higher risk subgroups is important, as these patients may benefit from earlier intervention. Exercise treadmill testing is reasonable in asymptomatic patients to identify those who actually do have symptoms with exercise, have ST-segment changes on ECG, or have an abnormal blood pressure response (lack of increase in systolic blood pressure by at least 20 mm Hg above baseline), as these patients may benefit from earlier surgery. Patients must be closely monitored during exercise testing. Additional factors that may predict more rapid progression and thus indicate closer follow-up include elevated B-type natriuretic peptide level, LV ejection fraction below 50%, pulmonary hypertension, and moderate to severe valve calcification. Appropriate follow-up of asymptomatic patients is based on lesion severity (see Table 35).

Aortic valve replacement is indicated for asymptomatic **H** patients with severe aortic stenosis and LV systolic dysfunction (LV ejection fraction <50%) as well as for those patients with severe aortic stenosis who are undergoing coronary artery bypass grafting or surgery on the aorta or other heart valves.

Surgical aortic valve replacement is the treatment of choice for most patients with symptomatic severe aortic stenosis. It is associated with low mortality for patients younger than 70 years (1%-3%) and for selected patients who are older than 80 years. Balloon aortic valvuloplasty (BAV) has a limited role in the treatment of adult aortic stenosis. Whereas BAV does result in reduction in gradient and increase in valve area, these results typically last only for a few months. Recently, BAV in the adult has been used successfully as a bridge to definitive treatment (surgical or transcatheter aortic valve replacement [TAVR]) or to differentiate symptoms in high-risk patients with comorbid conditions such as COPD.

Medical therapy has limited benefit in the treatment of aortic stenosis. Statins do not delay the progression of aortic stenosis but should be prescribed as indicated to patients with

CONT.
hyperlipidemia or atherosclerotic risk factors. In patients with heart failure, ACE inhibitors, diuretics, angiotensin receptor blockers, and digoxin may be used as appropriate but have not been shown to be helpful in changing the natural history of aortic stenosis.

It is estimated that fewer than half of patients with symptomatic, severe aortic stenosis undergo surgical aortic valve replacement because of comorbid medical conditions that increase surgical risk. This population has become the target for TAVR. The 3-year follow-up results of the PARTNER trial indicate that TAVR has a survival benefit similar to that of surgical replacement for high-risk patients (PARTNER A cohort). TAVR is superior to medical therapy in patients thought not to be surgical candidates (PARTNER B cohort), as 1-year mortality was 30.7% in the TAVR arm versus 50.7% in the medical therapy arm. Complications include stroke and paravalvular aortic regurgitation. Currently, TAVR is indicated for patients who have been determined by a cardiac surgeon to be inoperable or at high risk for death or major morbidity with open aortic valve replacement and in whom existing comorbidities would not preclude the expected benefit from correction of the aortic stenosis. For high-risk patients who are surgical candidates, risk should be determined by a team of cardiologists and cardiac surgeons, with the use of objective measurements, such as the Society of Thoracic Surgeons adult cardiac risk score (STS score) (http://riskcalc.sts.org/STSWebRiskCalc273/de.aspx). Patients with an STS risk score of greater than or equal to 8% may be candidates for TAVR. TAVR is not approved in patients with a bicuspid aortic valve, significant aortic regurgitation, or mitral valve disease. **H**

KEY POINTS

- Once symptoms of aortic stenosis develop, prognosis is poor without intervention (valve replacement), with an average survival of only 2 to 3 years and a high risk of sudden death.

- Transcatheter aortic valve replacement is a treatment option for patients with aortic stenosis who are inoperable or at high risk for death or major morbidity with open aortic valve replacement.

Aortic Regurgitation

Clinical Presentation and Evaluation

Acute severe aortic regurgitation usually is caused by infective endocarditis or aortic dissection (typically in a setting of hypertension or Marfan syndrome). Chronic severe aortic regurgitation is most commonly associated with a dilated ascending aorta from hypertension or primary aortic disease, calcific aortic sclerosis, bicuspid aortic valve, or rheumatic disease. Calcific aortic sclerosis can progress to significant stenosis and is associated with a mild degree of aortic regurgitation.

Symptoms from acute aortic regurgitation result from the sudden large volume in a previously normal LV, resulting in a rapid increase in LV end-diastolic pressure and compensatory increase in heart rate and contractility to maintain cardiac output. When this compensation becomes inadequate, pulmonary edema, myocardial ischemia (due to decreased diastolic perfusion), and cardiogenic shock ensue. Conversely, chronic aortic regurgitation permits a compensatory increase in LV size with increased LV diastolic volume and LV hypertrophy (eccentric and concentric) due to increased volume and afterload. These compensatory mechanisms help maintain stroke volume and cardiac output, but eventually, the increase in volume leads to cardiac dysfunction and heart failure symptoms due to increased LV filling pressure as well as angina due to decreased coronary perfusion pressure and marked LV hypertrophy.

Quantifying the severity of aortic regurgitation is most often done with TTE. Markers of severe aortic regurgitation include wide vena contracta (or diameter of the regurgitant jet orifice), rapid equilibration of aortic and LV pressures during diastole, early mitral valve closure, and diastolic mitral regurgitation. TEE is useful in identifying leaflet anatomy, in further assessment of severity of aortic regurgitation and aortic root pathology, and in evaluation of subvalvular (for example, subaortic membrane) or supravalvular stenosis, and can aid in intraoperative repair and replacement. CMR imaging, including magnetic resonance angiography (MRA), can quantify severity of aortic regurgitation and assess aortic root and ascending aorta dilation. Cardiac CT may provide information such as coronary anomalies and leaflet anatomy.

Management

Urgent or emergent surgical valve replacement is indicated for acute severe aortic regurgitation. For chronic severe aortic regurgitation, valve replacement is indicated for symptomatic patients regardless of LV systolic function (see Table 34). Valve replacement also is indicated for asymptomatic patients with chronic severe aortic regurgitation and LV systolic dysfunction and for patients with chronic severe aortic regurgitation undergoing coronary artery bypass graft surgery or surgery on the aorta or other heart valves. Combined aortic root replacement with aortic valve replacement is used when there is an associated aortic root aneurysm. Follow-up of asymptomatic patients is based on severity of regurgitation and other factors (see Table 35).

Vasodilators and inotropic agents may benefit patients with acute severe aortic regurgitation and concomitant heart failure as short-term therapy before proceeding with surgery. ACE inhibitors or angiotensin receptor blockers may be used in patients with chronic severe aortic regurgitation and heart failure and in patients with hypertension; however, these agents, as well as dihydropyridine calcium channel blockers, have not been shown to delay need for surgery in asymptomatic patients without hypertension. **H**

- Urgent or emergent surgical valve replacement is indicated for patients with acute severe aortic regurgitation.

- Valve replacement is indicated for symptomatic patients with chronic severe aortic regurgitation regardless of left ventricular systolic function.

Bicuspid Aortic Valve

Bicuspid aortic valve is the most common congenital heart abnormality, affecting 0.5% to 2% of the total population. Although a bicuspid aortic valve may be suspected in patients with classic auscultatory findings (systolic ejection click at the left lower sternal border; murmur of aortic stenosis or aortic regurgitation in a young patient), it is most often diagnosed by TTE performed for some other indication. A bicuspid aortic valve may be diagnosed initially in a patient presenting with a complication, such as bacterial endocarditis or aortic dissection. Features that may raise suspicion include eccentric aortic regurgitation, enlarged sinuses of Valsalva, a dilated ascending aorta, or an elliptical valve opening. Calcification may obscure valve leaflets and make the diagnosis difficult. TEE may provide confirmatory information as to leaflet anatomy as well as the presence of associated conditions, including aortic aneurysms and aortic coarctation, and is appropriate when the diagnosis is uncertain.

The clinical course of patients with a bicuspid aortic valve varies widely. Although overall survival is similar to that of age-matched controls, approximately one in three patients with a bicuspid aortic valve may eventually require valve surgery for either stenosis or regurgitation. Stenosis proceeds at a faster rate when the aortic valve is bicuspid, and valve replacement may be required in the fifth or sixth decade of life. Some degree of regurgitation is common with a bicuspid aortic valve but is less likely than stenosis to lead to valve replacement. The presence of a bicuspid aortic valve carries an increased risk of infective endocarditis, and good dental care is important in these patients. Current guidelines no longer recommend antibiotic prophylaxis for this patient population (see Infective Endocarditis, later). The timing of follow-up TTE depends on many factors, including patient age and severity of the valve lesion. In general, older, asymptomatic patients with a bicuspid aortic valve and severe aortic valve stenosis or regurgitation require yearly echocardiography; those with mild stenosis or regurgitation should have echocardiography every 3 to 5 years.

A bicuspid aortic valve may occur with other cardiovascular and systemic abnormalities, such as aortic coarctation, aneurysm of the sinuses of Valsalva, and patent ductus arteriosus. Patients with a bicuspid aortic valve are predisposed to aortic aneurysm and dissection owing to aortic connective tissue abnormalities. For this reason, the ascending aortic diameter should be reassessed by echocardiography if the aortic root or ascending aorta dimension is greater than or equal to 4.0 cm, with the evaluation interval determined by degree and rate of aortic dilation and by family history. Annual evaluation should occur if the aortic diameter is greater than 4.5 cm. Multidetector CT or CMR imaging is appropriate for further assessment of aortic pathology when TTE or TEE is not conclusive and for long-term follow up of aortic dimensions when TEE images are inadequate. A bicuspid aortic valve may be present in patients with other thoracic aneurysm syndromes as well, such as Loeys-Dietz syndrome (hypertelorism, split uvula or cleft palate, and aortic aneurysms). Echocardiography of first-degree relatives of patients with a bicuspid aortic valve is indicated to screen for bicuspid aortic valve or aortic aneurysms.

As with calcific aortic stenosis, medical therapies for bicuspid aortic valve stenosis are limited. Aortic valve replacement is the only therapeutic option for adult patients with a stenotic bicuspid aortic valve, and recommendations regarding when to intervene are the same as for tricuspid aortic valves (see Table 34).

For patients with a regurgitant bicuspid aortic valve, valve replacement is the treatment of choice when regurgitation is clinically significant; however, repair may be performed in selected patients by experienced surgeons.

Surgery to repair the aortic root or replace the ascending aorta is indicated in patients with a bicuspid aortic valve when the aortic root diameter is greater than 5.5 cm. Surgery is reasonable if the diameter of the ascending aorta or aortic root is greater than 5.0 cm and a risk factor for dissection is present (family history of aortic dissection or if the rate of increase in diameter is ≥0.5 cm per year). Ascending aorta replacement is reasonable in patients who are undergoing aortic valve surgery because of severe aortic stenosis or aortic regurgitation if the diameter of the ascending aorta is greater than 4.5 cm. **H**

- In general, older, asymptomatic patients with a bicuspid aortic valve and severe aortic valve stenosis or regurgitation require yearly echocardiography; those with mild aortic stenosis or regurgitation require echocardiography every 3 to 5 years. **HVC**

- Echocardiography of first-degree relatives of patients with a bicuspid aortic valve is indicated to screen for bicuspid aortic valve or aortic aneurysms.

- Patients with a bicuspid aortic valve are predisposed to aortopathy, and aortic surgery is indicated when the aortic root diameter is greater than 5.5 cm.

Mitral Stenosis
Clinical Presentation and Evaluation

The primary cause of mitral stenosis is rheumatic carditis. Improved hygiene and the routine use of antibiotics for group A streptococcal pharyngitis have greatly reduced the incidence of rheumatic heart disease in the United States and developed countries. Rarely, functional mitral stenosis occurs as a result of outflow obstruction from tumor (such as myxoma) or left atrial thrombus. Other causes of mitral stenosis include congenital disease (such as parachute mitral valve, wherein the mitral chordae insert into one instead of two papillary muscles) and mitral annular calcification. Symptoms can be indolent, with patients remaining asymptomatic for years and then presenting with a gradual decrease in activity. Other symptoms include dyspnea, orthopnea, fatigue, and, less commonly, hemoptysis or systemic embolization. Symptoms typically are not present until the mitral valve area is less than 1.5 cm², although tachycardia may precipitate symptoms at larger valve areas. The decrease in mitral valve area results in a diastolic pressure gradient between the left atrium and ventricle. This increase in left atrial pressure causes left atrial enlargement, with development of atrial fibrillation and a significantly increased risk of left atrial/left atrial appendage thrombus, as well as exertional dyspnea and eventual pulmonary edema owing to increased pulmonary venous pressure. In addition, chronic pulmonary venous pressure elevation may result in pulmonary hypertension. The risk of thromboembolism increases with age and the presence of atrial fibrillation. Warfarin remains the anticoagulant of choice for these patients with concomitant atrial fibrillation as they were excluded from trials of novel oral anticoagulants.

TTE is used to assess disease severity of mitral stenosis by measuring valve area and transvalvular gradient (see Table 35). Typical echocardiographic findings of rheumatic mitral stenosis include a domed or "hockey stick" appearance to the mitral valve, with thickened, calcified subvalvular apparatus and marked left atrial enlargement. Gradients are heart-rate dependent and can vary greatly in patients who are tachycardic or have atrial fibrillation. Echocardiography is essential for assessment of valve morphology, including factors such as valve calcification and thickening, leaflet motion, and subchordal thickening. These factors, taken together, help predict the likelihood of successful percutaneous mitral balloon valvuloplasty. TEE provides better visualization for assessment of mitral regurgitation severity as well as the presence of left atrial appendage thrombus. Multidetector CT may provide additional information by valve planimetry as well as visualization of the coronary anatomy. This may be helpful for patients whose valve is not well imaged on TTE and are unable to tolerate TEE.

H **Management**

Percutaneous mitral balloon valvotomy is indicated for symptomatic patients (New York Heart Association [NYHA] functional class II, III, or IV) with severe mitral stenosis (see Table 34) and favorable valve morphology. TEE plays an important role in assessment of patients being considered for percutaneous balloon valvotomy to evaluate for potential contraindications, including left atrial appendage clot or significant (moderate to severe) mitral regurgitation. Mitral valve surgery (repair if possible) is indicated in patients with symptomatic (NYHA functional class III-IV) severe mitral stenosis when balloon

valvotomy is unavailable, unsuccessful, or contraindicated or when the valve morphology is unfavorable.

Medical therapy for mitral stenosis consists of diuretics or long-acting nitrates, which may help improve symptoms such as dyspnea. In addition, β-blockers or nondihydropyridine calcium channel blockers can lower heart rate and improve LV diastolic filling time. **H**

KEY POINT

- Mitral valvotomy or surgery is indicated for symptomatic patients (New York Heart Association functional class II-IV) with severe mitral stenosis and favorable valve morphology.

Mitral Regurgitation

Clinical Presentation and Evaluation

Abnormalities in any of the structures of the mitral valve apparatus, including anterior and posterior mitral leaflets, the annulus, the papillary muscles, and the chordae tendineae, can result in mitral regurgitation. Organic, or primary, mitral regurgitation refers to processes involving the leaflets, such as mitral valve prolapse, myxomatous degeneration (the abnormal accumulation of proteoglycans), collagen vascular disease, and infective endocarditis. Processes that affect the support structures, such as coronary artery disease and LV remodeling in the setting of LV dysfunction, result in functional, or secondary, mitral regurgitation.

Acute severe mitral regurgitation is associated with papillary muscle rupture following acute myocardial infarction, flail mitral valve (dissociation of the valve leaflet from the chordae), and infective endocarditis with leaflet perforation. The sudden large volume in the left atrium and ventricle results in rapid increases in LV end-diastolic pressure and left atrial pressure, which leads to elevated pulmonary artery pressure and pulmonary edema. The diminished LV stroke volume leads to hypotension and shock. **H**

Patients with chronic mild to moderate mitral regurgitation may remain asymptomatic for many years. Progression is variable and caused by either progression of lesions or increasing mitral annulus size. The increase in volume and subsequent increase in left atrial pressure lead to compensatory dilation of the left atrium and LV. Left atrial dilation predisposes to atrial fibrillation. A chronic increase in preload and resultant eccentric hypertrophy, in the setting of increased stroke volume (normal forward stroke volume and regurgitant volume) lead to contractile dysfunction and increased end-diastolic volume, which lead to pulmonary congestion and pulmonary hypertension. Appropriate follow-up of asymptomatic patients with mitral regurgitation is outlined in Table 35.

TTE serves as the main imaging modality in the evaluation and management of mitral regurgitation. TTE allows diagnosis of the mechanism of mitral regurgitation, qualitative and quantitative measurement of disease severity, and measurement of chamber sizes and function and pulmonary artery pressures. In severe mitral regurgitation, echocardiographic findings may include left atrial dilation, left ventricular dilation and/or reduced ejection fraction, abnormal mitral leaflet mobility, high-volume regurgitant flow, and/or evidence of pulmonary hypertension. TEE provides additional information if TTE image quality is suboptimal or equivocal. Three-dimensional echocardiography can provide additional information on leaflet morphology and mitral regurgitation quantification. Multidetector CT and CMR imaging may be helpful in some patients by providing similar quantification and assessment of coronary anatomy. These modalities are most helpful when TTE and TEE do not provide adequate information.

H Management

The only definitive therapy for severe mitral regurgitation is mitral valve surgery. Indications are shown in Table 34. Options are mitral valve repair, mitral valve replacement with preservation of part or all of the mitral apparatus, and mitral valve replacement with removal of the mitral apparatus. In general, mitral valve repair is preferred to valve replacement, as it is associated with improved survival in retrospective studies. Chordal preservation is preferred when replacement is needed, as it is associated with improved left ventricular geometry and long-term function.

Many patients who could benefit from mitral valve repair are denied surgery owing to high surgical risk, advanced age, or other comorbidities. A catheter-based device has recently been approved by the FDA that repairs the mitral valve by delivering a clip percutaneously to approximate the valve leaflet edges and improve leaflet coaptation at the origin of the mitral regurgitation jet. The device is approved for patients with significant symptomatic degenerative mitral regurgitation for whom mitral valve surgery poses a prohibitive risk.

Medical therapy is used to stabilize decompensated heart failure in patients with acute or chronic mitral regurgitation. Nitrates and diuretics reduce filling pressures in patients with acute severe mitral regurgitation; sodium nitroprusside reduces afterload and regurgitant fraction, as does an intra-aortic balloon pump. Inotropic agents, an intra-aortic balloon pump, or other means of circulatory support may be added in patients with hypotension. Vasodilators, including ACE inhibitors and angiotensin receptor blockers, have not been shown effective in preventing progression of LV dysfunction and may mask the development of symptoms in asymptomatic patients. Medical therapy should not be considered a substitute for surgery when the patient is thought to be a surgical candidate. In symptomatic patients with primary mitral regurgitation, medical treatment should aim to reduce blood pressure. In patients with secondary mitral regurgitation, standard treatment for LV systolic dysfunction is appropriate. **H**

- In patients with severe mitral regurgitation, mitral valve repair is the treatment of choice when the valve is suitable for repair and appropriate surgical skill is available.

- Nitrates and diuretics reduce filling pressures in patients with acute severe mitral regurgitation, and sodium nitroprusside and an intra-aortic balloon pump reduce afterload and regurgitant fraction.

Tricuspid Valve Disease
Tricuspid Regurgitation

Mild tricuspid regurgitation is frequently detected as an incidental finding in patients undergoing echocardiography for another cause. Primary causes include endocarditis, rheumatic and carcinoid disease, myxomatous disease, and congenital diseases such as Ebstein anomaly. More significant tricuspid regurgitation is often caused by nonvalvular factors, such as annular dilatation and leaflet tethering due to right ventricular pressure or volume overload. Severe tricuspid regurgitation may be well tolerated for a long period of time; therefore, the main symptoms are usually those of associated valve diseases, such as shortness of breath from mitral regurgitation and mitral stenosis. Clinical signs of right-sided heart failure are an indication of severity. Echocardiography is used to define the etiology and differentiate primary from secondary tricuspid regurgitation. Echocardiographic findings of severe tricuspid regurgitation include right atrial and right ventricle dilatation, large color flow jet into the right atrium with dense Doppler velocity profile, and bowing of the interatrial septum into the left atrium.

Although data are limited, current experience favors **H** placement of an annular ring (either prosthetic or biologic) for severe tricuspid regurgitation related to isolated tricuspid annular dilatation, with bioprostheses favored over mechanical valves. Timing of surgical intervention remains controversial, mostly because of the limited available data and heterogeneous nature of tricuspid valve disease. The only class I recommendation for treatment of tricuspid regurgitation is tricuspid valve surgery in patients with severe tricuspid regurgitation who are undergoing left-sided valve surgery, although surgery can be considered in patients with severe primary tricuspid regurgitation refractory to medical therapy. **H**

Tricuspid Stenosis

Tricuspid stenosis is largely caused by rheumatic disease. Surgery is indicated for patients with severe symptomatic tricuspid stenosis. Biologic prostheses are preferred for valve replacement owing to a significantly higher risk of thrombosis with mechanical valves.

- Tricuspid valve surgery is indicated in patients with severe tricuspid regurgitation who are undergoing left-sided valve surgery and can be considered in patients with severe primary tricuspid regurgitation refractory to medical therapy.

Infective Endocarditis

Diagnosis and Management

Infective endocarditis, a bacterial or fungal infection of the endocardium that affects both native and prosthetic valves and other endocardial surfaces, as well as implantable cardiac devices, is an uncommon but life-threatening infection. Despite advances in diagnosis, antimicrobial therapy, surgical techniques, and management of complications, patients with infective endocarditis still have high morbidity and mortality rates.

In patients with a cardiac murmur suggestive of organic valvular or congenital heart disease or patients with a prosthetic heart valve, infective endocarditis should be suspected in the presence of fever, anemia, hematuria, and typical physical findings suggestive of embolization. The diagnosis is often imprecise; bacteremia can occur without endocardial infection, and endocarditis can occur with negative blood cultures, especially if a patient has received antibiotics for another febrile illness. Echocardiography is integral in the diagnosis as well as for detecting complications. Echocardiographic findings that favor a vegetation rather than a thrombus or other lesion include an irregularly shaped mass with ultrasound intensity less than that of myocardium that is upstream of the affected valve and has independent motion. TTE is generally sufficient to rule out endocarditis when the probability of endocarditis is low based on clinical suspicion; however, TEE is necessary to confirm the diagnosis in patients with a high likelihood of endocarditis (based on preexisting valve disease, positive blood cultures, or suspected severe valvular regurgitation), those with suspected prosthetic valve endocarditis, and those with other intracardiac devices (such as a pacemaker). TEE is also needed to evaluate for paravalvular abscess and fistula formation. Chest MRI is helpful in assessing for the presence of aortic root abscess when TEE is inconclusive. CT scan is helpful to identify areas of peripheral embolization, such as kidney, spine, spleen, and brain.

Patients at risk for infective endocarditis who have unexplained fever for more than 48 hours should have at least two sets of blood cultures obtained from different sites. In addition, stable patients with known valve disease or valve prosthesis with unexplained fever should not receive antibiotics before blood cultures are obtained.

Diagnosis of infective endocarditis is made by use of the modified Duke criteria (**Table 36**), which define major and minor criteria. A definitive diagnosis may be made with positive blood cultures and characteristic echocardiographic findings.

In patients with an intermediate to high likelihood of infective endocarditis, empiric antibiotic therapy is appropriate and should be given after blood cultures have been drawn (**Table 37**). Antibiotic therapy for infective endocarditis should be based on organisms and sensitivities. Nosocomial endocarditis is often defined as infective endocarditis diagnosed more than 72 hours after hospital admission in patients with no evidence of infective endocarditis on admission, or occurring

TABLE 36. Clinical Criteria for the Diagnosis of Endocarditis	
Definite Endocarditis	
Presence of any pathologic criteria[a] *or*	
2 major criteria *or*	
1 major and 3 minor criteria *or*	
5 minor criteria	
Major Criteria	**Minor Criteria**
Persistently positive blood cultures of organisms typical for endocarditis[b]	Predisposing condition or injection drug use
	Fever
Endocardial involvement (new valvular regurgitation or positive echocardiogram)	Embolic vascular phenomena
	Immunologic phenomena (e.g., glomerulonephritis, rheumatoid factor)
	Positive blood cultures not meeting major criteria

[a]Organisms demonstrated by culture or histologic examination of a vegetation, a vegetation that has embolized, or an intracardiac abscess specimen; or a vegetation or abscess showing active endocarditis.

[b]Or a single positive culture for *Coxiella burnetii* or IgG antibody titer >1:800.

Information from Li JS, Sexton DJ, Mick N, et al. Proposed modifications to the Duke criteria for the diagnosis of infective endocarditis. Clin Infect Dis. 2000;30(4):633-638. [PMID: 10770721]

TABLE 37.	Empiric Therapy for Infective Endocarditis
Condition	**Therapy**
Community-acquired native valve IE	Consider vancomycin + gentamicin
Nosocomial-associated IE	Consider vancomycin + gentamicin + rifampin or vancomycin + gentamicin + a carbapenem or cefepime
Prosthetic valve IE	Consider vancomycin + gentamicin + rifampin

IE = infective endocarditis.

CONT. within 60 days of a hospital admission that was associated with a risk for bacteremia or infective endocarditis. For nosocomial infections, coverage for multidrug-resistant bacteria, particularly coagulase-negative staphylococci, is recommended.

Surgery for native valve endocarditis usually entails resection of the vegetation and valve repair or replacement if appropriate. Early surgery (during initial hospitalization and before completion of a full course of antibiotics) is indicated for patients with acute infective endocarditis presenting with valve stenosis or regurgitation resulting in heart failure; left-sided infective endocarditis caused by *Staphylococcus aureus*, fungal, or other highly resistant organisms; infective endocarditis complicated by heart block, annular or aortic abscess, or destructive penetrating lesion; and infective endocarditis with persistent bacteremia or fever lasting longer than 5 to 7 days after starting antibiotic therapy. Surgery is recommended for patients with relapsing prosthetic valve endocarditis. In patients with infective endocarditis who have documented infection of pacemaker or defibrillator systems, complete removal of these systems (all leads and generator) is indicated. Early surgery is reasonable in patients with infective endocarditis who have recurrent emboli and persistent vegetations on antibiotic therapy, and may be considered in patients with native valve endocarditis who have mobile vegetations greater than 10 mm in length. The Early Surgery versus Conventional Treatment in Infective Endocarditis (EASE) trial compared the clinical outcomes of early surgery with a conventional treatment strategy in patients with left-sided infective endocarditis and a high risk of embolism. In this study, early surgery (within 48 hours after diagnosis and randomization) in patients with large vegetations (>10 mm) significantly reduced embolic events with similar in-hospital and 6-month mortality rates compared with delayed surgery. **H**

Prophylaxis

The significant morbidity and mortality associated with infective endocarditis underscore the importance of appropriate administration of antibiotics before procedures expected to produce bacteremia. The American College of Cardiology/American Heart Association (ACC/AHA) recommendations and the European Society of Cardiology (ESC) recommendations,

which changed significantly in recent years, may contradict long-standing expectations of patients and practice patterns of health care providers. However, infective endocarditis is more likely to result from frequent exposure to random bacteremia associated with daily activities than from bacteremia caused by dental, gastrointestinal tract, or genitourinary procedures; additionally, the risk of antibiotic-associated adverse effects may exceed the benefit (if any) from prophylactic antibiotic therapy.

Infective endocarditis prophylaxis is currently recommended for patients with cardiac conditions with the highest risk for adverse outcomes from infective endocarditis (rather than those with an increased lifetime risk for infective endocarditis). Prophylaxis is recommended for patients with (1) a prosthetic cardiac valve; (2) a previous episode of infective endocarditis; (3) congenital heart disease, including unrepaired cyanotic congenital heart disease, a completely repaired congenital heart defect with prosthetic material or device during the first 6 months after the procedure, and repaired congenital heart disease with residual defects; or (4) valvulopathy following cardiac transplantation.

Unless there is a history of infective endocarditis, prophylaxis is not recommended for patients with native valve disease, including rheumatic heart disease, mitral valve prolapse with regurgitation, or a bicuspid aortic valve.

In patients who meet the criteria, prophylaxis should be administered prior to dental procedures that involve manipulation of gingival tissue or the periapical region of the teeth or perforation of the oral mucosa (**Table 38**). Infective endocarditis prophylaxis is not recommended prior to nondental procedures, such as TEE, genitourinary procedures, or gastrointestinal procedures. Antimicrobial prophylaxis is recommended for procedures involving incision or biopsy of the respiratory tract mucosa, such as bronchial biopsy, tonsillectomy, and adenoidectomy.

KEY POINTS

- In patients with a cardiac murmur suggestive of organic valvular or congenital heart disease or patients with a prosthetic heart valve, infective endocarditis should be suspected in the presence of fever, anemia, hematuria, and physical findings suggestive of embolization.

- Early surgery is indicated for patients with acute infective endocarditis presenting with valve stenosis or regurgitation resulting in heart failure; left-sided infective endocarditis caused by *Staphylococcus aureus*, fungal, or other highly resistant organisms; infective endocarditis complicated by heart block, annular or aortic abscess, or destructive penetrating lesion; and infective endocarditis with persistent bacteremia or fever lasting longer than 5 to 7 days after starting antibiotic therapy.

- Surgery is recommended for patients with prosthetic valve endocarditis and relapsing infection.

(Continued)

TABLE 38. Prophylactic Infective Endocarditis Regimens for Adults Before a Dental Procedure

Situation	Agent[a]	Dosage
Oral	Amoxicillin	2 g
Unable to take oral medication	Ampicillin	2 g IM or IV
	or	
	Cefazolin or ceftriaxone	1 g IM or IV
Allergic to penicillin or ampicillin - oral	Cephalexin	2 g
	or	
	Clindamycin	600 mg
	or	
	Azithromycin or clarithromycin	500 mg
Allergic to penicillin or ampicillin and unable to take oral medication	Cefazolin or ceftriaxone	1 g IM or IV
	or	
	Clindamycin	600 mg IM or IV

IM = intramuscular; IV = intravenous.

[a]Regimen consists of a single dose 30 to 60 minutes before the dental procedure, or, if inadvertently not administered, drug may be given up to 2 hours after the procedure.

Adapted from Wilson W, Taubert KA, Gewitz M, et al; American Heart Association. Prevention of infective endocarditis: guidelines from the American Heart Association: a guideline from the American Heart Association Rheumatic Fever, Endocarditis and Kawasaki Disease Committee, Council on Cardiovascular Disease in the Young, and the Council on Clinical Cardiology, Council on Cardiovascular Surgery and Anesthesia, and the Quality of Care and Outcomes Research Interdisciplinary Working Group. J Am Dent Assoc. 2008 Jan;139 Suppl:3S-24S. Review. Erratum in: J Am Dent Assoc. 2008 Mar;139(3):253. [PMID: 18167394]. Copyright 2008 American Dental Association.

KEY POINTS *(continued)*

HVC
- Infective endocarditis prophylaxis should be limited to those with a prosthetic cardiac valve; a history of infective endocarditis; unrepaired cyanotic congenital heart disease or repaired congenital heart defect with prosthesis or shunt (≤6 months post-procedure) or residual defect; or valvulopathy following cardiac transplantation.

Prosthetic Valves

The choice of prosthesis for patients requiring valve replacement must account for various considerations, including the patient's age, any comorbid factors, and the patient's preference and ability to adhere to medical therapy post-implantation. The ACC/AHA and ESC have published recommendations regarding valve selection (**Table 39**). In general, patient factors that favor a mechanical prosthesis include younger age, an absence of contraindications to long-term anticoagulation, a risk of accelerated bioprosthetic structural valve deterioration (for example, with pregnancy or kidney failure), and a reasonable life expectancy in patients for whom future redo valve surgery would be high risk. Conversely, factors that would favor a bioprosthetic valve include older age; patients in whom adequate long-term anticoagulation is unlikely (for example, owing to adherence problems or anticoagulation agents not being readily available) or contraindicated because of high bleeding risk (prior major bleed, lifestyle or occupation issues); patients requiring reoperation for mechanical valve thrombosis despite good long-term anticoagulant control; and young women contemplating pregnancy (although a mechanical prosthesis requiring anticoagulation is not a contraindication to pregnancy).

TABLE 39. Summary of Recommendations for Prosthetic Valve Choice

Type of Valve	Recommendation
Bioprosthesis	Recommended: patients of any age for whom anticoagulant therapy is contraindicated, cannot be managed appropriately, or is not desired
	Reasonable: patients >70 y of age
Mechanical prosthesis	Reasonable: AVR or MVR in patients <60 y of age who do not have a contraindication to anticoagulation
Either bio- or mechanical prosthesis	Reasonable: patients between 60 y and 70 y of age

AVR = aortic valve replacement; MVR = mitral valve replacement.

NOTE: The guideline recommends that the choice of valve intervention and prosthetic valve type should be a shared decision-making process.

Recommendations from Nishimura RA, Otto CM, Bonow RO, et al; American College of Cardiology/American Heart Association Task Force on Practice Guidelines. 2014 AHA/ACC guideline for the management of patients with valvular heart disease: executive summary: a report of the American College of Cardiology/American Heart Association Task Force on Practice Guidelines. J Am Coll Cardiol. 2014 Jun 10;63(22):2438-88. Erratum in: J Am Coll Cardiol. 2014 Jun 10;63(22):2489. [PMID: 24603192]

Lifelong oral anticoagulation with warfarin is recommended for all patients with a mechanical prosthesis and those with bioprostheses with other indications for anticoagulation. The target INR is based upon prosthesis location, with a target of 2.5 for patients with a mechanical aortic prosthetic valve and 3.0 for patients with a mechanical mitral prosthetic valve and those patients with a mechanical aortic prosthetic valve and risk factors (atrial fibrillation, LV dysfunction, previous thromboembolism, hypercoagulable condition, or older-generation mechanical aortic valve replacement). The addition of aspirin, 75 to 100 mg/d, is recommended as well. Ongoing studies are evaluating various anticoagulation regimens for newer and potentially less thrombogenic valves.

The need for anticoagulation for those with bioprosthetic valves is less clear. Oral anticoagulation should be considered for the first 3 months after implantation of a mitral or tricuspid bioprosthesis and for the first 3 months after bioprosthetic mitral valve repair. Low-dose aspirin or anticoagulation should be considered for the first 3 months after implantation of an aortic bioprosthesis. Long-term aspirin use is reasonable for all patients with bioprosthetic valves. ⊞

Patients with prosthetic valves require lifelong cardiology follow-up, including annual clinical examination. For baseline assessment, all patients undergoing valve replacement surgery should have TTE performed 2 to 3 months after implantation as a baseline study. Patients with bioprosthetic valves may be considered for annual echocardiograms after the first 10 years in the absence of a change in clinical status. Routine echocardiography is not recommended for patients with mechanical valves or those with recently implanted biologic valves in the absence of any change in symptoms or examination findings.

KEY POINTS

- Lifelong oral anticoagulation with warfarin is recommended for all patients with a mechanical prosthetic heart valve.
- Oral anticoagulation should be considered for the first 3 months after implantation for patients with a bioprosthetic mitral or tricuspid valve and for the first 3 months after bioprosthetic mitral valve repair.
- Routine echocardiography is not recommended for patients with mechanical valves or those with recently implanted biologic valves in the absence of any change in symptoms or examination findings.

Adult Congenital Heart Disease

Introduction

Advances in care of patients with congenital heart disease over the past six decades have resulted in more adults than children living in North America with these conditions. Cardiovascular residua are common in patients with previous intervention for congenital cardiac lesions, underscoring the importance of peri-

odic informed follow-up by a team consisting ideally of the internist and an adult or pediatric cardiologist trained in adult congenital heart disease. Specialized care is particularly important for patients with complex and cyanotic congenital cardiac disease. Congenital heart conditions may be first identified during pregnancy or symptom status may be worsened by the physiologic changes of pregnancy. Decisions regarding the safety of pregnancy in patients with congenital cardiac disease and management during pregnancy should be made on an individual basis in consultation with a congenital heart disease specialist.

Patent Foramen Ovale

The foramen ovale allows transfer of oxygenated placental blood to the fetal circulation and usually closes within the first few weeks of life. In 25% to 30% of the population, however, the foramen ovale remains patent (**Figure 27**). Patent foramen ovale (PFO) is usually asymptomatic and identified incidentally. No treatment or follow-up is needed for the PFO found incidentally in an asymptomatic patient.

PFO is diagnosed by visualizing the interatrial septum by echocardiography and demonstrating shunting of blood across the defect by color flow Doppler imaging or by using agitated saline injected intravenously and subsequent transfer through the PFO from right to left atrium. If transthoracic echocardiography (TTE) is nondiagnostic, transesophageal echocardiography (TEE) usually provides improved visualization of the atrial septum.

Antiplatelet therapy is recommended as first-line therapy for patients with PFO and cryptogenic stroke. Results of randomized controlled trials of device closure for cryptogenic stroke and PFO have not demonstrated benefit compared with medical therapy for secondary stroke prevention. Patients with cryptogenic stroke and PFO may be treated with antiplatelet or anticoagulant therapy and should be encouraged to participate in one of the ongoing trials comparing closure with medical therapy. There is no indication for PFO closure or for antiplatelet therapy in asymptomatic patients.

Observational studies have suggested an association between PFO and migraine. However, randomized studies of PFO closure to prevent migraine recurrence have not shown beneficial effect, and PFO closure should not be performed for the prophylaxis of migraine.

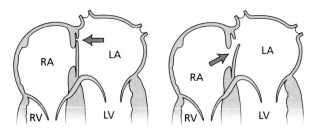

FIGURE 27. Patent foramen ovale. The *arrows* demonstrate the mechanism of right-to-left shunt through the patent foramen ovale. LA = left atrium; LV = left ventricle; RA = right atrium; RV = right ventricle.

Redrawn from original supplied courtesy of Dr. William D. Edwards, Department of Laboratory Medicine and Pathology, Mayo Clinic, Rochester, MN.

Rarely, a PFO may be associated with the platypnea-orthodeoxia syndrome. Platypnea-orthodeoxia syndrome is an acquired disorder characterized by cyanosis and dyspnea in the upright position. These symptoms are related to right-to-left shunting across a PFO or atrial septal defect and are caused by a transient increase in right atrial pressure, which occurs as a complication of right ventricular myocardial infarction, pulmonary embolism, tricuspid regurgitation, or acute right heart failure. Device PFO closure in these patients may decrease hypoxemia and cyanosis.

Atrial septal aneurysm is redundant and mobile atrial septal tissue. No treatment is needed when atrial septal aneurysm is discovered incidentally. Atrial septal aneurysm in conjunction with a PFO reportedly increases the risk of stroke compared with a PFO alone. Antiplatelet therapy is recommended for patients with cryptogenic stroke and an isolated atrial septal aneurysm. In patients with atrial septal aneurysm and recurrent stroke on antiplatelet therapy, anticoagulant therapy is recommended if no other cause of stroke is identified. Rarely, surgical excision of an atrial septal aneurysm and defect closure is considered if antiplatelet or warfarin therapy fails to prevent stroke recurrence.

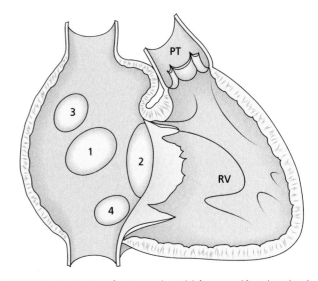

FIGURE 28. Positions of various atrial septal defects viewed from the right side of the heart. (1) ostium secundum; (2) ostium primum; (3) sinus venosus; (4) inferior vena cava. PT = pulmonary trunk; RV = right ventricle.

Redrawn from original supplied courtesy of Dr. William D. Edwards, Department of Laboratory Medicine and Pathology, Mayo Clinic, Rochester, MN.

KEY POINTS

- Antiplatelet therapy is recommended as first-line therapy for patients with patent foramen ovale and cryptogenic stroke.

HVC • There is no indication for patent foramen ovale closure or for antiplatelet therapy in asymptomatic patients.

HVC • Randomized trials do not support patent foramen ovale closure to reduce risk of recurrent stroke or migraine.

Atrial Septal Defect
Pathophysiology and Genetics

An atrial septal defect (ASD) is a communication between the atria. Left-to-right shunt occurs and, over time, causes right-sided cardiac chamber dilatation. Defects are classified according to location (**Figure 28**). Ostium secundum ASDs are the most common type (75% of cases). These are located in the middle portion of the atrial septum and are usually isolated anomalies. Ostium primum defects (15%-20% of cases) are located in the lowest portion of the atrial septum; they are commonly associated with a cleft mitral valve, ventricular septal defect, and subaortic stenosis, a collection of abnormalities termed endocardial cushion defect. Sinus venosus defects (5%-10% of cases) are usually located near the superior vena cava or, rarely, near the inferior vena cava. More than 90% of patients with sinus venosus ASD have associated anomalies of pulmonary venous connection. A coronary sinus ASD (<1% of cases) is a communication between the coronary sinus and the left atrium. These defects are commonly associated with complex congenital heart lesions or a persistent left-sided superior vena cava.

Most ASDs occur sporadically; however, several genetic syndromes associated with ASDs are recognized. The Holt-Oram syndrome involves bilateral upper extremity bone abnormalities and congenital heart defects, most commonly an ASD. Familial ostium secundum ASDs have also been described and may be autosomal dominant or are linked to chromosome 5. Down syndrome is commonly associated with congenital heart disease, most commonly a form of atrioventricular septal defect, including ostium primum ASD.

Clinical Presentation

ASDs may initially be identified in adulthood; the age of presentation depends on the shunt size and associated defects. Common presenting features include fatigue; exertional dyspnea; atrial fibrillation; paradoxical embolism; and abnormalities on the physical examination, including a pulmonary outflow murmur or fixed splitting of S_2 or, less commonly, findings that are consistent with a genetic syndrome involving an ASD. Occasionally, an ASD is identified as the cause for right heart enlargement found incidentally on an echocardiogram. Rarely, patients with isolated ASDs present with pulmonary arterial hypertension (PAH); this usually occurs in young women, suggesting the coexistence of idiopathic PAH.

Clinical findings in ASD include jugular venous distention, a parasternal impulse, and a systolic flow murmur at the second left intercostal space. Large shunts may cause a diastolic flow rumble across the tricuspid valve owing to a large left-to-right shunt. Fixed splitting of the S_2 is the characteristic auscultatory finding in patients with an ASD.

Diagnostic Evaluation

The electrocardiogram (ECG) and chest radiograph findings in patients with ASDs are outlined in **Table 40**. Complete heart block may occur in familial ASD.

TTE is the diagnostic imaging modality of choice for identification of ostium primum and secundum ASDs. Additional

TABLE 40.	Imaging Findings and Late Complications in Adult Congenital Heart Disease	
Lesion	**ECG and CXR Findings**	**Late Complications**
Patent foramen ovale	Normal	Paradoxical embolism, platypnea-orthodeoxia syndrome
Ostium secundum ASD	ECG: Incomplete RBBB, RA enlargement, right axis deviation	Right heart enlargement, atrial fibrillation, PAH (rare)
	CXR: Right heart enlargement, prominent pulmonary artery, increased pulmonary vascularity	Post repair: residual shunt (rare)
Ostium primum ASD	ECG: Left axis deviation, 1st-degree atrioventricular block	Right heart enlargement, atrial fibrillation, mitral regurgitation (from mitral valve cleft), PAH (rare)
	CXR: Right heart enlargement, prominent pulmonary artery, increased pulmonary vascularity	Post repair: residual shunt (rare), mitral regurgitation (from mitral valve cleft), left ventricular outflow tract obstruction
Sinus venosus ASD	ECG: Abnormal P axis	Right heart enlargement, atrial fibrillation, PAH (rare)
	CXR: Right heart enlargement, prominent pulmonary artery, increased pulmonary vascularity	Post repair: residual shunt (rare), residual anomalous pulmonary venous connection
Small VSD	Normal	Endocarditis
Large VSD	ECG: RV or RV/LV hypertrophy	Left heart enlargement, PAH, Eisenmenger syndrome
	CXR: LA and LV enlargement, increased pulmonary vascular markings; with PAH: prominent central pulmonary arteries, reduced peripheral pulmonary vascular markings	Post repair: residual VSD, residual shunt (rare)
Small PDA	Normal	Endocarditis
Large PDA	ECG: LA enlargement, LV hypertrophy; with PAH: RV hypertrophy	Endocarditis, heart failure, PAH, Eisenmenger syndrome
	CXR: Cardiomegaly, increased pulmonary vascular markings; calcification of PDA (occasional); with PAH: prominent central pulmonary arteries, reduced peripheral pulmonary vascular markings	Post repair: residual shunt (rare)
Pulmonary valve stenosis	ECG: Normal when RV systolic pressure <60 mm Hg; if RV systolic pressure >60 mm Hg: RA enlargement, right axis deviation, RV hypertrophy	Post repair: Severe pulmonary valve regurgitation after pulmonary valvotomy or valvuloplasty
	CXR: Pulmonary artery dilatation, calcification of pulmonary valve (rare); RA enlargement may be noted	
Aortic coarctation	ECG: LV hypertrophy and ST-T wave abnormalities	Hypertension (75% of cases), bicuspid aortic valve (>50% of cases), increased risk of aortic aneurysm and intracranial aneurysm
	CXR: Dilated ascending aorta, "figure 3 sign" beneath aortic arch, rib notching from collateral vessels	Post repair: Recoarctation, hypertension, aortic aneurysm
Repaired tetralogy of Fallot	ECG: RBBB, increased QRS duration (QRS duration reflects degree of RV dilatation)	Post repair: Increased atrial and ventricular arrhythmia risk, pulmonary valve regurgitation or stenosis; tricuspid regurgitation
	CXR: Cardiomegaly with pulmonary or tricuspid valve regurgitation; right aortic arch in 25% of cases	QRS >180 msec increases risk of ventricular tachycardia and sudden death
Eisenmenger syndrome	ECG: Right axis deviation, RA enlargement, RV hypertrophy	Right heart failure, hemoptysis, stroke
	CXR: RV dilatation, prominent pulmonary artery, reduced pulmonary vascularity	

ASD = atrial septal defect; CXR = chest radiograph; ECG = electrocardiogram; LA = left atrium; LV = left ventricle; PAH = pulmonary arterial hypertension; PDA = patent ductus arteriosus; RA = right atrium; RBBB = right bundle branch block; RV = right ventricle; VSD = ventricular septal defect.

findings on TTE include right-sided cardiac chamber enlargement, tricuspid regurgitation related to annular dilatation, and increased right ventricular systolic pressure. Agitated saline contrast injection may help identify a right-to-left atrial shunt if Eisenmenger syndrome is suspected (see Adults with Cyanotic Congenital Heart Disease, later). Sinus venosus and coronary sinus ASDs are less readily diagnosed by TTE in adults and often require TEE, MRI, or CT imaging.

MRI and CT can be used to quantify right ventricular volumes and ejection fraction. These studies are rarely used as the primary imaging modality when ASD is suspected but may help quantify right heart enlargement in a patient with ASD. In addition, a CT or MRI performed for another reason may be the first imaging study to demonstrate the ASD. MRI, CT, and TEE are useful for identifying anomalous pulmonary veins.

Cardiac catheterization is the only reliable method to calculate the pulmonary-to-systemic blood flow ratio (Qp:Qs) but is rarely required for uncomplicated ASDs. Cardiac catheterization may be recommended in the patient with an ASD and PAH to aid in determining whether ASD closure is indicated.

Treatment

Symptoms and right-sided cardiac chamber enlargement are the main indications for ASD closure. Closure should also be considered for patients with platypnea-orthodeoxia syndrome and patients with intracardiac shunt before pacemaker placement because of the increased risk of systemic thromboembolism. Other considerations include patient age, defect size and location, and associated abnormalities such as right heart enlargement, moderate (or less) hypertension, and tricuspid regurgitation. A small ASD (Qp:Qs <1.5:1.0) with no associated symptoms or right heart enlargement can be followed clinically.

Percutaneous intervention involves closure of the ASD using a device delivered via the venous system in the catheterization laboratory. This is the preferred treatment for patients with an isolated ostium secundum ASD and right-sided cardiac chamber enlargement but no other associated cardiovascular abnormality that requires operative intervention. Surgical closure is indicated for very large ostium secundum ASDs or insufficient septal anatomy for device closure; for all other types of ASDs; and for patients with any type of ASD when there is coexistent cardiovascular disease that requires operative intervention, such as coronary artery disease or tricuspid valve regurgitation.

Patients with severe PAH and an ASD may be considered for closure providing there is persistent left-to-right shunt and no evidence of fixed pulmonary vascular disease. Standard medical therapy for PAH should also be considered. ◨

Patients with an isolated anomalous pulmonary venous connection may present with clinical and TTE features similar to an ASD, but no atrial-level shunt during agitated saline contrast study. A high clinical index of suspicion should prompt focused imaging with TEE, CT, or MRI.

Patients with small ASDs do not need any limitation of physical activity. In patients with large left-to-right shunts, exercise is often self-limited owing to decreased cardiopulmonary function. If pulmonary vascular disease is present, patients should be advised against isometric or competitive exercise.

Pregnancy in patients with ASD is generally well tolerated in the absence of PAH. The risk of congenital heart disease transmission in patients with sporadic ASD is estimated to be less than 10%. Genetic syndromes have variable inheritance; a family history should be taken. Holt-Oram syndrome is inherited in an autosomal dominant fashion.

Follow-up After Atrial Septal Defect Closure

Clinical follow-up is recommended for all adult patients after surgical or device ASD closure; the frequency of follow-up should be individualized. TTE imaging is generally recommended within the first year after closure and then periodically after that. Pre- and post-closure atrial fibrillation occurs more frequently the older the patient is at the time of ASD closure. Rare complications after device closure include device migration, erosion into the aorta or pericardium, and sudden death. Chest pain or syncope after device closure warrants urgent evaluation for device erosion.

KEY POINTS

- Fixed splitting of the S_2 is the characteristic auscultatory finding in patients with an atrial septal defect.
- A small atrial septal defect (pulmonary-to-systemic blood flow ratio [Qp:Qs] <1.5:1) with no associated symptoms or right heart enlargement can be followed clinically.
- Symptoms and right-sided cardiac chamber enlargement are the main indications for atrial septal defect closure.

HVC

Ventricular Septal Defect

Pathophysiology

Ventricular septal defects (VSDs) are common at birth, but the frequency decreases by adulthood because of spontaneous closure of small defects. VSDs are defined by their location on the ventricular septum (**Figure 29**). The most common type of VSD is perimembranous, comprising 80% of cases; these are usually isolated abnormalities. Subpulmonary VSDs (also called outlet or supracristal VSDs) account for approximately 6% of defects in the non-Asian population and 33% in Asians. Spontaneous closure of these defects is rare, and progressive aortic valve regurgitation is common owing to aortic cusp distortion. Muscular VSDs (10% of cases) can be located anywhere in the ventricular septum and may be single or multiple; these defects usually close spontaneously. Inlet defects (4%) occur in the superior-posterior portion of the ventricular septum adjacent to the tricuspid valve. These defects occur as

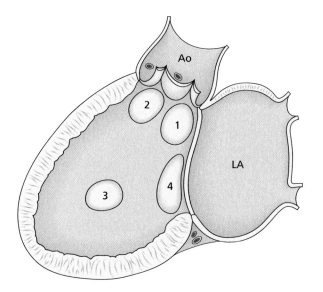

FIGURE 29. Positions of various ventricular septal defects viewed from the left side of the heart. (1) perimembranous; (2) subpulmonary; (3) muscular; (4) inlet. Ao = aorta; LA = left atrium.

Redrawn from original supplied courtesy of Dr. William D. Edwards, Department of Laboratory Medicine and Pathology, Mayo Clinic, Rochester, MN.

part of the atrioventricular septal defect complex and are characteristically seen in patients with Down syndrome.

Clinical Presentation

Clinical presentation of an isolated VSD depends on the defect size and pulmonary vascular resistance. Patients with a small VSD and no PAH present with a loud holosystolic murmur located at the left sternal border that often obliterates the S_2 and may be palpable. Small VSDs do not cause left heart enlargement or PAH.

A moderate-sized VSD with a moderate left-to-right shunt may cause left ventricular volume overload and PAH. Patients remain asymptomatic for many years but eventually present with symptoms of heart failure. The left ventricular impulse may be displaced, suggesting volume overload. A holosystolic murmur is noted at the left sternal border; the duration and quality depend on the pressure gradient between the left and right ventricles. Progressive PAH results in shortening of the murmur.

Large VSDs associated with moderate or large left-to-right shunts are usually detected in childhood by the presence of a murmur, heart failure, and failure to thrive. Unless closure is performed early in life, fixed PAH will ensue within several years, resulting in Eisenmenger syndrome and right-to-left shunt reversal.

Diagnostic Evaluation

The ECG and chest radiograph findings in patients with VSDs are outlined in Table 40. TTE is the primary diagnostic test for patients in whom a VSD is suspected. TTE allows determination of the location, size, and hemodynamic impact of the VSD in most patients, along with the presence or absence of associated valve regurgitation, PAH, and left heart enlargement. MRI or CT imaging may be used in select patients for delineation of cardiac anatomy in patients with limited echocardiographic images and measurement of ventricular volumes. Cardiac catheterization is rarely performed to confirm the diagnosis but is helpful in delineating pulmonary vascular disease and the Qp:Qs ratio.

Treatment

Although percutaneous device closure is possible for select VSDs, most patients are treated surgically. Closure of a VSD is generally indicated when there is a significant shunt (Qp:Qs ratio is 2.0 or greater), and there is evidence of left ventricular volume overload; an additional indication for closure is a history of endocarditis.

For small VSDs with a small left-to-right shunt and no left heart enlargement or valve disease, observation is appropriate with periodic clinical evaluation and imaging. Large VSDs with right-to-left shunt reversal and PAH (Eisenmenger syndrome) should not be closed; closure will result in clinical deterioration due to reduction in cardiac output.

Patients with a small VSD require no activity restrictions. If pulmonary vascular disease is present (pulmonary artery systolic pressure >50 mm Hg), patients should be advised against isometric or competitive exercise.

In the absence of PAH, pregnancy in women with VSDs is generally well tolerated. Women with VSDs and associated PAH should be counseled against pregnancy.

Follow-up After Ventricular Septal Defect Closure

Complications following VSD repair include residual or recurrent VSD, arrhythmias, PAH, endocarditis, and aortic or tricuspid valve regurgitation. Cardiovascular evaluation with TTE imaging is recommended within 1 year of VSD closure. Subsequent clinical and TTE follow-up frequency depends on clinical and cardiac status. Anticoagulation is not routinely recommended following VSD closure.

KEY POINTS

- For small ventricular septal defects with a small left-to-right shunt and no left heart enlargement or valve disease, observation is appropriate with periodic clinical evaluation and imaging.

- Closure of a ventricular septal defect is indicated when the pulmonary–to–systemic blood flow ratio (Qp:Qs) is 2.0 or greater, and there is evidence of left ventricular volume overload or a history of endocarditis.

- Large ventricular septal defects with right-to-left shunt reversal and pulmonary arterial hypertension (Eisenmenger syndrome) should not be closed as closure will result in clinical deterioration.

HVC

Patent Ductus Arteriosus

Pathophysiology

Patent ductus arteriosus (PDA) is the persistence of the arterial duct that connects the aorta and the pulmonary artery in the fetus. Maternal rubella and neonatal prematurity predispose to PDA. The PDA may be an isolated abnormality or associated with other congenital cardiac defects.

Clinical Presentation

A PDA produces an arteriovenous fistula, usually resulting in a continuous murmur that envelops the S_2. A tiny PDA is generally asymptomatic and inaudible. Patients with a moderate-sized PDA may present with symptoms of dyspnea and heart failure. A continuous "machinery" murmur is heard beneath the left clavicle. Bounding pulses and a wide pulse pressure may also be noted.

A large PDA causes a large left-to-right shunt and, if unrepaired, may cause PAH with eventual shunt reversal from right-to-left (Eisenmenger syndrome). A characteristic feature of an Eisenmenger PDA is clubbing and oxygen desaturation that affects the feet but not the hands owing to desaturated blood reaching the lower part of the body preferentially (differential cyanosis).

Diagnostic Evaluation

The ECG and chest radiograph findings in patients with PDA are outlined in Table 40. TTE with color flow Doppler imaging usually confirms the presence of a PDA. In patients with severe PAH, the PDA may be difficult to visualize owing to equalization of pressures in the aorta and pulmonary artery. In patients with a PDA and elevated pulmonary artery pressures, cardiac catheterization is used to determine reversibility and shunt size. Angiography confirms the size and shape of the PDA and helps to determine whether percutaneous closure is feasible. Cardiac CT and MRI may identify a PDA but are not used as primary diagnostic techniques.

Treatment

Closure of a PDA is indicated for left-sided cardiac chamber enlargement in the absence of severe PAH. Closure may be performed surgically or percutaneously; however, surgical closure of a calcified PDA may be challenging. Referral to a congenital cardiac center for consideration of closure options is appropriate for these patients.

A tiny PDA requires no intervention. In patients with a small PDA and prior endocarditis, closure is suggested. A moderate-sized PDA is generally closed percutaneously. A large PDA with severe PAH and shunt reversal should be observed, as closure may be detrimental. In these patients, medical therapy for PAH should be considered.

Patients with a small PDA without PAH do not need any limitation of physical activity. Anticoagulation is not routinely recommended for patients with PDA or following PDA closure.

Pulmonary Valve Stenosis

Pathophysiology

Pulmonary valve stenosis is usually an isolated congenital cardiac lesion, causing obstruction to right ventricular outflow. Noonan syndrome, an autosomal dominant disorder, is often associated with isolated pulmonary valve stenosis or other congenital cardiac defects. Additional features of Noonan syndrome include short stature, variable intellectual impairment, unique facial features, neck webbing, and hypertelorism.

Clinical Presentation

Patients with mild or moderate pulmonary valve stenosis are generally asymptomatic, whereas those with severe stenosis may have exertional dyspnea. On physical examination, mild pulmonary valve stenosis is characterized by a normal jugular venous waveform and precordial impulse. A pulmonary ejection click decreases with inspiration. Moderate or severe pulmonary valve stenosis results in right ventricular hypertrophy with a resultant prominent a wave on the jugular venous pressure waveform and a right ventricular lift. An ejection click may be audible, but as the severity of pulmonary valve stenosis progresses, the click disappears owing to loss of valve pliability. An ejection systolic murmur, heard at the left sternal border, increases in intensity and duration as the severity of pulmonary valve stenosis worsens. The pulmonary valve component of S_2 is delayed and eventually disappears with increasing severity. A right ventricular S_4 is heard in severe pulmonary valve stenosis.

Diagnostic Evaluation

The ECG and chest radiograph findings in patients with pulmonary valve stenosis are outlined in Table 40. TTE with Doppler confirms the presence of pulmonary valve stenosis and allows assessment of its severity. Pulmonary valve stenosis is considered severe if the peak gradient is 60 mm Hg or greater. Pulmonary cusp mobility, calcification, and the effects of obstruction on the right ventricle may affect treatment options. Right ventricular hypertrophy is expected in patients with pulmonary valve stenosis, but when right heart enlargement occurs, an associated lesion, such as pulmonary regurgitation or an ASD, should be suspected. Cardiac catheterization is primarily used when percutaneous intervention is considered. MRI and CT are not routinely used in patients with pulmonary valve stenosis.

Treatment

Pulmonary balloon valvuloplasty is the treatment of choice for pulmonary valve stenosis and is indicated for asymptomatic patients with appropriate pulmonary valve morphology who have a peak instantaneous Doppler gradient of at least 60 mm Hg or a mean gradient greater than 40 mm Hg and pulmonary valve regurgitation that is less than moderate. Balloon valvuloplasty is also recommended for symptomatic patients with appropriate valve morphology who have a peak instantaneous Doppler gradient of greater than 50 mm Hg or a mean gradient greater than 30 mm Hg. Operative intervention is recommended for pulmonary valve stenosis associated with a small pulmonary annulus, more than moderate pulmonary regurgitation, severe subvalvar or supravalvar pulmonary stenosis, or another cardiac lesion that requires operative intervention. H

Patients with previous pulmonary balloon or surgical valvuloplasty rarely have residual pulmonary stenosis but are at increased risk for pulmonary valve regurgitation. Long-term clinical and TTE follow-up is recommended after intervention; the frequency depends on the severity of pulmonary valve regurgitation.

Patients with pulmonary valve stenosis and a peak gradient below 50 mm Hg do not require exercise restriction. Patients with more severe stenosis should participate only in low-intensity sports.

Pregnancy is generally well tolerated in women with pulmonary valve stenosis unless the lesion is severe. Percutaneous valvotomy has been performed during pregnancy.

> **KEY POINT**
> - Pulmonary balloon valvuloplasty is the treatment of choice for severe pulmonary valve stenosis.

Aortic Coarctation

Pathophysiology

Aortic coarctation is a discrete aortic narrowing, usually located just beyond the left subclavian artery, causing hypertension proximal and reduced blood pressure distal to the aortic narrowing.

Clinical Presentation

Patients with aortic coarctation may be asymptomatic or present with hypertension, symptoms of exertional leg fatigue, or headaches. Upper extremity hypertension and reduced blood pressure and pulse amplitude in the lower extremities are characteristic findings and cause a radial artery–to–femoral artery pulse delay. More than 50% of patients with aortic coarctation have a bicuspid aortic valve.

Turner syndrome is a chromosomal abnormality (45,X) characterized by a female with short stature, a broad chest with widely spaced nipples, webbed neck, and aortic coarctation. Aortic coarctation is also associated with bicuspid aortic valve, aortic valve and subaortic stenosis, parachute mitral valve, VSD, and cerebral artery aneurysms.

The characteristic murmur of aortic coarctation is a systolic murmur heard in the left infraclavicular region or over the back. When severe, the murmur may be continuous, and a murmur from collateral intercostal vessels may also be audible and palpable over the chest wall. In patients with aortic coarctation and a bicuspid aortic valve, an ejection click or a systolic murmur may be heard. An S_4 is often audible.

Diagnostic Evaluation

The ECG and chest radiograph findings in patients with aortic coarctation are outlined in Table 40. The "figure 3 sign" on chest radiograph (**Figure 30**) is caused by dilatation of the aorta above and below the area of coarctation. Dilatation of intercostal arteries may result in the radiographic appearance of "rib notching."

TTE is usually the initial diagnostic test in patients with suspected aortic coarctation and allows identification of associated features, such as bicuspid aortic valve and left ventricular hypertrophy. MRI and CT are recommended to identify coarctation severity, the presence of collateral vessels, and associated abnormalities such as aortic aneurysm. Cardiac catheterization is reserved for patients who are being considered for percutaneous intervention. H

Treatment

Severe aortic coarctation is associated with reduced survival. Common causes of morbidity and mortality include systemic

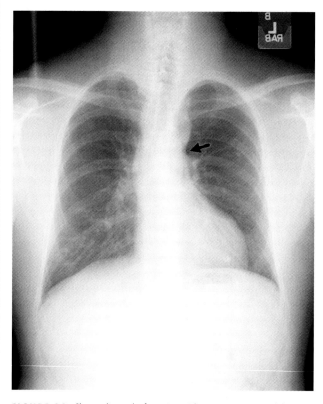

FIGURE 30. Chest radiograph of a patient with aortic coarctation exhibiting the "figure 3 sign," caused by dilatation of the aorta above and below the area of coarctation (*arrow*).

hypertension, coronary artery disease, stroke, aortic dissection, and heart failure.

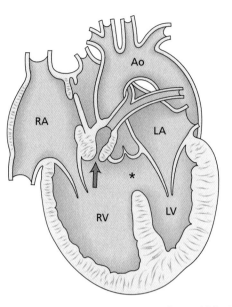

Intervention for coarctation is recommended when the coarctation systolic peak (peak-to-peak) pressure gradient is 20 mm Hg or higher (measured by TTE Doppler or cardiac catheterization) or if there is radiologic evidence of severe coarctation with collateral flow. Surgical and percutaneous intervention options are available, and selection depends on the length, location, and severity of the coarctation as well as the presence of associated lesions.

Patients with severe residual or unrepaired coarctation, aortic stenosis, or a dilated aorta should be counseled to avoid contact sports and isometric exercise.

Women with repaired aortic coarctation and no significant residua generally tolerate pregnancy well. A comprehensive prepregnancy evaluation is warranted to evaluate for residua. Women with severe unoperated coarctation should avoid pregnancy prior to intervention. Patients with mild or moderate residual or unoperated coarctation will generally tolerate pregnancy well but should undergo blood pressure monitoring during pregnancy and receive cardiovascular follow-up.

Follow-up After Aortic Coarctation Repair

Hypertension occurs in up to 75% of patients following coarctation repair. Blood pressure control is recommended to reduce hypertension-related morbidity. Intervention is often required for bicuspid aortic valve, aortic aneurysm, aortic dissection, recoarctation, coronary artery disease, systolic or diastolic heart failure, and intracranial aneurysm. Age at the time of repair is the most important predictor of long-term survival. Regular follow-up should include evaluation with a congenital cardiologist as well as TTE and aortic imaging.

KEY POINTS

- Upper extremity hypertension and reduced blood pressure and pulse amplitude in the lower extremities are characteristic findings of aortic coarctation and cause a radial artery–to–femoral artery pulse delay.

- Intervention for aortic coarctation is recommended when the coarctation systolic peak (peak-to-peak) pressure gradient is 20 mm Hg or higher or if there is radiologic evidence of severe coarctation with collateral flow.

- Patients with severe residual or unrepaired aortic coarctation, aortic stenosis, or a dilated aorta should be counseled to avoid pregnancy, contact sports, and isometric exercise.

Tetralogy of Fallot

Tetralogy of Fallot is the most common cyanotic congenital cardiac lesion and includes a large subaortic VSD, infundibular or valvular pulmonary stenosis, aortic override, and right ventricular hypertrophy (**Figure 31**). Unoperated adult patients are rarely encountered.

FIGURE 31. Tetralogy of Fallot. A subarterial ventricular septal defect (*asterisk*) and pulmonary stenosis (*arrow*) are associated with secondary aortic override and right ventricular hypertrophy. Ao = aorta; LA = left atrium; LV = left ventricle; RA = right atrium; RV = right ventricle.

Redrawn from original supplied courtesy of Dr. William D. Edwards, Department of Laboratory Medicine and Pathology, Mayo Clinic, Rochester, MN.

Approximately 15% of patients with tetralogy of Fallot have the 22q11.2 chromosome microdeletion. This increases the chance of congenital heart disease inheritance to approximately 50% compared with 5% in patients without the microdeletion. Genetic testing is recommended for all patients with tetralogy of Fallot who are planning reproduction. Tetralogy of Fallot is also common in persons with Down syndrome.

Surgical repair of tetralogy of Fallot involves patch closure of the VSD and relief of right ventricular outflow tract obstruction by patch enlargement. The transannular patch procedure invariably disrupts the integrity of the pulmonary valve, causing severe pulmonary valve regurgitation, the most common reason for reoperation in patients after repair of tetralogy of Fallot. Over many years, pulmonary regurgitation causes progressive right heart enlargement, tricuspid regurgitation, exercise limitation, and increased risk for arrhythmias. Annual follow-up by a congenital cardiologist is recommended to monitor these sequelae and determine optimal timing for intervention. Current surgical techniques include attempted relief of pulmonary valve stenosis with preservation of native pulmonary valve function.

Diagnostic Evaluation After Repair of Tetralogy of Fallot

The ECG and chest radiograph findings in patients with repaired tetralogy of Fallot are outlined in Table 40. Presence of an arrhythmia should prompt a search for right heart chamber enlargement from pulmonary valve regurgitation. The QRS duration on the ECG reflects the degree of right ventricular dilatation. A QRS duration of 180 msec or longer and non-

CONT.
sustained ventricular tachycardia are risk factors for sudden cardiac death.

TTE can confirm the presence of pulmonary or tricuspid valve regurgitation, right ventricular outflow tract obstruction, residual VSD, aortic regurgitation, and aortic dilatation. MRI is used to assess right ventricular size and function, which helps determine appropriate timing for pulmonary valve replacement. Diagnostic catheterization may be required to assess hemodynamics and residual shunts and delineate coronary artery and pulmonary artery anatomy. **H**

Treatment of Tetralogy of Fallot Residua

Pulmonary valve replacement is recommended in patients with repaired tetralogy of Fallot who have severe pulmonary valve regurgitation with symptoms, decreased exercise tolerance, more than moderate right heart enlargement or dysfunction, or arrhythmias. Long-standing pulmonary valve regurgitation may result in tricuspid regurgitation, and repair of the tricuspid valve may also be needed. Percutaneous pulmonary valve replacement is now available for select patients with previous operative intervention for tetralogy of Fallot.

Patients with repaired tetralogy of Fallot and residual sequelae should be cautioned regarding participation in contact sports and heavy isometric exercise.

KEY POINT

- Pulmonary valve replacement is recommended in patients with repaired tetralogy of Fallot who have severe pulmonary valve regurgitation with symptoms, decreased exercise tolerance, more than moderate right heart enlargement or dysfunction, or arrhythmias.

Adults with Cyanotic Congenital Heart Disease

General Management

Right-to-left cardiac shunts, such as unrepaired or palliated tetralogy of Fallot, truncus arteriosus, tricuspid atresia, and Eisenmenger syndrome, result in hypoxemia, erythrocytosis, and cyanosis. Erythrocyte mass is increased in patients with cyanosis as a compensatory response to improve oxygen transport.

Physical features include central cyanosis and digital clubbing. Patients with cyanotic congenital heart disease are predisposed to scoliosis, arthropathy, gallstones, pulmonary hemorrhage or thrombus, paradoxical cerebral emboli or cerebral abscess, kidney dysfunction, and hemostatic problems. Because of these problems, a congenital cardiac specialist should evaluate patients with cyanotic congenital heart disease at least annually.

H
Patients with cyanotic or complex congenital heart disease are at increased risk for endocarditis; therefore, antimicrobial prophylaxis is recommended prior to certain nonsterile procedures. In patients who are hospitalized with a right-to-

left intracardiac shunt, filters on intravenous lines should be used to prevent paradoxical air embolism. Early ambulation, pneumatic compression devices, or anticoagulation is also recommended for prevention of venous stasis and potential venous thrombosis and paradoxical embolism. Because perioperative cardiac complications are common in these patients, elective operations should be performed at centers that care for such patients with a coordinated multidisciplinary team approach. Consultation with a congenital cardiac specialist is recommended when patients are hospitalized. **H**

Most patients with cyanosis have compensated erythrocytosis and stable hemoglobin levels. Occasionally, hyperviscosity symptoms occur, including headaches and reduced concentration. Phlebotomy is recommended for a hemoglobin level greater than 20 g/dL (200 g/L) and a hematocrit level greater than 65% associated with hyperviscosity symptoms in the absence of dehydration. Phlebotomy should be performed no more than two to three times each year. Dehydration should be excluded before considering the procedure, and it should be followed by intravenous fluid administration. Repeated phlebotomies deplete iron stores and may result in the production of iron-deficient erythrocytes or microcytosis, increasing the risk of stroke. Iron deficiency in a patient with destabilized erythropoiesis is treated with oral iron therapy for a short time. Iron therapy is discontinued when serum ferritin and transferrin saturation values are within the normal range.

Maternal cyanosis impairs normal fetal growth and development and increases the risk of intrauterine growth retardation and miscarriage. Maternal and fetal morbidity and mortality are increased, related to the degree of cyanosis, ventricular function, and pulmonary pressures. If pregnancy occurs in a patient with cyanotic heart disease, physical activity should be curtailed and supplemental oxygen is recommended. Preventive measures to decrease the risk of venous thrombosis and paradoxical embolism also are recommended.

Eisenmenger Syndrome

Eisenmenger syndrome is severe PAH and reversal of a congenital cardiac shunt caused by VSD, PDA, or, less commonly, ASD. Eisenmenger syndrome has become increasingly rare owing to medical screening, including TTE and appropriate intervention.

Conservative medical measures are recommended in the management of Eisenmenger syndrome. Persons with Eisenmenger syndrome should be cautioned regarding iron deficiency, dehydration, acute exposure to excess heat, and moderate or severe strenuous or isometric exercise. Routine phlebotomy based on hemoglobin or hematocrit level is not recommended because iron deficiency and microcytosis may lead to increased symptoms; rather, phlebotomy should be performed only when symptoms of hyperviscosity occur and with saline volume replacement. In addition, chronic high altitude exposure should be avoided, as it further reduces oxygen saturation. Women should be cautioned to avoid pregnancy because of the high risk for maternal mortality.

All patients with Eisenmenger syndrome should be evaluated annually by a congenital cardiac specialist. Noncardiac surgery should be performed at centers with expertise in the care of patients with complex congenital cardiac disease whenever possible. Meticulous care of intravenous lines with filters to avoid paradoxical air embolism is imperative. Patients with progressive symptoms may benefit from pulmonary vasodilator therapy.

Long-distance air travel should be approached with caution and occur in pressurized aircrafts. Select patients may benefit from supplemental oxygen during prolonged air travel.

KEY POINT

- In patients with Eisenmenger syndrome, meticulous care of intravenous lines with filters to avoid paradoxical air embolism is imperative.

Diseases of the Aorta

Introduction

Aortic disease includes acute life-threatening conditions such as aortic dissection, chronic conditions such as aortic atheroma that may lead to embolism, and aortic aneurysms that carry the risk of rupture. Appropriate surveillance and treatment of aortic disease are crucial to preventing catastrophic vascular events.

Imaging of the Thoracic Aorta

Using imaging to screen asymptomatic patients for abnormalities of the thoracic aorta is not recommended, except in patients with underlying vascular pathology (such as Marfan or Ehlers-Danlos syndrome), a bicuspid aortic valve, or a family history of aortic disease. Abnormalities of the thoracic aorta are sometimes discovered incidentally on chest radiography performed for other purposes. An acute aortic syndrome may produce a widening of the mediastinal silhouette, enlargement of the aortic knob, or displacement of the trachea from midline (**Figure 32**). If an abnormality is identified, additional noninvasive imaging of the aorta may be useful to determine aortic cross-sectional area, which may predict the risk of aneurysm rupture or dissection. Echocardiography, CT, and MRI can be used to cross-sectionally image the aorta (**Table 41**). There is substantial variance in measured aortic dimension according to image technique based on measurement of either internal or external aortic diameter. Care must be taken to measure the dimension perpendicular to the long axis of the aorta because oblique or tangential measurements may overestimate the true aortic diameter.

Maximum aortic diameter at a specific location is generally reported by imaging results. Dilation above the upper limits for normal may represent an aneurysm, but a patient with a larger body size may have a larger absolute aortic diameter. The maximum ascending aortic diameter may be indexed to body surface area (z-score).

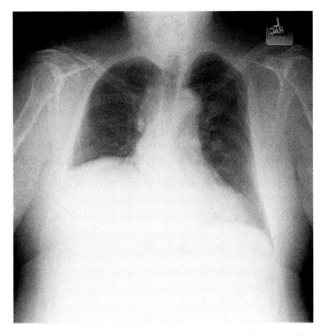

FIGURE 32. Chest radiograph shows a widened superior mediastinum and a right pleural effusion consistent with aortic dissection.

Echocardiography, CT, and MRI have similar sensitivity and specificity for diagnosis of acute thoracic aorta disease, although each has advantages and disadvantages. Transthoracic echocardiography (TTE) and transesophageal echocardiography (TEE) have the advantages of being performed at the patient's bedside and providing results within several minutes. However, although TTE may be useful in identifying an intimal flap, enlarged aortic root, or aortic insufficiency, it is limited in evaluating the mid-distal ascending aorta, transverse aorta, or descending thoracic aorta. TEE overcomes the shortcomings of TTE but requires conscious sedation. The primary advantages of TEE compared with CT imaging of suspected aortic dissection include its portability in the unstable patient and lack of contrast injection.

Invasive imaging of the aorta by angiography is rarely indicated for the diagnosis of acute disease. It may be helpful in determining the length of an aneurysm and involvement of branch vessels and should be reserved for patients in whom a percutaneous intervention is planned.

KEY POINTS

- Screening of asymptomatic patients for abnormalities of the thoracic aorta should be reserved for patients with underlying vascular pathology (such as Marfan or Ehlers-Danlos syndrome), a bicuspid aortic valve, or a family history of aortic disease. **HVC**

- Invasive imaging of the aorta by angiography is rarely necessary for the diagnosis of acute disease; it should be reserved for patients in whom a percutaneous intervention is planned. **HVC**

TABLE 41. Comparison of Thoracic Aortic Imaging Modalities

Modality	Advantages	Disadvantages
Transthoracic echocardiography (TTE)	Good visualization of aortic root/proximal ascending aorta	Limited visualization of the distal ascending aorta and aortic arch with branches of the great vessels
	No exposure to radiation or contrast dye	Requires experienced operator
	Allows definition of valvular pathology, myocardial function, pericardial disease	A negative TTE does not rule out aortic dissection, and other imaging techniques must be considered.
	Bedside diagnosis	
Transesophageal echocardiography (TEE)	TEE has superior imaging quality versus TTE	Requires experienced operator
	Excellent visualization of the aorta from its root to the descending aorta	Invasive procedure
	No exposure to radiation or contrast dye	
	Allows definition of valvular pathology, myocardial function, pericardial disease	
	Bedside diagnosis	
CT	Visualization of entire aorta and side branches	Exposes patient to radiation, iodinated contrast dye
	Rapid imaging	
	Multiplanar reconstruction	
MRI	Visualization of entire aorta and side branches	For acute disease, prolonged image acquisition away from acute care area
	No exposure to radiation or iodinated contrast dye	Contraindicated in patients with implanted pacemaker or defibrillator
		Gadolinium contrast dye contraindicated in patients with kidney disease

Thoracic Aortic Aneurysm

Thoracic aortic aneurysms may involve the aortic root, ascending aorta, aortic arch, or descending aorta. Aneurysms of the aortic root and ascending aorta are most common and usually occur as a consequence of underlying medial degeneration. Thoracic aortic aneurysms often are asymptomatic and are frequently detected incidentally during evaluation for another problem. Rarely, thoracic aortic aneurysms may be discovered because of compressive symptoms, such as hoarseness, stridor, or dysphagia. If rupture occurs, patients may have severe chest pain, back pain, sudden shortness of breath, or sudden death. A diastolic heart murmur or symptoms of heart failure may occur with aneurysmal dilatation of the aortic root and subsequent aortic valve regurgitation.

Causes of thoracic aortic aneurysms are listed in **Table 42**. These aneurysms typically result from cystic medial degeneration that leads to loss of smooth muscle cells and elastic fiber degeneration, resulting in a weakening of the aortic wall. Cystic medial degeneration occurs normally with aging and is exacerbated by hypertension. In younger patients, aneurysm is most often related to a connective tissue disorder (such as Marfan or Ehlers-Danlos syndrome). Bicuspid aortic valve is an important risk factor for aneurysm involving the aortic root and ascending thoracic aorta. Approximately 50% of patients with bicuspid aortic valves have enlargement of the proximal aorta that may be independent of the severity of aortic valve

disease. The vast majority of aneurysms affecting the descending thoracic aorta are associated with atherosclerosis. Other causes of thoracic aortic aneurysm include acquired infection and inflammatory conditions, such as syphilis, Takayasu arteritis, and giant cell arteritis.

The leading cause of death in patients with thoracic aortic aneurysm is rupture (60%). Several studies have shown an increasing risk of rupture after the aneurysm has surpassed 5.0 cm in diameter (4.0-5.0 cm in patients with genetically mediated disorders), and a rapid rate of expansion is an independent risk factor for rupture. Pregnancy also is associated with an increased risk of aortic dissection, particularly in women with Marfan syndrome, in whom dissection may occur at aortic diameters that are smaller than would usually be considered for elective repair.

Smaller thoracic aortic aneurysms can be medically managed with aggressive blood pressure control. β-Blockers may be of particular benefit for reducing the rate of aortic growth in patients with Marfan syndrome, although their benefit in treating aneurysms of other etiologies has not been proved. Losartan, an angiotensin receptor blocker, has also been associated with slower progression of aortic root dilation in patients with Marfan syndrome.

In any patient with a thoracic aortic aneurysm that does not require immediate intervention, regular surveillance is important for identifying the development of signs and

TABLE 42.	Causes of Thoracic Aortic Aneurysms
Category	**Syndrome**
Atherosclerosis	
Connective tissue disorders	Marfan syndrome
	Ehlers-Danlos syndrome, type IV
	Loeys-Dietz syndrome
Other genetic and/or congenital conditions	Familial thoracic aortic aneurysms and aortic dissections (TAAD) syndrome
	Bicuspid aortic valve
	Turner syndrome
Vasculitis	Takayasu arteritis
	Giant cell arteritis
	Nonspecific (idiopathic) aortitis
	Other autoimmune conditions (Behçet syndrome, systemic lupus erythematosus)
Infectious	Septic embolism
	Direct bacterial inoculation
	Bacterial seeding
	Contiguous infection
	Syphilis
Aortic injury	Prior acute aortic syndrome
	Chest trauma

symptoms. Annual echocardiography should be performed to monitor aortic growth. Earlier re-evaluation is indicated for changes in symptoms or physical examination findings and for hemodynamic assessment related to pregnancy. When the aortic dimension nears the threshold for intervention, patients should be referred to an appropriate specialist for evaluation. Because patients with a bicuspid aortic valve have an increased risk of aortic aneurysm and dissection, these patients should undergo echocardiography of the aorta annually if the aortic root or ascending aorta dimension is greater than 4.5 cm. In those with an aortic diameter between 4.0 and 4.5 cm, the examination interval depends on the rate of progression of dilation and the family history.

Familial thoracic aortic aneurysms and aortic dissections (TAAD) is an inherited autosomal dominant condition. Screening is recommended for first-degree relatives of persons with TAAD once a year or at least every few years. If the mutation is known, genetic testing can identify those relatives who should be screened with aortic imaging.

In patients with Marfan syndrome, follow-up imaging is recommended 6 months after diagnosis with annual surveillance thereafter if the aortic root is less than 4.5 cm in diameter and otherwise stable. If the aortic diameter is 4.5 cm or greater or shows significant growth over time, then more frequent surveillance is suggested (for example, twice yearly). Most patients with Marfan syndrome present with enlargement of the ascending aorta; therefore, serial examination is focused mainly on assessing this portion of aorta, and transthoracic ultrasound is the preferred imaging modality in these patients.

The repair of a thoracic aortic aneurysm is often recommended prophylactically to prevent the morbidity and mortality associated with aneurysm rupture. In asymptomatic patients, elective thoracic aortic repair is recommended if the aortic root or ascending aorta is greater than 5.5 cm (5.5–6.0 cm for the descending aorta) or has rapid growth (>0.5 cm/year). For genetically mediated disorders (such as Marfan syndrome), a lower threshold of 5.0 cm (4.0–5.0 cm in certain patients) may be used for repair. For patients with a bicuspid aortic valve, repair is indicated if the aortic diameter is greater than 5.5 cm and is reasonable if the diameter is greater than 5.0 cm and the patient has an increased risk of dissection (family history of dissection or rapid growth).

Repair of ascending aortic and aortic arch aneurysms requires surgery and may include aortic valve replacement or repair in patients with significant annular dilatation or associated aortic valve pathology. A conservative procedure whereby the aneurysm is replaced with a Dacron graft and the aortic valve is preserved has gained widespread use. If the aortic valve needs replacement and the patient has a dilated aortic root, a composite aortic valve and aortic root and ascending aorta graft replacement (Bentall operation) may be performed. The Bentall operation includes re-implantation of the coronary arteries into the ascending aortic graft. Thoracic endovascular aortic repair (TEVAR) with stent grafting has emerged as a promising alternative to open repair for

H CONT. aneurysm of the descending thoracic aorta. TEVAR has been associated with shorter hospital stays and lower hospital morbidity and has the potential advantages of avoiding thoracotomy, aortic cross-clamping, and extracorporeal support. Adverse events following TEVAR include stroke, spinal ischemia, access complications, and endoleaks. **H**

KEY POINTS

- Patients with a thoracic aortic aneurysm should undergo annual echocardiography to monitor aortic aneurysm growth.

- Patients with a bicuspid aortic valve should undergo annual echocardiography of the aorta if the aortic root or ascending aorta dimension is greater than 4.5 cm.

- In asymptomatic patients, elective thoracic aortic repair is recommended if the aortic root or ascending aorta is greater than 5.5 cm (5.5-6.0 cm for the descending aorta) or has rapid growth (>0.5 cm/year); for patients with genetically mediated disorders, the threshold for repair is lower.

Acute Aortic Syndromes

H Acute aortic syndromes include aortic dissection, intramural hematoma, penetrating atherosclerotic ulcer, and trauma-induced aortic rupture (**Figure 33**). Acute aortic syndromes threaten central aortic pressure, critical organ perfusion, and survival. Prompt recognition and delivery of appropriate medical and interventional care are critical determinants of outcome. **H**

Pathophysiology

In aortic dissection, blood passes through a tear in the aortic intima, creating a false lumen that separates layers of the aorta. Propagation of the dissection can proceed in an anterograde or retrograde fashion from the initial tear, involving side branches and causing complications such as tamponade, aortic valve insufficiency, or malperfusion syndromes. An intramural hematoma may result from rupture of the vasa vasorum or "microtears" in the intima, resulting in a crescent of hematoma within the media without identifiable interruption of the intima. Penetrating atherosclerotic ulcers are most likely caused by atherosclerosis with subsequent erosion across the internal elastic membrane of the aorta, allowing for a blood-filled false space within the wall of the aorta.

The Stanford classification describes type A dissections as originating within the ascending aorta or arch, whereas type B dissections originate distal to the left subclavian artery. This nomenclature has been generalized to all of the acute aortic syndromes, although most intramural hematomas and penetrating ulcers are type B lesions.

Diagnosis and Evaluation

H The diagnosis of an acute aortic syndrome requires a high index of suspicion because of its life-threatening

Acute aortic dissection

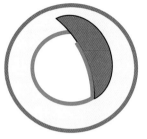

Acute intramural hematoma

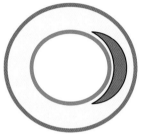

Penetrating atherosclerotic ulcer

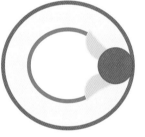

FIGURE 33. Cross-sectional representation of acute aortic syndromes. Acute aortic dissection: interruption of intima (*blue*) with creation of an intimal flap and false lumen formation within the media (*red*). Color flow by Doppler echocardiography or intravenous (IV) contrast by CT is present within the false lumen in the acute phase. Acute intramural hematoma: crescent-shaped hematoma contained within the media without interruption of the intima (*blue*). No color flow by Doppler echocardiography or IV contrast by CT within crescent. Penetrating atherosclerotic ulcer: atheroma (*yellow*) with plaque rupture disrupting intimal integrity; blood pool contained within intima-medial layer (pseudoaneurysm). Color flow by Doppler echocardiography or IV contrast by CT enters the ulcer crater.

complications. The classic presentation consists of "aortic chest pain" described as severe ripping or tearing pain that may radiate to the anterior chest or back, jaw, or abdomen, depending on which segment of the aorta is involved. Hypertension is the most important risk factor; other risk factors include smoking and atherosclerosis. In the setting of an acute aortic dissection, hypertension and an aortic regurgitation murmur that is faint, short in duration, and low in pitch may be present. Other findings on physical examination that may increase the index of suspicion include pulsus paradoxus, asymmetric blood pressure in the upper extremities, and an asymmetric pulse examination. A low D-dimer level

(<0.5 µg/mL [0.5 mg/L]) suggests against an acute aortic syndrome. In aortic dissection, chest radiography may demonstrate a widening of the mediastinum. An electrocardiogram is often abnormal, but nondiagnostic. Clinical suspicion should be high, and CT, MRI, or TEE for confirmation of the diagnosis should not be delayed.

Treatment

Patients with a suspected acute aortic syndrome who are not in cardiogenic shock should receive medical therapy to control heart rate and blood pressure. Intravenous β-blockers should be used to target a heart rate of below 70/min. In patients requiring additional blood pressure control, a rapidly titratable antihypertensive medication, such as sodium nitroprusside, labetalol, enalaprilat, hydralazine, or nicardipine, should be given intravenously, with a goal of decreasing the mean arterial pressure to the lowest level that still allows visceral and cerebral perfusion.

Emergency surgery is recommended for all patients with type A aortic dissection as well as for type A intramural hematoma. Any delays to surgery should be avoided or addressed, as type A dissection has a very high short-term mortality rate. Concomitant aortic arch reconstruction, coronary artery reimplantation, aortic valve repair or replacement, or branch vessel repair may be required depending on the anatomy and pathology of the lesion.

Uncomplicated type B aortic syndromes may be treated medically. The INSTEAD trial, which enrolled subjects with uncomplicated chronic type B dissection, showed no difference in clinical or aortic outcomes at 2 years for patients treated with TEVAR versus medical therapy alone. Among patients who survived at 2 years, additional long-term follow-up of the INSTEAD trial demonstrated that TEVAR in addition to optimal medical treatment was associated with improved long-term aorta-specific survival and delayed disease progression. Surgery is indicated for complicated type B aortic dissection defined by refractory pain or hypertension, rapid aneurysmal expansion, rupture, or malperfusion syndrome. **H**

KEY POINTS

- The classic presentation of an acute aortic syndrome consists of "aortic chest pain"—severe ripping or tearing pain that may radiate to the anterior chest or back, jaw, or abdomen, depending on which segment of the aorta is involved.

- Findings that increase the index of suspicion for an acute aortic syndrome include pulsus paradoxus, asymmetric blood pressure in the upper extremities, and an asymmetric pulse examination.

- Type A aortic dissection has a very high short-term mortality rate, and emergency surgery is recommended for all patients without delay.

Aortic Atheroma

Aortic atherosclerotic plaques are a manifestation of systemic atherosclerosis. Aortic atheroma may be detected incidentally during imaging (**Figure 34**). The risk of embolism and stroke in patients with aortic atheroma is significantly increased for plaques that are mobile or protruding, particularly if the plaque is greater than 4 mm in size. Thromboembolism may also result from dislodgment of debris from the aortic wall occurring as a complication of an invasive cardiovascular procedure, such as catheterization, intra-aortic balloon pump placement, or vascular surgery.

Noncoronary atherosclerotic disease, including aortic atheroma, is a coronary heart disease risk equivalent and, therefore, should be aggressively treated to reduce the risk of future cardiovascular events, including treatment with antiplatelet agents and statins. In an observational study, statin therapy was associated with a 17% absolute reduction in thromboembolic events in patients with aortic atheroma.

KEY POINT

- Aortic atheroma is a coronary heart disease risk equivalent, and patients should be aggressively treated with antiplatelet agents and statins to reduce their cardiovascular risk.

Abdominal Aortic Aneurysm
Screening and Surveillance

An abdominal aortic aneurysm (AAA) is considered to be present when the minimum anteroposterior diameter of the aorta reaches 3.0 cm. The most important risk factors for AAA are increasing age, smoking, and male sex (men with AAA outnumber women by up to 6:1). Other risk factors include atherosclerosis, hypertension, and family history of AAA.

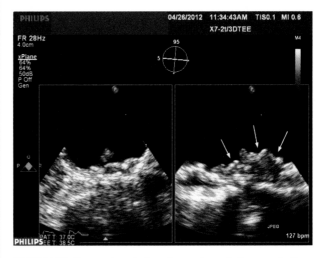

FIGURE 34. Transesophageal echocardiogram demonstrating an aortic atheroma in the descending aorta (*arrows*). *Left panel*: short axis view; *right panel*: long axis view.

Based on randomized data, the U.S. Preventive Services Task Force guidelines recommend a one-time ultrasonographic screening in men aged 65 to 75 years who are active or former smokers (see MKSAP 17 General Internal Medicine). The sensitivity and specificity of ultrasonography for detection of AAA are excellent.

AAA rupture has an exceedingly high mortality rate, yet most AAAs never rupture. Thus, deciding when and in whom to intervene and electively repair an AAA is of major importance. The strongest risk factor for the rupture of an AAA is maximal aortic diameter; this measurement is the dominant indication for repair. Estimated annual rupture risk according to AAA diameter is shown in **Table 43**.

After AAA has been identified, surveillance imaging results determine the timing of repair. The frequency of surveillance is dependent on baseline aneurysm size; larger aneurysms expand faster than smaller ones and may require more frequent surveillance. If AAA maximum diameter is 3.5 to 4.4 cm, repeat ultrasonography is recommended annually; if maximum diameter is 4.5 to 5.4 cm, repeat ultrasonography should be performed every 6 to 12 months. Elective repair should be considered for AAA of 5.5 cm in diameter, for those that increase in diameter by more than 0.5 cm within a 6-month interval, and for those that are symptomatic (tenderness or abdominal or back pain). For women, elective repair may be considered for an AAA that reaches 5.0 cm in diameter.

Treatment

Medical therapies for AAA focus on targeting modifiable risk factors for AAA and cardiovascular disease with the goals of reducing aneurysm expansion or rupture, reducing morbidity and mortality associated with repair, and reducing cardiovascular morbidity and mortality. Smoking cessation is the cornerstone of therapy for active smokers.

If repair is being considered, the choice between open surgical or endovascular aneurysm repair (EVAR) is individualized based on the patient's age, comorbidities, patient preference, and aortic anatomy. Randomized trials comparing open repair with EVAR have found significantly improved short-term (30-day) morbidity and mortality for EVAR, but no significant differences in long-term mortality. Moreover, in the long term, EVAR was associated with increased complication rates (including endovascular leaks, device migration and failure, and post-implantation syndrome) and the need for reinterventions. Because of these potential complications, patients who have undergone EVAR of AAA require diligent follow-up with imaging studies performed annually to evaluate the status of the graft. Additional long-term data from prospective randomized trials are needed to fully evaluate the benefit/risk profile of open AAA repair versus EVAR. In patients with severe comorbid disease considered not eligible for open surgical correction, a trial of EVAR versus medical therapy demonstrated no difference in all-cause mortality at 8 years, but greater cost and increased complications were associated with endovascular repair. ◨

KEY POINTS

- The most important risk factors for abdominal aortic aneurysm are increasing age, smoking, and male sex; one-time ultrasonographic screening is recommended for men ages 65 to 75 years who have ever smoked.
- Elective repair should be considered for an abdominal aortic aneurysm of 5.5 cm in diameter, for those that increase in diameter by more than 0.5 cm within a 6-month interval, and for those who are symptomatic.
- Medical therapies for abdominal aortic aneurysm focus on targeting modifiable risk factors for abdominal aortic aneurysm and cardiovascular disease; smoking cessation is the cornerstone of therapy for active smokers.

Peripheral Arterial Disease
Epidemiology and Screening

Lower extremity peripheral arterial disease (PAD) is a disorder of the aortic bifurcation or arteries of the lower limbs. The most common cause of PAD is atherosclerosis, and PAD shares the primary atherosclerotic risk factors of smoking, diabetes mellitus, and increasing age. However, unlike other types of arterial disease, the population burden of PAD is higher in women than in men. PAD is defined noninvasively by calculation of the ankle-brachial index (ABI). PAD is common, with an estimated unselected adult prevalence in the United States of approximately 6% in persons aged 40 years and older.

There is a wide spectrum of clinical manifestations for PAD:

- Asymptomatic patients found to have PAD from a screening ABI (20%-50%)
- Atypical symptoms associated with exercise limitation (40%-50%)

TABLE 43. Annual Rupture Risk of Abdominal Aortic Aneurysm by Diameter

Aneurysm Diameter	Annual Rupture Risk
<4.0 cm	<0.5%
4.0-4.9 cm	0.5%-5%
5.0-5.9 cm	3%-15%
6.0-6.9 cm	10%-20%
7.0-7.9 cm	20%-40%
≥8.0 cm	30%-50%

Adapted with permission of Elsevier Science and Technology Journals, from Brewster DC, Cronenwett JL, Hallett JW Jr, et al; Joint Council of the American Association for Vascular Surgery and Society for Vascular Surgery. Guidelines for the treatment of abdominal aortic aneurysms. Report of a subcommittee of the Joint Council of the American Association for Vascular Surgery and Society for Vascular Surgery. J Vasc Surg. 2003 May;37(5):1106-17. [PMID:12756363]; permission conveyed through Copyright Clearance Center, Inc.

- Classic intermittent claudication (10%-35%)
- Ischemic pain and ulceration in a lower extremity from chronic limb ischemia (1%-2%)

PAD is associated with reduced exercise capacity and functional status regardless of the symptomatic state. Limb-specific outcomes (such as limb ischemia or amputation) occur less frequently than systemic manifestations of atherosclerosis (myocardial infarction or stroke). Both asymptomatic and symptomatic patients with PAD are at increased risk of cardiovascular morbidity and mortality, and PAD is considered a coronary heart disease risk equivalent. Patients with PAD are likely to have concomitant vascular disease in other arterial beds and have an annual cardiovascular event rate of 5% to 7%. Thus, early recognition of PAD provides a unique opportunity to identify persons at early increased risk for a cardiovascular event and to modify risk factors. However, the U.S. Preventive Services Task Force concluded that the current evidence is insufficient to assess the balance of benefits and harms of screening for PAD and cardiovascular disease risk assessment with the ABI in adults. Initial testing may be considered in persons with the following characteristics that signify high risk:

- Exertional leg discomfort
- Nonhealing wounds
- Age 50 years or older with a history of smoking or diabetes

KEY POINTS

- Patients with peripheral arterial disease are likely to have concomitant vascular disease in other arterial beds and have an annual cardiovascular event rate of 5% to 7%.
- Initial testing for peripheral arterial disease may be considered in persons with exertional leg discomfort, nonhealing wounds, or aged 50 years or older with a history of smoking or diabetes mellitus.

Evaluation

History and Physical Examination

Patients at risk for PAD should undergo a vascular review of symptoms to assess walking impairment, claudication, and ischemic pain while at rest. Patients with PAD may have symptoms of leg ischemia, but many are asymptomatic. Among symptomatic patients, the perception of symptoms can vary from minimal to severe and may not necessarily correlate with severity of disease. Discriminating claudication from pseudoclaudication (a result of narrowing of the lumbar spinal canal) is important (**Table 44**). In severe PAD or critical limb ischemia, patients may describe discomfort that worsens with elevation of the leg and improves with dependent positioning, such as dangling the leg off the foot of the bed.

Components of the physical examination of patients with suspected PAD are shown in **Table 45**. Patients at risk for lower extremity PAD should undergo comprehensive pulse examination and inspection of the feet. Shoes and socks are removed and the feet inspected for skin changes. Physical examination may reveal diminished, absent, or asymmetric pulses below the level of stenosis, with occasional bruits over stenotic lesions and evidence of poor wound healing. Other physical findings seen in PAD include a unilaterally cool extremity; a prolonged venous filling time (>20 seconds); shiny atrophied skin; ulceration; and thickened, ridged, and brittle nails. Most patients with upper extremity PAD are asymptomatic, and PAD may be detected only by the finding of asymmetric arm blood pressures, with a typical differential in systolic blood pressures of greater than 15 mm Hg.

Diagnostic Testing

There are several diagnostic modalities to choose from to assess for PAD. Measurement of the ABI is a simple, inexpensive, and noninvasive technique that correlates well with angiographic disease severity and functional symptoms. Patients should rest for 5 to 10 minutes before measuring the ankle pressure and should be lying flat for an accurate ABI measurement, with the head and heels fully supported. The study is performed by applying a blood pressure cuff to the calf and measuring the systolic blood pressure by palpation or Doppler at the ankle. The blood pressure is recorded for both the dorsalis pedis (DP) and the posterior tibial (PT) arteries, and the higher of the two is used as the ankle pressure. This procedure is repeated for the opposite ankle. The brachial artery systolic blood pressure is measured in a similar fashion in both arms. For the measurement of ABI, measuring the limb pressures in the following order is recommended: first

TABLE 44.	Discriminating Claudication from Pseudoclaudication	
Characteristic	**Claudication**	**Pseudoclaudication**
Nature of discomfort	Cramping, tightness, aching, fatigue	Same as claudication plus tingling, burning, numbness, weakness
Location of discomfort	Buttock, hip, thigh, calf, foot	Same as claudication; most often bilateral
Exercise-induced	Yes	Variable
Walking distance at onset of symptoms	Consistent	Variable
Discomfort occurs with standing still	No	Yes
Action for relief	Stand or sit	Sit, flexion at the waist
Time to relief	<5 minutes	≤30 minutes

TABLE 45. Clinical Examination of Patients for Peripheral Arterial Disease

Measure blood pressure in both arms (systolic blood pressure difference >15 mm Hg is suggestive of subclavian stenosis)

Auscultate for presence of arterial bruits (e.g., femoral artery)

Palpate for presence of an abdominal aortic aneurysm

Palpate and record pulses (radial, brachial, carotid, femoral, popliteal, posterior tibial, dorsalis pedis)

Evaluate for elevation pallor and dependent rubor

Inspect feet for ulcers, fissures, calluses, tinea, and tendinous xanthoma; evaluate overall skin care

arm, first PT artery, first DP artery, other PT artery, other DP artery, and other arm. If the systolic blood pressure of the first arm exceeds the systolic blood pressure of the other arm by more than 10 mm Hg, measurement of the blood pressure of the first arm should be repeated (to temper the "white coat effect" of the first measurement), and the first measurement of the first arm should be disregarded. For each leg, the ABI is calculated by dividing the ankle pressure by the higher of the two brachial pressures. In healthy persons, the ankle and arm systolic pressures are approximately the same or slightly higher in the ankle. Thus, a normal resting ABI is between 1.00 and 1.40 (**Table 46**). However, if a fixed obstruction of the arterial lumen supplying the lower extremity is present, a pressure gradient occurs, resulting in a reduced downstream pressure and concomitant reduction in the ABI (ABI <0.90). ABI values between 0.91 and 0.99 are considered borderline, and while equivocal for PAD, these patients are at increased risk for adverse cardiovascular events. An ABI greater than 1.40 is associated with calcification of the arterial wall and may occur in patients with medial calcinosis, diabetes mellitus, or end-stage kidney disease. This finding is uninterpretable, and therefore a toe-brachial index may be useful for diagnosing PAD in patients who are at risk for PAD and have an ABI above 1.40. A toe-brachial index below 0.70 is considered diagnostic of PAD. This test is typically performed in a vascular laboratory.

The sensitivity of the ABI is increased when it is measured after exercise. A common exercise protocol involves walking on a treadmill at 2 mph at a 12% incline for 5 minutes or until the patient is forced to stop because of leg pain. Alternatively,

repetitive active pedal plantar flexion ("toe ups") while standing has been proposed for an office-based assessment of postexercise ABI. In patients with even mild PAD, the ankle pressure decreases more during treadmill exercise compared with healthy patients, and the recovery time to the pre-exercise value after exercise cessation is prolonged, proportional to the severity of PAD. A decrease of the ABI by 20% after exercise suggests significant PAD.

A common procedure in many vascular laboratories is measurement of multiple or segmental pressures in the lower extremities along with pulse volume recordings, which measure the magnitude and contour of the blood pulse volume. Once a patient is placed in a supine position for 5 to 10 minutes, blood pressures are obtained at successive levels of the extremity, localizing the level of disease fairly accurately.

Noninvasive angiography may be performed for anatomic delineation of PAD in patients requiring surgical or endovascular intervention. CT angiography (CTA) is rapid and easily available but requires the administration of intravenous contrast dye. The risk of dye-induced nephropathy must be considered in patients with chronic kidney disease, especially if an endovascular repair is being contemplated, because this would entail repeat administration of iodinated contrast dye. Magnetic resonance angiography (MRA) requires intravenous gadolinium for PAD definition; gadolinium has been associated with nephrogenic systemic fibrosis in patients with severe kidney disease. Additionally, MRA may be contraindicated in patients with implanted pacemakers or cardioverter-defibrillators. Both CTA and MRA compare favorably with digital subtraction (invasive) angiography for the detection of occlusive arterial disease. CTA has additional benefits of demonstrating vascular calcification, has higher spatial resolution than MRA, and allows visualization of adjacent soft tissues and of endovascular stent grafts. Invasive angiography, in most instances, is used only as part of an interventional procedure. **H**

KEY POINTS

- An ankle-brachial index of 0.90 or below is diagnostic for peripheral arterial disease.

- An ankle-brachial index greater than 1.40 is uninterpretable, and a toe-brachial index should be obtained for diagnosing peripheral arterial disease.

- An exercise ankle-brachial index (ABI) may help establish the diagnosis of peripheral arterial disease (PAD) in patients in whom the resting ABI is equivocal; a decrease of the ABI by 20% after exercise suggests significant PAD.

Medical Therapy

The treatment of PAD has evolved over the past decade to include a broad approach, focusing on the reduction of adverse cardiovascular events, improving symptoms in claudication, and preventing tissue loss in critical limb ischemia.

TABLE 46. Interpretation of the Ankle-Brachial Index

Ankle-Brachial Index	Interpretation
>1.40	Noncompressible (calcified) vessel (uninterpretable result)
1.00-1.40	Normal
0.91-0.99	Borderline
0.41-0.90	Mild to moderate PAD
0.00-0.40	Severe PAD

PAD = peripheral arterial disease.

Cardiovascular Risk Reduction

Cigarette smoking is the strongest risk factor for PAD and for subsequent complications, and smoking cessation is imperative for patients with PAD. Smokers with PAD who quit have lower risks for myocardial infarction and stroke and an improved long-term survival versus those who continue to smoke. Cessation of cigarette smoking is also associated with a lower amputation rate, lower incidence of rest ischemia, improvement in maximal treadmill walking distance, and improved bypass graft patency rates.

A moderate- or high-intensity statin is indicated in all patients with PAD. Although no prospective statin trials have focused singularly on PAD, the Heart Protection Study (HPS) studied 6748 patients with PAD. Use of simvastatin was associated with relative reduction in overall mortality by 12%, vascular mortality by 17%, and cardiovascular events by 24% at a mean follow-up of 5 years.

Antihypertensive therapy is effective at reducing cardiovascular events in patients with PAD. Current guidelines recommend a brachial blood pressure goal of less than 140/90 mm Hg for patients with PAD. Whereas cardiovascular groups have advocated a lower target of 130/80 mm Hg for patients with PAD and diabetes or kidney disease, the recently released report of the Eighth Joint National Committee (JNC 8) suggests a therapeutic target of 140/90 mm Hg with or without diabetes or kidney disease. Data are insufficient to recommend use of one class of antihypertensive agents over another. Concern has been raised regarding the use of β-blockers in the treatment of hypertension in the setting of intermittent claudication; however, data have not supported this concern. Thus, β-blockers are not contraindicated in patients with PAD and should be used when appropriate. Nonetheless, thiazide diuretics, ACE inhibitors or angiotensin receptor blockers, and calcium channel blockers remain first-line therapy in patients with hypertension. In the Heart Outcomes Prevention Evaluation (HOPE) trial, ramipril (5 to 10 mg/d) decreased cardiovascular events in subjects with PAD with or without hypertension. The use of an ACE inhibitor is reasonable in patients with lower-extremity PAD to reduce the risk of adverse cardiovascular events.

Current guidelines recommend antiplatelet therapy in patients with PAD. Because most patients with PAD have concomitant coronary artery disease or cerebrovascular disease, aspirin is an acceptable antiplatelet agent in this setting despite the lack of good-quality evidence supporting improved outcomes in PAD. In addition to aspirin, clopidogrel (as monotherapy, not with aspirin) is a reasonable alternative strategy, and some data suggest clopidogrel may be particularly effective in patients with PAD.

Oral anticoagulation with warfarin has not been established to reduce cardiovascular events in patients with PAD because it is no more effective than antiplatelet therapy and confers a higher risk of bleeding. There are no data to suggest using newer anticoagulants in patients with PAD for the reduction of cardiovascular events.

Diabetes is one of the strongest risk factors for PAD. Although intensive diabetic control (hemoglobin $A_{1c} \leq 7\%$) can be effective to reduce microvascular complications, no prospective studies have demonstrated that this strategy reduces macrovascular complications, including PAD. In general, diabetes treatment of patients with PAD should follow current national treatment guidelines, with meticulous attention paid to foot care.

Symptom Relief

Exercise rehabilitation is a class I, level of evidence A, recommendation for the treatment of claudication in patients with PAD. Either treadmill exercise or resistance training improves functional performance, but treadmill exercise has shown greater increases in the 6-minute walk distance and in the maximum treadmill walking time compared with resistance training. Although supervised exercise therapy has statistically significant benefit on treadmill walking distance compared with non-supervised regimens, a randomized trial found benefit in both a supervised exercise and a home-based exercise program in patients with claudication. The National Institutes of Health-funded CLEVER trial evaluated the relative efficacy, safety, and health economic impact of noninvasive and endovascular treatment strategies for patients with aortoiliac PAD and claudication. Whereas supervised exercise provided a superior improvement in walking outcomes, patients undergoing endovascular repair had greater improvements in self-reported physical function.

Cilostazol is a phosphodiesterase inhibitor with antiplatelet activity and vasodilatory properties. A meta-analysis of eight randomized trials that included 2702 patients with PAD with claudication found that cilostazol improved maximum and pain-free treadmill walking distance and quality-of-life measures. Cilostazol may have an additional benefit of reducing restenosis and repeat revascularization following endovascular therapy. Because milrinone, another phosphodiesterase inhibitor, increased mortality in patients with heart failure, cilostazol should not be used in this population. In the absence of heart failure, a therapeutic trial of cilostazol should be considered in all patients with lifestyle-limiting claudication.

Pentoxifylline is a xanthine derivative that affects platelet adhesiveness and whole-blood viscosity. A meta-analysis demonstrated a modestly improved walking distance with pentoxifylline, but it was substantially less effective than either cilostazol or a supervised exercise program.

Some data have shown that therapy with statins and ACE inhibitors leads to substantial improvements in pain-free walking time and maximal walking time.

KEY POINTS

- Smoking cessation, lipid control, antiplatelet medications, and antihypertensive therapy are important components of cardiovascular risk reduction in patients with peripheral arterial disease.

- Exercise therapy and cilostazol are effective treatments for claudication.

Interventional Therapy

Endovascular or surgical revascularization is indicated for patients with significant disability due to claudication who have had an inadequate response to exercise or pharmacologic therapy, provided the benefits outweigh the risks. Revascularization should be considered in the following settings:

- The patient is significantly disabled by claudication, resulting in an inability to perform normal work or other activities that are important to the patient.

- The patient has not had an adequate response in symptom alleviation to exercise rehabilitation and pharmacologic therapy.

- The patient is able to benefit from an improvement in claudication; that is, exercise is not limited by another cause, such as angina, heart failure, lung disease, or orthopedic problems.

In addition, the characteristics of the lesion should permit appropriate intervention at low risk with a high likelihood of initial and long-term success. Inflow (aortoiliac artery) and outflow (infrapopliteal artery) should always be assessed before revascularization. Inflow lesions should be revascularized first followed by outflow lesions if bothersome symptoms persist.

Endovascular options are minimally invasive and confer a lower risk of perioperative adverse events than open surgery. The most common endovascular options include balloon angioplasty with or without stenting; other options include drug-coated balloons, lasers, atherectomy devices, and thermal devices. Endovascular treatment has become the revascularization modality of choice for aortoiliac disease in all but the most complex lesions. Endovascular procedures have high rates of procedural success, low restenosis rates, and decreased morbidity and mortality compared with open surgical repair. In patients with aortoiliac disease, primary stenting is associated with a 43% reduction in long-term failure compared with angioplasty alone. Infrainguinal (femoral, popliteal, and infrapopliteal arteries) revascularization offers less robust clinical benefit than aortoiliac revascularization. As a general rule, excellent long-term results can be achieved with intervention for short focal lesions, whereas longer lesions are associated with less durable primary patency rates following intervention. In patients with infrainguinal disease, balloon angioplasty is usually performed without stenting, as the latter procedure has significant reocclusion and restenosis rates and does not appear to improve outcomes after intervention. Recent trials suggest that use of drug-coated balloons may be an effective endovascular approach; however, long-term data are needed. Lesions with complex anatomy (for example, long-segment stenosis, multifocal stenosis, eccentric/calcified stenosis, or long-segment occlusions) may be better treated surgically.

Patients with critical limb ischemia (ABI <0.40, a flat waveform on pulse volume recording, and low or absent pedal flow on duplex ultrasonography) should be considered for immediate revascularization, either surgical or endovascular. **H**

KEY POINTS

- Endovascular or surgical revascularization is indicated for patients with significant disability due to claudication who have had an inadequate response to exercise or pharmacologic therapy.

- Patients with critical limb ischemia should be considered for immediate revascularization, either surgical or endovascular.

Acute Limb Ischemia **H**

Acute limb ischemia is an uncommon manifestation of PAD that carries significant risk of morbidity and mortality. Physical findings are characterized by the "6Ps"—Paresthesia, Pain, Pallor, Pulselessness, Poikilothermia (coolness), and Paralysis. Acute limb ischemia is caused by acute thrombosis of a limb artery or bypass graft, embolism, dissection, or trauma. Limb viability is determined by clinical findings and by the viability of tissues at the time of potential revascularization (**Table 47**). The onset of acute limb ischemia represents a true emergency. Complication rates of acute limb ischemia are high; despite urgent revascularization, amputation occurs in 10% to 15% of patients during hospitalization. Approximately 15% to 20% of patients die within 1 year after presentation.

Anticoagulation should be started as soon as the diagnosis has been made. Early consultation with a vascular specialist is appropriate. Patients with acute limb ischemia and a salvageable extremity should undergo emergent angiography to define the anatomic level of occlusion and assess treatment options. Treatment consists of surgical or percutaneous revascularization or, in selected patients, thrombolytic therapy. Catheter-directed thrombolysis is an adjunctive approach that may be useful in patients with a viable or marginally threatened limb, recent occlusion (no more than 2 weeks' duration), thrombosis of a synthetic graft or an occluded stent, and at least one identifiable distal runoff vessel. Although many patients will require revascularization following thrombolysis, the procedure is frequently less complex than if thrombolysis was not performed.

Following limb reperfusion, close monitoring is required for limb edema and tissue swelling that may cause a compartment syndrome. Symptoms and signs include severe pain, hypoesthesia, and weakness of the affected limb; myoglobinuria and increased serum creatine kinase levels often occur. If the compartment syndrome occurs, surgical fasciotomy is indicated to prevent irreversible neurologic and soft-tissue damage. **H**

TABLE 47. Categories and Prognosis of Acute Limb Ischemia

Category	Sensory Loss	Muscle Weakness	Arterial Doppler Signals	Prognosis
Viable	None	None	Audible	Not immediately threatened
Marginally threatened	None to minimal (toes)	None	Inaudible	Salvageable with prompt treatment
Immediately threatened	More than toes	Mild to moderate	Inaudible	Salvageable only with immediate revascularization
Irreversible	Profound anesthesia	Profound/paralysis	Inaudible	Not viable; major tissue loss inevitable

Adapted from Hirsch AT, Haskal ZJ, Hertzer NR, etal; American Association for Vascular Surgery; Society for Vascular Surgery; Society for Cardiovascular Angiography and Interventions; Society for Vascular Medicine and Biology; Society of Interventional Radiology; ACC/AHA Task Force on Practice Guidelines Writing Committee to Develop Guidelines for the Management of Patients With Peripheral Arterial Disease; American Association of Cardiovascular and Pulmonary Rehabilitation; National Heart, Lung, and Blood Institute; Society for Vascular Nursing; TransAtlantic Inter-Society Consensus; Vascular Disease Foundation. ACC/AHA 2005 Practice Guidelines for the management of patients with peripheral arterial disease (lower extremity, renal, mesenteric, and abdominal aortic): a collaborative report from the American Association for Vascular Surgery/Society for Vascular Surgery, Society for Cardiovascular Angiography and Interventions, Society for Vascular Medicine and Biology, Society of Interventional Radiology, and the ACC/AHA Task Force on Practice Guidelines (Writing Committee to Develop Guidelines for the Management of Patients With Peripheral Arterial Disease): endorsed by the American Association of Cardiovascular and Pulmonary Rehabilitation; National Heart, Lung, and Blood Institute; Society for Vascular Nursing; TransAtlantic Inter-Society Consensus; and Vascular Disease Foundation. Circulation. 2006 Mar 21;113(11):e488. [PMID: 16549646]

KEY POINTS

- Physical findings of acute limb ischemia are characterized by the "6Ps"—Paresthesia, Pain, Pallor, Pulselessness, Poikilothermia (coolness), and Paralysis.

- Patients with acute limb ischemia should receive immediate anticoagulation therapy; those with a salvageable extremity should undergo an emergent evaluation that defines the anatomic level of occlusion and leads to prompt endovascular or surgical revascularization.

- Following limb reperfusion in patients with acute limb ischemia, close monitoring is required for limb edema and tissue swelling that may cause a compartment syndrome.

Cardiovascular Disease in Cancer Survivors

Cardiotoxicity of Radiation Therapy to the Thorax

Chest radiation therapy is associated with significant cardiotoxicity, which can manifest as a complex, life-threatening disorder. Radiation-induced toxicity can affect nearly every component of the cardiovascular system, with manifestations such as pericarditis (acute or chronic), cardiomyopathy, aortitis, conduction system disease, valvulopathy, and coronary artery disease (**Table 48**). These pathologic alterations are likely caused by the generation of reactive oxygen species from irradiation, which leads to blood vessel injury and a cascade of inflammation, ischemia with loss of capillary density, and fibrosis of the cardiovascular structures.

Although pericarditis may occur acutely with chest radiation, manifestations of radiation-induced cardiotoxicity frequently develop after a long indolent period (5 to 20 years or later) owing to the chronic nature of the pathology and therefore require a high index of suspicion in at-risk patients. The clinical manifestations are related to the affected portion of the cardiovascular system. Myocardial fibrosis leads to a restrictive cardiomyopathy, resulting in poor chamber compliance and diastolic heart failure (see Myocardial Disease). Signs of restrictive cardiomyopathy have been reported in 15% to 50% of patients with previously treated Hodgkin lymphoma and are more evident in those who have received therapy with cardiotoxic drugs. Constrictive pericarditis also frequently is present. The potential for coexistent constrictive pericarditis and restrictive cardiomyopathy presents significant challenges in the management of these patients, as the clinical manifestations frequently overlap while the treatments for these two disorders vary considerably (that is, pericardiectomy versus cardiac transplantation). Pericardial effusion is particularly common in patients treated for esophageal cancer (approximately 25%), with a median presentation time of 5 months after therapy in one report. Any cardiac valve can be affected by radiation injury (5%-40% of patients), although left-sided lesions predominate and frequently occur with mixed stenosis and regurgitation. Coronary artery disease typically is ostial or proximal in location; microvasculopathy (disease involving vessels that are not epicardial in location) also can occur.

Recognition of the potential for cardiotoxicity has led to reductions in radiation exposure in the treatment of chest malignancy. Most contemporary studies have demonstrated significant decreases in cardiac mortality in comparison with historical studies. However, the increased risk of cardiotoxicity and death due to vascular complications attributable to radiation therapy remains. Thus, lifetime clinical monitoring for

TABLE 48.	Cardiotoxicity of Radiation Therapy to the Thorax	
Manifestations	**Clinical Onset After Radiation Therapy**	**Comments**
Acute pericarditis or pericardial effusion	As early as 2 months, but 5 months on average	A common cardiac complication historically (25%), less common now (2%) owing to methods minimizing mediastinal irradiation
Pericardial fibrosis and constriction	As early as 1.5 years, but often 10 to 15 years or more	Risk persists for >25 years
		RV more extensively involved, leading to marked findings of RV failure
Accelerated coronary atherosclerosis	Average onset 7 years	Predilection for involvement of ostia or proximal segments of coronary arteries
		Patients with traditional risk factors for CAD are at higher risk
		May manifest as myocardial infarction
		Sudden death may occur rarely
Valvular fibrosis and regurgitation	10 to 25 years or more	Frequency greater in left- vs. right-sided valves
		Clinically significant aortic regurgitation may occur in ≥25% of long-term survivors
		Slowly progressive and requires lifelong monitoring
		Concomitant anthracycline use increases risk
Myocardial fibrosis, diastolic dysfunction, and restrictive cardiomyopathy	Years	Concomitant anthracycline use increases risk for heart failure
Fibrosis of conduction pathways leading to bradycardia, dysrhythmias, or heart block	Years or decades	

CAD = coronary artery disease; RV = right ventricle.

radiation-induced cardiotoxicity is warranted owing to the chronic, lethal nature of this complication. Propensity for radiation-induced injury is related to younger age at treatment, female sex, radiation exposure (total dose, dose per fraction, and cardiac chamber affected), the use of concomitant cardiotoxic drugs (such as anthracyclines), and the presence of cardiac risk factors (hypertension, smoking, hyperlipidemia). There is no clearly defined threshold of radiation exposure for cardiotoxicity risk. In all patients with a history of significant chest radiation, aggressive management of risk factors for atherosclerosis is warranted owing to the heightened risk of ischemic heart disease in these patients.

Although contemporary studies have shown a lower incidence of radiation-induced cardiotoxicity, the follow-up in these studies has been relatively short (frequently 5 to 10 years) and thus may be inadequate to ascertain the indolent effects of radiation-induced cardiotoxicity. Recent analyses frequently have focused on mortality rates without detailed examinations of other complications, such as myopathy, valvular disease, and constrictive pericarditis. The timing and clinical methods for serial monitoring have not been defined, but cardiotoxicity should be considered in any patient with symptoms or signs of cardiovascular disease and a history of chest radiation.

Owing to the frequent multiple cardiac pathologies in these patients, management of radiation-induced heart disease can be challenging. Treatment is directed primarily toward the predominant pathology, although it is recognized that concomitant abnormalities increase the surgical procedural risk. For example, patients undergoing pericardiectomy will be at significant operative risk owing to the propensity for increased surgical bleeding and myopathy in these patients. Thus, a high degree of individualization of the treatment plan for patients with radiation-induced heart disease is recommended.

KEY POINTS

- In all patients with a history of significant chest radiation, aggressive management of risk factors for atherosclerosis is warranted owing to the heightened risk of ischemic heart disease in these patients.
- Cardiotoxicity should be considered in any patient with a history of chest radiation who develops symptoms or signs of cardiovascular disease.

Cardiotoxicity of Chemotherapy

Cardiotoxicity from chemotherapy can result from traditional cytotoxic chemotherapy agents, such as anthracyclines (doxorubicin, daunorubicin, mitoxantrone), as well as from newer agents, such as monoclonal antibodies (trastuzumab) and tyrosine kinase inhibitors. Cardiotoxicity can occur in patients with normal hearts but is more common in patients with preexisting cardiac disease. Cardiotoxicity from these agents can manifest as dilated cardiomyopathy, myocardial ischemia from coronary vasospasm, or arrhythmias (**Table 49**).

The cardiotoxic effects of chemotherapy can be short-term, intermediate, or long-term. 5-Fluorouracil is associated with a high incidence of acute chest pain and electrocardiographic changes (70% within 72 hours of the first treatment cycle), resulting in death in 2% to 8% of patients affected by 5-fluorouracil toxicity.

Early manifestations of anthracycline toxicity are relatively uncommon (3%) and include high-grade heart block, supraventricular and ventricular arrhythmias, heart failure, myocarditis, and pericarditis, with resolution in many patients

occurring within 1 week after presentation. Chronic cardiotoxicity due to anthracyclines, which begins with a subclinical decline in systolic and diastolic function, manifests with symptoms usually within months after completion of chemotherapy. However, cardiotoxicity from anthracyclines can have long latency periods (10 years or more).

The strongest risk factor for cardiotoxicity related to anthracycline agents is cumulative dose. The incidence of cardiotoxicity for doxorubicin or daunorubicin has been reported to be less than 1% for cumulative dose of less than 400 mg/m^2, but 26% for cumulative doses of 550 mg/m^2 or more. It is generally accepted that maximum cumulative doses for these drugs should be limited to 450 to 500 mg/m^2, but the doses

TABLE 49. Late-Onset Cardiotoxicity of Chemotherapeutic Agents[a]	
Drug	**Cardiotoxicity**
Anthracyclines	Synergistic toxicity when administered with nonanthracycline agents
Doxorubicin	Heart failure (1.6%-5%)
	Higher in elderly women
	Typically irreversible
	Improved by aggressive treatment (resynchronization therapy)
	Left ventricular dysfunction (progression slowed by standard treatment)
	Dilated cardiomyopathy (odds ratio: 6.25[b])
	Cardiac death (odds ratio: 4.94[b])
Daunorubicin	Presumably similar to doxorubicin
Epirubicin	Heart failure (<5% with appropriate dosing)
Mitoxantrone	Heart failure
	Incidence significantly increased with dose >160 mg/m^2
	Survival improved by standard heart failure treatment
	Left ventricular dysfunction
Alkylating agents	
Cyclophosphamide	Heart failure (dose dependent)
	Left ventricular dysfunction (3%-5% with dose >100 mg/kg)
Cisplatin	Heart failure
Mitomycin	Cardiomyopathy
5-Fluorouracil	Vasospasm (common) and heart failure (rare) from myocardial infarction occurring during treatment
Paclitaxel	Heart failure (if given with doxorubicin)
Trastuzumab	Heart failure
	0.6% (NYHA class III or IV)
	1.5% (NYHA class II at 2 y)
	Left ventricular dysfunction (3%; asymptomatic and reversible)
	Not dose dependent
Interleukin-2	Heart failure from previous cardiomyopathy, myocarditis, or myocardial infarction occurring during treatment (rare)
Interferon-α	Heart failure from previous myocardial infarction during treatment (rare)

NYHA = New York Heart Association.

[a]Cardiotoxicity emerging 1 year or more after chemotherapy.

[b]When an anthracycline is added to chemotherapy regimen.

that lead to toxic responses vary considerably among individual patients. Other risk factors for cardiotoxicity include age at treatment, concomitant therapy with other cardiotoxic agents, chest radiation, and preexisting cardiac disease. The toxic responses to anthracyclines can be modified by liposome encapsulation of the molecule, infusional rather than bolus administration, use of structural analogues (epirubicin and mitoxantrone), and adjunctive cardioprotective agents. Dexrazoxane is an EDTA chelator that reduces the risk of chronic cardiotoxicity associated with doxorubicin and epirubicin and may be considered in patients being treated with high anthracycline doses (>300 mg/m^2).

Cardiotoxicity due to trastuzumab typically causes a chronic, asymptomatic decline in ventricular function with a low frequency of overt heart failure (3%-7%). Older patients (age >50 years) and those with prior or concomitant exposure to anthracyclines are at increased risk of trastuzumab-induced cardiotoxicity. In most patients, cardiotoxicity due to trastuzumab is related to changes in contractility and is reversible. Unlike anthracyclines, trastuzumab-related cardiotoxicity is not dose related and patients can be successfully rechallenged after recovery of ventricular function.

Kinase inhibitors, such as tyrosine kinase inhibitors, are a relatively new approach to tumor receptor–targeted therapy. Hypertension is a potential adverse effect that may require dose adjustment or, in patients with severe hypertension, discontinuation of the kinase inhibitor.

In adult patients being considered for chemotherapy with anthracyclines, baseline evaluation of left ventricular function should be considered before initiation of therapy, although the need for this assessment is controversial in patients with no symptoms or signs of abnormal left ventricular function and in whom the cumulative dose is expected to be low (<300 mg/m^2). For patients who receive treatment with trastuzumab, a baseline evaluation of left ventricular function should be performed, particularly if there is a history of anthracycline use. Routine surveillance of cardiac function using echocardiography should be performed in all patients with assessment of left ventricular ejection fraction as well as indices of diastolic function. The timing intervals for these assessments are individualized based on the patient's baseline function, chemotherapeutic regimen, risk profile, and evidence of change in function in serial evaluations.

In adults undergoing doxorubicin therapy, the drug should be discontinued if there is evidence of heart failure, a 10% or greater decline in left ventricular ejection fraction to below the lower limit of normal, an absolute left ventricular ejection fraction of less than 45%, or a 20% decline in left ventricular ejection fraction to any level. Owing to the reversible nature of cardiotoxicity related to trastuzumab, this therapy can be resumed after recovery of left ventricular function in selected patients.

Although other echocardiographic indices (such as strain imaging or volume measurements) and serum markers (cardiac troponin, B-type natriuretic peptide) have been proposed for serial monitoring of patients who have undergone chemotherapy, the thresholds for these markers as well as the appropriate timing for their measurement remain uncertain. Patients who have left ventricular dysfunction should receive appropriate therapy with β-blockers, vasodilators, and diuretics as in patients with heart failure disorders not related to chemotherapy toxicity.

KEY POINTS

- Hypertension is a potential adverse effect of kinase inhibitors that may require dose adjustment or, in patients with severe hypertension, discontinuation of the kinase inhibitor.

- Cardiotoxicity related to trastuzumab is not dose related and is reversible.

- Chronic cardiotoxicity with anthracyclines is dose related and is not reversible.

- In patients who have undergone chemotherapy, baseline evaluation and routine surveillance of cardiac function using echocardiography should be performed with assessment of left ventricular ejection fraction as well as indices of diastolic function.

Pregnancy and Cardiovascular Disease

Cardiovascular Changes During Pregnancy

Understanding the normal physiologic changes of pregnancy is important in the interpretation of signs and symptoms in the pregnant patient (**Table 50**). During a normal pregnancy, there is an increase in plasma volume and a lesser increase in erythrocyte mass, resulting in increased total blood volume and relative anemia. The systemic vascular resistance decreases during pregnancy, but the heart rate and cardiac output rise; as a result, there is generally a slight reduction in mean arterial pressure. Maternal cardiac output peaks at approximately 40% above the prepregnancy level by the 32nd week of pregnancy and then plateaus until delivery. During delivery, heart rate and blood pressure increase, leading to a rise in cardiac output to as much as 80% above the prepregnancy level.

Prepregnancy Evaluation

Prepregnancy evaluation is recommended for all women with cardiovascular disease who are anticipating pregnancy. Patients with congenital heart disease should consult with a cardiologist specializing in congenital conditions and a high-risk obstetrician to discuss the need for genetic counseling, evaluate the risks of future pregnancy, and develop a plan for management during labor and the postpartum period.

TABLE 50. Normal Versus Abnormal Cardiac Symptoms and Signs in Pregnancy

Symptom or Sign	Normal	Pathologic
Shortness of breath	Mild, with exertion	Orthopnea, PND, cough
Palpitations	Atrial and ventricular premature beats	Atrial fibrillation or flutter; ventricular tachycardia
Chest pain	No	Chest pressure, heaviness, or pain
Murmur	Basal systolic murmur grade 1/6 or 2/6 present in 80% of pregnant women	Systolic murmur grade ≥3/6; any diastolic murmur
Tachycardia	Heart rate increased by 20%-30%	Heart rate >100/min
Low blood pressure	Blood pressure typically is modestly decreased (~10 mm Hg)	Low blood pressure associated with symptoms
Edema	Mild peripheral	Pulmonary edema
Gallop	S_3	S_4

PND = paroxysmal nocturnal dyspnea.

The CARPREG index is used to estimate risk for cardiovascular complications during pregnancy in women with cardiovascular disease (**Table 51**). Women with severe pulmonary hypertension (pulmonary artery pressure ≥ two-thirds systemic pressure) are at high risk during pregnancy, with an estimated maternal mortality rate between 30% and 50%. Systolic ventricular dysfunction (ejection fraction <40%) with New York Heart Association (NYHA) functional class III or IV heart failure confers a high risk of maternal and fetal complications and is considered a contraindication to pregnancy.

Patients with severe obstructive cardiac disease, such as mitral or aortic valve stenosis, are generally considered for intervention before pregnancy, even if asymptomatic.

KEY POINTS

- Women with severe pulmonary hypertension are at high risk for pregnancy-related death.
- Systolic ventricular dysfunction (ejection fraction <40%) with New York Heart Association (NYHA) functional class III or IV heart failure is considered a contraindication to pregnancy.

Management of Cardiovascular Disease During Pregnancy

Because pregnancy involves an increase in blood volume and cardiac output, women with severe obstructive cardiac lesions

TABLE 51. Predictors of Maternal Cardiac Events in Women with Congenital or Acquired Cardiac Disease (CARPREG Index)

Risk Factor (Predictor)	Operational Definition
Previous cardiac event or arrhythmia	Heart failure, transient ischemic attack, stroke, arrhythmia
Baseline NYHA functional class III or IV or cyanosis	Mild symptoms (mild shortness of breath and/or angina) and slight limitation during ordinary activity
Left-sided heart obstruction	Mitral valve area <2 cm²; aortic valve area <1.5 cm² or resting peak left ventricular outflow tract gradient >30 mm Hg
Reduced systemic ventricular systolic function	Ejection fraction <40%

Estimated Risk for Cardiac Events[a]		
No. of Predictors	**Estimated Risk (%)**	**Recommendation**
0	4	Consider preconception cardiac intervention for specific lesions; increase frequency of follow-up; delivery at community hospital
1	31	Consider preconception cardiac intervention for specific lesions; refer to regional center for ongoing care
>1	69	Consider preconception cardiac intervention for specific lesions; refer to regional center for ongoing care

NYHA = New York Heart Association.

[a]Pulmonary edema, tachyarrhythmia, embolic stroke, cardiac death.

Data and recommendations from Siu SC, Sermer M, Colman JM, et al. Cardiac Disease in Pregnancy (CARPREG) Investigators. Prospective multicenter study of pregnancy outcomes in women with heart disease. Circulation. 2001;104(5):515-521. [PMID: 11479246] generally develop symptoms during pregnancy, whereas women with regurgitant valve lesions tolerate pregnancy reasonably well.

Vaginal delivery is generally preferred for patients with cardiovascular disease because it results in a shorter and less marked hemodynamic derangement than cesarean delivery. To reduce the risk of fetal intracranial hemorrhage, cesarean delivery is recommended in women receiving warfarin anticoagulation therapy. Cesarean delivery is also recommended for obstetric reasons and in select patients with severe pulmonary hypertension or a markedly dilated aorta.

Peripartum Cardiomyopathy

Left ventricular systolic dysfunction identified toward the end of pregnancy or in the months following delivery in the absence of another identifiable cause is known as peripartum cardiomyopathy. This occurs with increased frequency in women who are multiparous, older (age >30 years), and black; in those with multifetal pregnancy, gestational hypertension, or preeclampsia; and in those treated with tocolytic agents.

The leading cause of pregnancy-related maternal death in North America is peripartum cardiomyopathy. Death in women with peripartum cardiomyopathy results from heart failure, thromboembolic events, and arrhythmias. Half of women who develop peripartum cardiomyopathy show improvement in left ventricular function within 6 months of delivery, and 20% to 40% have normalization of ventricular function.

Prompt initiation of medical therapy is recommended for women with peripartum cardiomyopathy and includes β-blockers, digoxin, hydralazine, nitrates, and diuretics. ACE inhibitors, angiotensin receptor blockers, and aldosterone antagonists should be avoided until after delivery owing to teratogenicity. Anticoagulation with warfarin is recommended for women with peripartum cardiomyopathy with left ventricular ejection fraction below 35%, owing to the increased risk of thromboembolism related to this disorder; the duration of anticoagulation is individualized, and anticoagulation is discontinued when the ejection fraction improves.

In women with acute severe peripartum cardiomyopathy, bromocriptine, which blocks prolactin secretion, has been shown to improve left ventricular ejection fraction and clinical outcomes when added to peripartum-related heart failure therapy. Bromocriptine inhibits lactation and may increase risk of thromboembolism; therefore, anticoagulation is suggested in conjunction with bromocriptine. For these reasons, discussion with the patient is an important precursor to initiating therapy. Referral for ventricular assist device or heart transplantation should be considered for women with refractory severe heart failure related to peripartum cardiomyopathy.

Women with peripartum cardiomyopathy with persistent left ventricular dysfunction should be counseled to avoid subsequent pregnancy since another pregnancy is often associated with recurrent or further reduction of left ventricular function, which can result in clinical deterioration or even death.

Other Cardiovascular Disorders

Women with Marfan syndrome have been reported to have an increased risk of aortic dissection during pregnancy. Women with Marfan syndrome and an ascending aortic diameter of 4.5 cm or greater are recommended to have aortic repair surgery before considering pregnancy to reduce this risk. Some women with Marfan syndrome and aortic diameter less than 4.5 cm are at high risk for dissection during pregnancy and are counseled to have aortic valve replacement before pregnancy; these include patients with rapid dilatation of the ascending aorta or a family history of aortic dissection.

Spontaneous coronary artery dissections in women without risk factors for coronary artery disease may occur in the peripartum setting. Spontaneous healing may occur with conservative medical therapy, but revascularization, either percutaneous or bypass surgery, has been utilized as well.

Cardiovascular Medication Use During Pregnancy

Limited data are available on the safety of cardiovascular medications administered during pregnancy. The FDA categorizes drugs by their fetal effects during pregnancy (see MKSAP 17 General Internal Medicine, Women's Health). Most cardiovascular drugs are not FDA-approved for use during pregnancy. General guidelines for the use of several cardiovascular drugs during pregnancy are provided in **Table 52**. Cardiovascular medications should be used only when needed and at the lowest possible dose, and the desired therapeutic effect should outweigh the risk.

When β-blockers are used during pregnancy or lactation, periodic fetal and newborn heart rate monitoring and initial newborn blood glucose assessment are indicated because β-blockers cross the placenta and are present in human breast milk. Atenolol is usually avoided during pregnancy because it has been reported to cause small fetal gestational size, early delivery, and low birth weight. Patients taking atenolol are usually transitioned to a different β-blocker.

The treatment of choice for acute symptomatic supraventricular tachycardia during pregnancy is adenosine. Recurrent tachycardia symptoms are often treated with β-blockers and digoxin; sotalol and flecainide have also been safely used. Amiodarone is rarely used owing to toxicity concerns.

Spironolactone is considered compatible with breastfeeding; although spironolactone and its active metabolite, canrenone, appear in breast milk, the concentrations are pharmacologically insignificant. ACE inhibitors, angiotensin receptor blockers, and aldosterone antagonists are teratogenic and should be avoided during pregnancy. Some ACE inhibitors are safe to use while breastfeeding. Angiotensin receptor blockers are generally avoided during lactation because data are inconclusive regarding infant risk when used during breastfeeding.

TABLE 52. Drugs for Cardiac Disorders in Pregnancy			
Drug	**Use in Pregnancy**	**Compatibility with Breastfeeding**	**Comments**
ACE inhibitors			
Captopril, enalapril	No	Yes	Teratogenic in first trimester; cause fetal/neonatal kidney failure with second or third trimester exposure; scleroderma renal crisis is only indication
Lisinopril	No	?	Same as above
ARBs	No	?	Teratogenic in first trimester; cause fetal/neonatal kidney failure with second or third trimester exposure
Adenosine	Yes	?	No change in fetal heart rate when used for supraventricular tachycardia
Amiodarone	No	No	Fetal hypothyroidism, prematurity
Antiplatelet agents			
Dipyridamole, clopidogrel	Yes	?	Second-line agent; no evidence of harm in animal clopidogrel studies; no human data
Aspirin (≤81 mg)	Yes	Yes	
β-Blockers			
Atenolol	Yes	No	Second-line agent; low birth weight, intrauterine growth restriction
Esmolol	Yes	?	Second-line agent; more pronounced bradycardia
Labetalol	Yes	Yes	Preferred drug in class
Metoprolol	Yes	Yes	Shortened half-life
Propranolol	Yes	Yes	Second-line agent; intrauterine growth restriction
Sotalol	Yes	?	Second-line agent; insufficient data; reserve use for arrhythmia not responding to alternative agent
Calcium channel blockers			
Diltiazem, verapamil	Yes	Yes	Second-line agent; maternal hypotension with rapid intravenous infusion; used for fetal supraventricular tachycardia
Digoxin	Yes	Yes	Second-line agent; shortened half-life
Disopyramide	Yes	Yes	Second-line agent; case reports of preterm labor
Diuretics	Yes	Yes	Second-line agent; use when needed for maternal volume overload only
Flecainide	Yes	?	Second-line agent; inadequate data but used for fetal arrhythmia; case report of fetal hyperbilirubinemia
Hydralazine	Yes	Yes	Vasodilator of choice
Lidocaine	Yes	Yes	Treatment of choice for ventricular arrhythmias
Sodium nitroprusside	No	No	Potential fetal thiocyanate toxicity
Organic nitrates	Yes	?	No apparent increased risk
Phenytoin	No	Yes	Known teratogenicity and bleeding risk; last resort for arrhythmia
Procainamide	Yes	Yes	Used for fetal arrhythmia
Propafenone	Yes	?	Second-line agent; used for fetal arrhythmia
Quinidine	Yes	Yes	Preferred drug in class; increases digoxin levels

ARB = angiotensin receptor blocker; ? = unknown.

Adapted from Rosene-Montella K, Keely EJ, Lee RV, Barbour LA. Medical Care of the Pregnant Patient. 2nd Edition. Philadelphia, PA: American College of Physicians; 2008. p 356-357. Copyright 2008, American College of Physicians.

Anticoagulation Therapy During Pregnancy

Pregnancy is a hypercoagulable state, and anticoagulation is often indicated during pregnancy; regimens and levels of anticoagulation depend on the specific indication (**Table 53**). Prepregnancy counseling is recommended for all women receiving chronic warfarin anticoagulation to help them understand maternal and fetal risk and to make an informed decision regarding which anticoagulation regimen to use during their pregnancy.

Unfractionated heparin, low-molecular-weight heparin (LMWH), and warfarin can all be used for anticoagulation during pregnancy. Meticulous monitoring and dose adjustment are recommended for all anticoagulation regimens. Warfarin is stopped before delivery owing to the risk of fetal intracranial hemorrhage if spontaneous labor occurs while the mother, and thus the fetus, is anticoagulated with warfarin.

Women with mechanical valve prostheses represent a high-risk subset of patients during pregnancy, with excess risk of valve thrombosis, bleeding, and fetal morbidity and mortality. The optimal anticoagulation regimen for this patient group has not been established. Warfarin anticoagulation during pregnancy may be the safest agent for prevention of maternal prosthetic valve thrombosis; however, warfarin poses an

TABLE 53. Anticoagulation Regimens During Pregnancy	
Weeks of Gestation	**Recommended Regimen**
Venous Thromboembolism	
Weeks 6-12	Warfarin (if dose to attain INR 2-3 is ≤5 mg)
	UFH (IV or SQ; aPTT 2 × control)
	Weight-based LMWH
Weeks 13-37	UFH (SQ; aPTT 2 × control)
	Weight-based LMWH
	Warfarin (INR 2-3)
Weeks 37 to term	UFH (IV; aPTT 2 × control)
Atrial Fibrillation	
Weeks 6-12	Warfarin (if dose to attain INR 2-3 is ≤5 mg)
	UFH (IV or SQ; aPTT 2 × control)
	Weight-based LMWH
Weeks 13-37	UFH (SQ; aPTT 2 × control)
	Weight-based LMWH
	Warfarin (INR 2-3)
Weeks 37 to term	UFH (IV; aPTT 2 × control)
Mechanical Valve Prosthesis	
Weeks 6-12	Warfarin dose ≤5 mg for therapeutic INR
	Continue warfarin (class IIa)
	UFH: IV; aPTT 2 × control (class IIb)
	Anti-factor Xa adjusted LMWH (class IIb)
	Warfarin dose >5 mg for therapeutic INR
	UFH: IV; aPTT 2 × control (class IIa)
	Anti-factor Xa adjusted LMWH (class IIa)
Weeks 13-37	Warfarin (therapeutic INR)
Weeks 37 to term	UFH (IV; aPTT 2 × control)

aPTT = activated partial thromboplastin time; IV = intravenous; LMWH = low-molecular-weight heparin; SQ = subcutaneous; UFH = unfractionated heparin.

Recommendations from Nishimura RA, Otto CM, Bonow RO, et al; American College of Cardiology/American Heart Association Task Force on Practice Guidelines. 2014 AHA/ACC guideline for the management of patients with valvular heart disease: executive summary: a report of the American College of Cardiology/American Heart Association Task Force on Practice Guidelines. J Am Coll Cardiol. 2014 Jun 10;63(22):2438-88. Erratum in: J Am Coll Cardiol. 2014 Jun 10;63(22):2489. [PMID: 24603192] and Bates SM, Greer IA, Middeldorp S, Veenstra DL, Prabulos AM, Vandvik PO; American College of Chest Physicians. VTE, thrombophilia, antithrombotic therapy, and pregnancy: Antithrombotic Therapy and Prevention of Thrombosis (9th edition): American College of Chest Physicians Evidence-Based Clinical Practice Guidelines. Chest. 2012 Feb;141(2 Suppl):e691S-736S. [PMID: 22315276] and Furie KL, Kasner SE, Adams RJ, et al; American Heart Association Stroke Council, Council on Cardiovascular Nursing, Council on Clinical Cardiology, and Interdisciplinary Council on Quality of Care and Outcomes Research. Guidelines for the prevention of stroke in patients with stroke or transient ischemic attack: a guideline for healthcare professionals from the American Heart Association/American Stroke Association. Stroke. 2011 Jan;42(1):227-276. [PMID: 20966421] increased fetal risk, with possible teratogenicity, miscarriage, and fetal loss due to intracranial hemorrhage. Data suggest that LMWH and unfractionated heparin are safer for the fetus than warfarin, but these therapies appear to increase the risk of maternal prosthetic valve thrombosis.

Guidelines from the American College of Cardiology/ American Heart Association on the management of anticoagulation during pregnancy conclude that intravenous unfractionated heparin, LMWH, or warfarin may be used for anticoagulation of pregnant women with mechanical heart valves. Intravenous unfractionated heparin is the drug of choice for patients with mechanical valve prostheses around the time of delivery.

KEY POINTS

- Women with Marfan syndrome and an ascending aortic diameter of 4.5 cm or greater are recommended to have aortic repair surgery before considering pregnancy to reduce the risk of aortic dissection.

- ACE inhibitors, angiotensin receptor blockers, and aldosterone antagonists are teratogenic and should be avoided during pregnancy.

- Unfractionated heparin, low-molecular-weight heparin, or warfarin may be used for anticoagulation of pregnant women with mechanical heart valves; unfractionated heparin is the drug of choice for patients with mechanical valve prostheses around the time of delivery.

Bibliography

Epidemiology and Risk Factors

Dhawan SS, Quyyumi AA. Rheumatoid arthritis and cardiovascular disease. Curr Atheroscler Rep. 2008 Apr;10(2):128-33. [PMID: 18417067]

Go AS, Mozaffarian D, Roger VL, et al; American Heart Association Statistics Committee and Stroke Statistics Subcommittee. Heart disease and stroke statistics--2013 update: a report from the American Heart Association. Circulation. 2013 Jan 1;127(1):e6-e245. Erratum in: Circulation. 2013 Jan 1;127 (1). Erratum in: Circulation. 2013 Jun 11;127(23):e841. [PMID: 23239837]

Greenland P, Alpert JS, Beller GA, et al; American College of Cardiology Foundation; American Heart Association. 2010 ACCF/AHA guideline for assessment of cardiovascular risk in asymptomatic adults: a report of the American College of Cardiology Foundation/American Heart Association Task Force on Practice Guidelines. J Am Coll Cardiol. 2010 Dec 14;56(25):e50-103. [PMID: 21144964]

Pignone M, Alberts MJ, Colwell JA, et al. Aspirin for primary prevention of cardiovascular events in people with diabetes: a position statement of the American Diabetes Association, a scientific statement of the American Heart Association, and an expert consensus document of the American College of Cardiology Foundation. Circulation. 2010 Jun 22;121(24):2694-701. [PMID: 20508178]

Schoenfeld SR, Kasturi S, Costenbaker KH. The epidemiology of atherosclerotic cardiovascular disease among patients with SLE: a systematic review. Semin Arthritis Rheum. 2013 Aug;43(1):77-95. [PMID: 23422269]

U.S. Preventive Services Task Force. Aspirin for the Prevention of Cardiovascular Disease. www.uspreventiveservicestaskforce.org/uspstf/ uspsasmi.htm. Updated October 2013. Accessed October 1, 2014.

Yusuf S, Hawken S, Ounpuu S, et al; INTERHEART Study Investigators. Effect of potentially modifiable risk factors associated with myocardial infarction in 52 countries (the INTERHEART study): case-control study. Lancet. 2004 Sep 11-17;364(9438):937-52. [PMID: 15364185]

Yusuf S, Reddy S, Ounpuu S, et al. Global burden of cardiovascular diseases. Part II: Variations in cardiovascular disease by specific ethnic groups and geographic regions and prevention strategies. Circulation. 2001 Dec 4;104(23):2855-64. [PMID: 11733407]

Diagnostic Testing in Cardiology

American College of Cardiology Foundation Task Force on Expert Consensus Documents, Hundley WG, Bluemke DA, Finn JP, et al. ACCF/ACR/AHA/ NASCI/SCMR 2010 expert consensus document on cardiovascular magnetic resonance: a report of the American College of Cardiology Foundation Task Force on Expert Consensus Documents. J Am Coll Cardiol. 2010 Jun 8;55(23):2614-62. [PMID: 20513610]

American College of Cardiology Foundation Task Force on Expert Consensus Documents, Mark DB, Berman DS, Budoff MJ, et al. ACCF/ACR/AHA/ NASCI/SAIP/SCAI/SCCT 2010 expert consensus document on coronary computed tomographic angiography: a report of the American College of Cardiology Foundation Task Force on Expert Consensus Documents. J Am Coll Cardiol. 2010 Jun 8;55(23):2663-99. [PMID: 20513611]

American College of Cardiology Foundation Appropriate Use Criteria Task Force; American Society of Echocardiography; American Heart Association; American Society of Nuclear Cardiology; Heart Failure Society of America; Heart Rhythm Society; Society for Cardiovascular Angiography and Interventions; Society of Critical Care Medicine; Society of Cardiovascular Computed Tomography; Society for Cardiovascular Magnetic Resonance, Douglas PS, Garcia MJ, Haines DE, et al. ACCF/ASE/AHA/ASNC/HFSA/ HRS/SCAI/SCCM/SCCT/SCMR 2011 Appropriate Use Criteria for Echocardiography. A Report of the American College of Cardiology Foundation Appropriate Use Criteria Task Force, American Society of Echocardiography, American Heart Association, American Society of Nuclear Cardiology, Heart Failure Society of America, Heart Rhythm Society, Society for Cardiovascular Angiography and Interventions, Society of Critical Care Medicine, Society of Cardiovascular Computed Tomography, and Society for Cardiovascular Magnetic Resonance Endorsed by the American College of Chest Physicians. J Am Coll Cardiol. 2011 Mar 1;57(9):1126-66. [PMID: 21349406]

Fihn SD, Blankenship JC, Alexander KP, et al. 2014 ACC/AHA/AATS/PCNA/ SCAI/STS Focused Update of the Guideline for the Diagnosis and Management of Patients With Stable Ischemic Heart Disease: A Report of the American College of Cardiology/American Heart Association Task Force on Practice Guidelines, and the American Association for Thoracic Surgery, Preventive Cardiovascular Nurses Association, Society for Cardiovascular Angiography and Interventions, and Society of Thoracic Surgeons. Circulation. 2014 Nov 4;130(19):1749-67. [PMID: 25070666]

Greenland P, Alpert JS, Beller GA, et al; American College of Cardiology Foundation; American Heart Association. 2010 ACCF/AHA guideline for assessment of cardiovascular risk in asymptomatic adults: a report of the American College of Cardiology Foundation/American Heart Association Task Force on Practice Guidelines. J Am Coll Cardiol. 2010 Dec 14;56(25):e50-103. [PMID: 21144964]

Greenland P, Bonow RO, Brundage BH, et al; American College of Cardiology Foundation Clinical Expert Consensus Task Force (ACCF/AHA Writing Committee to Update the 2000 Expert Consensus Document on Electron Beam Computed Tomography); Society of Atherosclerosis Imaging and Prevention; Society of Cardiovascular Computed Tomography. ACCF/AHA 2007 clinical expert consensus document on coronary artery calcium scoring by computed tomography in global cardiovascular risk assessment and in evaluation of patients with chest pain: a report of the American College of Cardiology Foundation Clinical Expert Consensus Task Force (ACCF/ AHA Writing Committee to Update the 2000 Expert Consensus Document on Electron Beam Computed Tomography) developed in collaboration with the Society of Atherosclerosis Imaging and Prevention and the Society of Cardiovascular Computed Tomography. J Am Coll Cardiol. 2007 Jan 23;49(3):378-402. [PMID: 17239724]

Hendel RC, Berman DS, Di Carli MF, et al; American College of Cardiology Foundation Appropriate Use Criteria Task Force; American Society of Nuclear Cardiology; American College of Radiology; American Heart Association; American Society of Echocardiology; Society of Cardiovascular Computed Tomography; Society for Cardiovascular Magnetic Resonance; Society of Nuclear Medicine. ACCF/ASNC/ACR/AHA/ASE/SCCT/SCMR/ SNM 2009 Appropriate Use Criteria for Cardiac Radionuclide Imaging: A Report of the American College of Cardiology Foundation Appropriate Use Criteria Task Force, the American Society of Nuclear Cardiology, the American College of Radiology, the American Heart Association, the American Society of Echocardiography, the Society of Cardiovascular Computed Tomography, the Society for Cardiovascular Magnetic Resonance, and the Society of Nuclear Medicine. J Am Coll Cardiol. 2009 Jun 9;53(23):2201-29. [PMID: 19497454]

Coronary Artery Disease

Amsterdam EA, Wenger NK, Brindis RG, et al; 2014 AHA/ACC Guideline for the Management of Patients With Non-ST-Elevation Acute Coronary Syndromes: Executive Summary: A Report of the American College of Cardiology/American Heart Association Task Force on Practice Guidelines. Circulation. 2014 Sep 23. [PMID: 25249586]

Bibliography

Antithrombotic Trialists' (ATT) Collaboration, Baigent C, Blackwell L, Collins R, et al. Aspirin in the primary and secondary prevention of vascular disease: collaborative meta-analysis of individual participant data from randomised trials. Lancet. 2009 May 30;373(9678):1849-60. [PMID: 19482214]

BARI 2D Study Group, Frye RL, August P, Brooks MM, et al. A randomized trial of therapies for type 2 diabetes and coronary artery disease. N Engl J Med. 2009 Jun 11;360(24):2503-15. [PMID: 19502645]

Farkouh ME, Domanski M, Sleeper LA, et al; FREEDOM Trial Investigators. Strategies for multivessel revascularization in patients with diabetes. N Engl J Med. 2012 Dec 20;367(25):2375-84. [PMID: 23121323]

Giugliano RP, White JA, Bode C, et al; EARLY ACS Investigators. Early versus delayed, provisional eptifibatide in acute coronary syndromes. N Engl J Med. 2009 May 21;360(21):2176-90. [PMID: 19332455]

Gulati M, Cooper-DeHoff RM, McClure C, et al. Adverse cardiovascular outcomes in women with nonobstructive coronary artery disease: a report from the Women's Ischemia Syndrome Evaluation Study and the St James Women Take Heart Project. Arch Intern Med. 2009 May 11;169(9):843-50. [PMID: 19433695]

Kaul S, Bolger AF, Herrington D, et al; American Heart Association; American College of Cardiology Foundation. Thiazolidinedione drugs and cardiovascular risks: a science advisory from the American Heart Association and the American College of Cardiology Foundation. J Am Coll Cardiol. 2010 Apr 27;55(17):1885-94. [PMID: 20413044]

Mehta SR, Granger CB, Boden WE, et al; TIMACS Investigators. Early versus delayed invasive intervention in acute coronary syndromes. N Engl J Med. 2009 May 21;360(21):2165-75. [PMID: 19458363]

O'Gara PT, Kushner FG, Ascheim DD, et al; American College of Cardiology Foundation/American Heart Association Task Force on Practice Guidelines. 2013 ACCF/AHA guideline for the management of ST-elevation myocardial infarction: a report of the American College of Cardiology Foundation/American Heart Association Task Force on Practice Guidelines. Circulation. 2013 Jan 29;127(4):e362-425. Erratum in: Circulation. 2013 Dec 24;128(25):e481. [PMID: 23247304]

Patel MR, Dehmer GJ, Hirshfeld JW, et al; ACCF/SCAI/STS/AATS/AHA/ASNC 2009 Appropriateness Criteria for Coronary Revascularization: A Report of the American College of Cardiology Foundation Appropriateness Criteria Task Force, Society for Cardiovascular Angiography and Interventions, Society of Thoracic Surgeons, American Association for Thoracic Surgery, American Heart Association, and the American Society of Nuclear Cardiology: Endorsed by the American Society of Echocardiography, the Heart Failure Society of America, and the Society of Cardiovascular Computed Tomography. Circulation. 2009 Mar 10;119(9):1330-52. Erratum in: Circulation. 2009 Apr 21;119(15):e488. [PMID: 19131581]

Qaseem A, Fihn SD, Williams S, et al; Clinical Guidelines Committee of the American College of Physicians. Diagnosis of stable ischemic heart disease: summary of a clinical practice guideline from the American College of Physicians/American College of Cardiology Foundation/American Heart Association/American Association for Thoracic Surgery/Preventive Cardiovascular Nurses Association/Society of Thoracic Surgeons. Ann Intern Med. 2012 Nov 20;157(10):729-34. [PMID: 23165664]

Qaseem A, Fihn SD, Dallas P, et al; Clinical Guidelines Committee of the American College of Physicians. Management of stable ischemic heart disease: summary of a clinical practice guideline from the American College of Physicians/American College of Cardiology Foundation/American Heart Association/American Association for Thoracic Surgery/Preventive Cardiovascular Nurses Association/Society of Thoracic Surgeons. Ann Intern Med. 2012 Nov 20;157(10):735-43. [PMID: 23165665]

Serruys PW, Morice MC, Kappetein AP, et al; SYNTAX Investigators. Percutaneous coronary intervention versus coronary-artery bypass grafting for severe coronary artery disease. N Engl J Med. 2009 Mar 5;360(10):961-72. Erratum in: N Engl J Med. 2013 Feb 7;368(6):584 [PMID: 19228612]

Shaw LJ, Bugiardini R, Merz CN. Women and ischemic heart disease: evolving knowledge. J Am Coll Cardiol. 2009 Oct 20;54(17):1561-75. [PMID: 19833255]

Sobel BE. Coronary revascularization in patients with type 2 diabetes and results of the BARI 2D trial. Coron Artery Dis. 2010 May;21(3):189-98. [PMID: 20308880]

Stone GW, Witzenbichler B, Guagliumi G, et al; HORIZONS-AMI Trial Investigators. Bivalirudin during primary PCI in acute myocardial infarction. N Engl J Med. 2008 May 22;358:2218-30. [PMID: 18499566]

Wallentin L, Becker RC, Budaj A, et al; PLATO Investigators, Freij A, Thorsen M. Ticagrelor versus clopidogrel in patients with acute coronary syndromes. N Engl J Med. 2009 Sep 10;361:1045-57. [PMID: 19717846]

Wiviott SD, Braunwald E, McCabe CH, et al; TRITON-TIMI 38 Investigators. Prasugrel versus clopidogrel in patients with acute coronary syndromes. N Engl J Med. 2007 Nov 15; 357(20):2001-15. [PMID: 17982182]

Heart Failure

Felker GM, Lee KL, Bull DA, et al; NHLBI Heart Failure Clinical Research Network. Diuretic strategies in patients with acute decompensated heart failure. N Engl J Med. 2011 Mar 3;364(9):797-805. [PMID: 21366472]

Heart Failure Society of America, Lindenfeld J, Albert NM, Boehmer JP, et al. HFSA 2010 Comprehensive Heart Failure Practice Guideline. J Card Fail. 2010 Jun;16(6):e1-194. [PMID: 20610207]

Mehra MR, Kobashigawa J, Starling R, et al. Listing criteria for heart transplantation: International Society for Heart and Lung Transplantation guidelines for the care of cardiac transplant candidates-2006. J Heart Lung Transplant. 2006 Sep;25(9):1024-42. [PMID: 16962464]

Russo AM, Stainback RF, Bailey SR, et al. ACCF/HRS/AHA/ASE/HFSA/SCAI/SCCT/SCMR 2013 appropriate use criteria for implantable cardioverter-defibrillators and cardiac resynchronization therapy: a report of the American College of Cardiology Foundation appropriate use criteria task force, Heart Rhythm Society, American Heart Association, American Society of Echocardiography, Heart Failure Society of America, Society for Cardiovascular Angiography and Interventions, Society of Cardiovascular Computed Tomography, and Society for Cardiovascular Magnetic Resonance. J Am Coll Cardiol. 2013 Mar 26;61(12):1318-68. [PMID: 23453819]

Yancy CW, Jessup M, Bozkurt B, et al; American College of Cardiology Foundation; American Heart Association Task Force on Practice Guidelines. 2013 ACCF/AHA guideline for the management of heart failure: a report of the American College of Cardiology Foundation/American Heart Association Task Force on Practice Guidelines. J Am Coll Cardiol. 2013 Oct 15;62(16):e147-239. [PMID: 23747642]

Myocardial Disease

Ammash NM, Seward JB, Bailey KR, Edwards WD, Tajik AJ. Clinical profile and outcome of idiopathic restrictive cardiomyopathy. Circulation. 2000 May 30;101(21):2490-6. [PMID: 10831523]

Gersh BJ, Maron BJ, Bonow RO, et al. 2011 ACCF/AHA guideline for the diagnosis and treatment of hypertrophic cardiomyopathy: executive summary: a report of the American College of Cardiology Foundation/American Heart Association Task Force on Practice Guidelines. J Am Coll Cardiol. 2011 Dec 13;58(25):2703-38. [PMID: 22075468]

Lee VH, Connolly HM, Brown RD Jr. Central nervous system manifestations of cardiac myxoma. Arch Neurol. 2007 Aug;64(8):1115-20. [PMID: 17698701]

Maron BJ. Hypertrophic cardiomyopathy and other causes of sudden cardiac death in young competitive athletes, with considerations for preparticipation screening and criteria for disqualification. Cardiol Clin. 2007 Aug;25(3):399-414, vi. [PMID: 17961794]

Maron BJ, Casey SA, Poliac LC, Gohman TE, Almquist AK, Aeppli DM. Clinical course of hypertrophic cardiomyopathy in a regional United States cohort. JAMA. 1999 Feb 17;281(7):650-5. Erratum in: JAMA 1999 Jun 23-30; 281(24):2288. [PMID: 10029128]

Maron BJ, Maron MS. Hypertrophic cardiomyopathy. Lancet. 2013 Jan 19; 381(9862):242-55. [PMID: 22874472]

Maron BJ, Spirito P, Shen WK, et al. Implantable cardioverter-defibrillators and prevention of sudden cardiac death in hypertrophic cardiomyopathy. JAMA. 2007 Jul 25;298(4):405-12. Erratum in: JAMA. 2007 Oct 3;298(13):1516. [PMID: 17652294]

Sorajja P, Ommen SR, Holmes DR Jr, et al. Survival after alcohol septal ablation for obstructive hypertrophic cardiomyopathy. Circulation. 2012 Nov 13;126(20):2374-80. [PMID: 23076968]

Sorajja P. Invasive hemodynamics of constrictive pericarditis, restrictive cardiomyopathy, and cardiac tamponade. Cardiol Clin. 2011 May;29(2):191-9. [PMID: 21459242]

Truong PT, Jones SO, Martens B, et al. Treatment and outcomes in adult patients with primary cardiac sarcoma: the British Columbia Cancer Agency experience. Ann Surg Oncol. 2009 Dec;16(12):3358-65. [PMID: 19830494]

Arrhythmias

Baddour LM, Epstein AE, Erickson CC, et al; American Heart Association Rheumatic Fever, Endocarditis, and Kawasaki Disease Committee; Council on Cardiovascular Disease in Young; Council on Cardiovascular Surgery and Anesthesia; Council on Cardiovascular Nursing; Council on Clinical Cardiology; Interdisciplinary Council on Quality of Care; American Heart Association. Update on cardiovascular implantable electronic device infections and their management: a scientific statement from the American Heart Association. Circulation. 2010 Jan 26;121(3):458-77. [PMID: 20048212]

Conen D, Adam M, Roche F, et al. Premature atrial contractions in the general population: frequency and risk factors. Circulation. 2012 Nov 6;126(19):2302-8. [PMID: 23048073]

Connolly SJ, Camm AJ, Halperin JL, et al; PALLAS Investigators. Dronedarone in high-risk permanent atrial fibrillation. N Engl J Med. 2011 Dec 15;365(24):2268-76. Erratum in: N Engl J Med. 2012 Feb 16;366(7):672. [PMID: 22082198]

Connolly SJ, Eikelboom J, Joyner C, et al; AVERROES Steering Committee and Investigators. Apixaban in patients with atrial fibrillation. N Engl J Med. 2011 Mar 3;364(9):806-17. [PMID: 21309657]

Connolly SJ, Ezekowitz MD, Yusuf S, et al; RE-LY Steering Committee and Investigators. Dabigatran versus warfarin in patients with atrial fibrillation. N Engl J Med. 2009 Sep 17;361(12):1139-51. Erratum in: N Engl J Med. 2010 Nov 4;363(19):1877. [PMID: 19717844]

Epstein AE, DiMarco JP, Ellenbogen KA, et al. 2012 ACCF/AHA/HRS focused update incorporated into the ACCF/AHA/HRS 2008 guidelines for device-based therapy of cardiac rhythm abnormalities: a report of the American College of Cardiology Foundation/American Heart Association Task Force on Practice Guidelines and the Heart Rhythm Society. Circulation. 2013 Jan 22;127(3):e283-352. [PMID: 23255456]

Friberg L, Rosenqvist M, Lip GY. Evaluation of risk stratification schemes for ischaemic stroke and bleeding in 182 678 patients with atrial fibrillation: the Swedish Atrial Fibrillation cohort study. Eur Heart J. 2012 Jun;33(12):1500-10. [PMID: 22246443]

Fuster V, Rydén LE, Cannom DS, et al; American College of Cardiology; American Heart Association Task Force; European Society of Cardiology Committee for Practice Guidelines; European Heart Rhythm Association; Heart Rhythm Society. ACC/AHA/ESC 2006 guidelines for the management of patients with atrial fibrillation: full text: a report of the American College of Cardiology/American Heart Association Task Force on practice guidelines and the European Society of Cardiology Committee for Practice Guidelines (Writing Committee to Revise the 2001 guidelines for the management of patients with atrial fibrillation) developed in collaboration with the European Heart Rhythm Association and the Heart Rhythm Society. Europace. 2006 Sep;8(9):651-745. Erratum in: Europace. 2007 Sep;9(9):856. [PMID: 16987906]

Goldschlager N, Epstein AE, Naccarelli G, et al. Practical guidelines for clinicians who treat patients with amiodarone. Practice Guidelines Subcommittee, North American Society of Pacing and Electrophysiology. Arch Intern Med. 2000 June 26;160(12):1741-8. [PMID: 10871966]

Greenspon AJ, Patel JD, Lau E, et al. 16-year trends in the infection burden for pacemakers and implantable cardioverter-defibrillators in the United States 1993 to 2008. J Am Coll Cardiol. 2011 Aug 30;58(10):1001-6. [PMID: 21867833]

Hart RG, Pearce LA. Current status of stroke risk stratification in patients with atrial fibrillation. Stroke. 2009 Jul;40(7):2607-10. [PMID: 19461030]

January CT, Wann LS, Alpert JS, et al. 2014 AHA/ACC/HRS Guideline for the Management of Patients With Atrial Fibrillation: A Report of the American College of Cardiology/American Heart Association Task Force on Practice Guidelines and the Heart Rhythm Society. Circulation. 2014 Apr 10. [PMID: 24682347]

Lee GK, Klarich KW, Grogan M, et al. Premature ventricular contraction-induced cardiomyopathy: a treatable condition. Circ Arrhythm Electrophysiol. 2012 Feb;5(1):229-36. [PMID: 22334430]

Nieuwlaat R, Connolly BJ, Hubers LM, et al; ACTIVE Investigators. Quality of individual INR control and the risk of stroke and bleeding events in atrial fibrillation patients: a nested case control analysis of the ACTIVE W study. Thromb Res. 2012 Jun;129(6):715-9. [PMID: 21924760]

Patel MR, Mahaffey KW, Garg J, et al; ROCKET AF Investigators. Rivaroxaban versus warfarin in nonvalvular atrial fibrillation. N Engl J Med. 2011 Sep 8;365(10):883-91. [PMID: 21830957]

Pericardial Disease

Antman EM, Cargill V, Grossman W. Low-pressure cardiac tamponade. Ann Intern Med. 1979 Sep;91(3):403-6. [PMID: 475168]

Bertog SC, Thambidorai SK, Parakh K, et al. Constrictive pericarditis: etiology and cause-specific survival after pericardiectomy. J Am Coll Cardiol. 2004 Apr 21;43(8):1445-52. [PMID: 15093882]

Burstow DJ, Oh JK, Bailey KR, Seward JB, Tajik AJ. Cardiac tamponade: characteristic Doppler observations. Mayo Clin Proc. 1989 Mar;64(3):312-24. [PMID: 2704254]

Ha JW, Oh JK, Schaff HV, et al. Impact of left ventricular function on immediate and long-term outcomes after pericardiectomy in constrictive pericarditis. J Thorac Cardiovasc Surg. 2008 Nov;136(5):1136-41. [PMID: 19026793]

Haley JH, Tajik AJ, Danielson GK, Schaff HV, Mulvagh SL, Oh JK. Transient constrictive pericarditis: causes and natural history. J Am Coll Cardiol. 2004 Jan 21;43(2):271-5. [PMID: 14736448]

Imazio M, Brucato A, Cemin R, et al; ICAP Investigators. A randomized trial of colchicine for acute pericarditis. N Engl J Med. 2013 Oct 17;369(16):1522-8. [PMID: 23992557]

Spodick DH. Acute cardiac tamponade. N Engl J Med. 2003 Aug 14;349(7):684-90. [PMID: 12917306]

Syed FF, Ntsekhe M, Mayosi BM, Oh JK. Effusive-constrictive pericarditis. Heart Fail Rev. 2013 May;18(3):277-87. [PMID: 22422296]

Talreja DR, Nishimura RA, Oh JK, Holmes DR. Constrictive pericarditis in the modern era: novel criteria for diagnosis in the cardiac catheterization laboratory. J Am Coll Cardiol. 2008 Jan 22;51(3):315-9. [PMID: 18206742]

Tsang TS, Freeman WK, Sinak LJ, Seward JB. Echocardiographically guided pericardiocentesis: evolution and state-of-the-art technique. Mayo Clin Proc. 1998 Jul;73(7):647-52. [PMID: 9663193]

Valvular Heart Disease

David TE. Surgical treatment of aortic valve disease. Nat Rev Cardiol. 2013 Jul;10(7):375-86. [PMID: 23670613]

Joint Task Force on the Management of Valvular Heart Disease of the European Society of Cardiology (ESC); European Association for Cardio-Thoracic Surgery (EACTS), Vahanian A, Alfieri O, Andreotti F, et al. Guidelines on the management of valvular heart disease (version 2012). Eur Heart J. 2012 Oct;33(19):2451-96. [PMID: 22922415]

Kang DH, Kim YJ, Kim SH, et al. Early surgery versus conventional treatment for infective endocarditis. N Engl J Med. 2012 Jun 28;366(26):2466-73. [PMID: 22738096]

Leong DP, Joseph MX, Selvanayagam JB. The evolving role of multimodality imaging in valvular heart disease. Heart. 2014 Feb;100(4):336-46. [PMID: 23574967]

Lindman BR, Bonow RO, Otto CM. Current management of calcific aortic stenosis. Circ Res. 2013 Jul 5;113(2):223-37. [PMID: 23833296]

Mordi I, Tzemos N. Bicuspid aortic valve disease: a comprehensive review. Cardiol Res Pract. 2012;2012:196037. [PMID: 22685681]

Nishimura RA, Otto CM, Bonow RO, et al; American College of Cardiology/American Heart Association Task Force on Practice Guidelines. 2014 AHA/ACC guideline for the management of patients with valvular heart disease: executive summary: a report of the American College of Cardiology/American Heart Association Task Force on Practice Guidelines. J Am Coll Cardiol. 2014 Jun 10;63(22):2438-88. Erratum in: J Am Coll Cardiol. 2014 Jun 10;63(22):2489. [PMID: 24603192]

Rogers JH, Franzen O. Percutaneous edge-to-edge MitraClip therapy in the management of mitral regurgitation. Eur Heart J. 2011 Oct;32(19):2350-7. [PMID: 21606080]

Wilson W, Taubert KA, Gewitz M, et al; American Heart Association Rheumatic Fever, Endocarditis, and Kawasaki Disease Committee; American Heart Association Council on Cardiovascular Disease in the Young; American Heart Association Council on Clinical Cardiology; American Heart Association Council on Cardiovascular Surgery and Anesthesia; Quality of Care and Outcomes Research Interdisciplinary Working Group. Prevention of infective endocarditis: guidelines from the American Heart Association: a guideline from the American Heart Association Rheumatic Fever, Endocarditis, and Kawasaki Disease Committee, Council on Cardiovascular Disease in the Young, and the Council on Clinical Cardiology, Council on Cardiovascular Surgery and Anesthesia, and the Quality of Care and Outcomes Research Interdisciplinary Working Group. Circulation. 2007 Oct 9;116(15):1736-54. Erratum in: Circulation. 2007 Oct 9;116(15):e376-7. [PMID: 17446442]

Adult Congenital Heart Disease

Brown ML, Burkhart HM, Connolly HM, et al. Coarctation of the aorta: lifelong surveillance is mandatory following surgical repair. J Am Coll Cardiol. 2013 Sep 10;62(11):1020-5. [PMID: 23850909]

D'Alto M, Romeo E, Argiento P, et al. Bosentan-sildenafil association in patients with congenital heart disease-related pulmonary arterial hypertension and Eisenmenger physiology. Int J Cardiol. 2012 Mar 22;155(3):378-82. [PMID: 21081251]

DeSimone CV, Friedman PA, Noheria A, et al. Stroke or transient ischemic attack in patients with transvenous pacemaker or defibrillator and echocardiographically detected patent foramen ovale. Circulation. 2013 Sep 24;128(13):1433-41. [PMID: 23946264]

European Society of Gynecology (ESG); Association for European Paediatric Cardiology (AEPC); German Society for Gender Medicine (DGesGM), Regitz-Zagrosek V, Blomstrom Lundqvist C, Borghi C, et al; ESC Committee for Practice Guidelines. ESC Guidelines on the management of cardiovascular diseases during pregnancy: the Task Force on the Management of Cardiovascular Diseases during Pregnancy of the European Society of Cardiology (ESC). Eur Heart J. 2011 Dec;32(24):3147-97. [PMID: 21873418]

Furie KL, Kasner SE, Adams RJ, et al; American Heart Association Stroke Council, Council on Cardiovascular Nursing, Council on Clinical Cardiology, and Interdisciplinary Council on Quality of Care and Outcomes Research.

Guidelines for the prevention of stroke in patients with stroke or transient ischemic attack: a guideline for healthcare professionals from the American Heart Association/American Stroke Association. Stroke. 2011 Jan;42(1):227-76. [PMID: 20966421]

Warnes CA, Williams RG, Bashore TM, et al; American College of Cardiology; American Heart Association Task Force on Practice Guidelines (Writing Committee to Develop Guidelines on the Management of Adults With Congenital Heart Disease); American Society of Echocardiography; Heart Rhythm Society; International Society for Adult Congenital Heart Disease; Society for Cardiovascular Angiography and Interventions; Society of Thoracic Surgeons. ACC/AHA 2008 guidelines for the management of adults with congenital heart disease: a report of the American College of Cardiology/American Heart Association Task Force on Practice Guidelines (Writing Committee to Develop Guidelines on the Management of Adults With Congenital Heart Disease). Developed in collaboration with the American Society of Echocardiography, Heart Rhythm Society, International Society for Adult Congenital Heart Disease, Society for Cardiovascular Angiography and Interventions, and Society of Thoracic Surgeons. J Am Coll Cardiol. 2008 Dec 2;52(23):e143-263. [PMID: 19038677]

Diseases of the Aorta

Baxter BT, Terrin MC, Dalman RL. Medical management of small abdominal aortic aneurysms. Circulation. 2008 Apr 8;117(14):1883-9. [PMID: 18391122]

Chaikof EL, Brewster DC, Dalman RL, et al. SVS practice guidelines for the care of patients with an abdominal aortic aneurysm: executive summary. J Vasc Surg. 2009 Oct;50(4):880-96. [PMID: 19786241]

De Bruin JL, Baas AF, Buth J, et al; DREAM Study Group. Long-term outcome of open or endovascular repair of abdominal aortic aneurysm. N Engl J Med. 2010 May 20;362(20):1881-9. [PMID: 20484396]

Hiratzka LF, Bakris GL, Beckman JA, et al; American College of Cardiology Foundation/American Heart Association Task Force on Practice Guidelines; American Association for Thoracic Surgery; American College of Radiology; American Stroke Association; Society of Cardiovascular Anesthesiologists; Society for Cardiovascular Angiography and Interventions; Society of Interventional Radiology; Society of Thoracic Surgeons; Society for Vascular Medicine. 2010 ACCF/AHA/AATS/ACR/ASA/SCA/SCAI/SIR/STS/SVM Guidelines for the diagnosis and management of patients with thoracic aortic disease. A Report of the American College of Cardiology Foundation/American Heart Association Task Force on Practice Guidelines, American Association for Thoracic Surgery, American College of Radiology, American Stroke Association, Society of Cardiovascular Anesthesiologists, Society for Cardiovascular Angiography and Interventions, Society of Interventional Radiology, Society of Thoracic Surgeons, and Society for Vascular Medicine. J Am Coll Cardiol. 2010 Apr 6;55(14):e27-e129. Erratum in: J Am Coll Cardiol. 2013 Sep 10;62(11):1039-40. [PMID: 20359588]

Jondeau G, Detaint D, Tubach F, et al. Aortic event rate in the Marfan population: a cohort study. Circulation. 2012 Jan 17;125(2):226-32. [PMID: 22133496]

Nienaber CA, Kische S, Rousseau H, et al; INSTEAD-XL trial. Endovascular repair of type B aortic dissection: long-term results of the randomized investigation of stent grafts in aortic dissection trial. Circ Cardiovasc Interv. 2013 Aug;6(4):407-16. [PMID: 23922146]

Nienaber CA, Rousseau H, Eggebrecht H, et al; INSTEAD Trial. Randomized comparison of strategies for type B aortic dissection: the INvestigation of STEnt Grafts in Aortic Dissection (INSTEAD) trial. Circulation. 2009 Dec 22;120(25):2519-28. [PMID: 19996018]

United Kingdom EVAR Trial Investigators, Greenhalgh RM, Brown LC, Powell JT, Thompson SG, Epstein D. Endovascular repair of aortic aneurysm in patients physically ineligible for open repair. N Engl J Med. 2010 May 20;362(20):1872-80. [PMID: 20382982]

United Kingdom EVAR Trial Investigators, Greenhalgh RM, Brown LC, Powell JT, Thompson SG, Epstein D, Sculpher MJ. Endovascular versus open repair of abdominal aortic aneurysm. N Engl J Med. 2010 May 20;362(20):1863-71. [PMID: 20382983]

Peripheral Arterial Disease

Aboyans V, Criqui MH, Abraham P, et al; American Heart Association Council on Peripheral Vascular Disease; Council on Epidemiology and Prevention; Council on Clinical Cardiology; Council on Cardiovascular Nursing; Council on Cardiovascular Radiology and Intervention, and Council on Cardiovascular Surgery and Anesthesia. Measurement and interpretation of the ankle-brachial index: a scientific statement from the American Heart Association. Circulation. 2012 Dec 11;126(24):2890-909. Erratum in: Circulation. 2013 Jan 1;127(1):e264. [PMID: 23159553]

Adam DJ, Beard JD, Cleveland T, et al; BASIL trial participants. Bypass versus angioplasty in severe ischaemia of the leg (BASIL): multicentre, randomised controlled trial. Lancet. 2005 Dec 3;366(9501):1925-34. [PMID: 16325694]

Anderson JL, Halperin JL, Albert NM, et al. Management of patients with peripheral artery disease (compilation of 2005 and 2011 ACCF/AHA guideline recommendations): a report of the American College of Cardiology Foundation/American Heart Association Task Force on Practice Guidelines. Circulation. 2013 Apr 2;127(13):1425-43. [PMID: 23457117]

Ankle Brachial Index Collaboration, Fowkes FG, Murray GD, Butcher I, et al. Ankle brachial index combined with Framingham Risk Score to predict cardiovascular events and mortality: a meta-analysis. JAMA. 2008 Jul 9;300(2):197-208. [PMID: 18612117]

Berger JS, Hiatt WR. Medical therapy in peripheral artery disease. Circulation. 2012 Jul 24;126(4):491-500. [PMID: 22825411]

Berger JS, Hochman J, Lobach I, Adelman MA, Riles TS, Rockman CB. Modifiable risk factor burden and the prevalence of peripheral artery disease in different vascular territories. J Vasc Surg. 2013 Sep;58(3):673-81.e1. [PMID: 23642926]

Creager MA, Kaufman JA, Conte MS. Clinical practice. Acute limb ischemia. N Engl J Med. 2012 Jun 7;366(23):2198-206. [PMID: 22670905]

McDermott MM, Ades P, Guralnik JM, et al. Treadmill exercise and resistance training in patients with peripheral arterial disease with and without intermittent claudication: a randomized controlled trial. JAMA. 2009 Jan 14;301(2):165-74. Erratum in: JAMA. 2012 Apr 25;307(16):1694. [PMID: 19141764]

Murphy TP, Cutlip DE, Regensteiner JG, et al; CLEVER Study Investigators. Supervised exercise versus primary stenting for claudication resulting from aortoiliac peripheral artery disease: six-month outcomes from the claudication: exercise versus endoluminal revascularization (CLEVER) study. Circulation. 2012 Jan 3;125(1):130-9. [PMID: 22090168]

Norgren L, Hiatt WR, Dormandy JA, et al; TASC II Working Group. Inter-Society Consensus for the Management of Peripheral Arterial Disease (TASC II). J Vasc Surg. 2007 Jan;45 Suppl S:S5-67. [PMID: 17223489]

Rooke TW, Hirsch AT, Misra S, et al; American College of Cardiology Foundation/American Heart Association Task Force on Practice Guidelines; Society for Cardiovascular Angiography and Interventions; Society of Interventional Radiology; Society for Vascular Medicine; Society for Vascular Surgery. 2011 ACCF/AHA focused update of the guideline for the management of patients with peripheral artery disease (updating the 2005 guideline): a report of the American College of Cardiology Foundation/American Heart Association Task Force on Practice Guidelines: developed in collaboration with the Society for Cardiovascular Angiography and Interventions, Society of Interventional Radiology, Society for Vascular Medicine, and Society for Vascular Surgery. J Vasc Surg. 2011 Nov; 54(5):e32-58. [PMID: 21958560]

Cardiovascular Disease in Cancer Survivors

Fiúza M. Cardiotoxicity associated with trastuzumab treatment of HER2+ breast cancer. Adv Ther. 2009 Jul;26 Suppl 1:S9-17. [PMID: 19669637]

Perez EA, Suman VJ, Davidson NE, et al. Cardiac safety analysis of doxorubicin and cyclophosphamide followed by paclitaxel with or without trastuzumab in the North Central Cancer Treatment Group N9831 adjuvant breast cancer trial. J Clin Oncol. 2008 Mar 10;26(8):1231-8. [PMID: 18250349]

Slamon D, Eiermann W, Robert N, et al; Breast Cancer International Research Group. Adjuvant trastuzumab in HER2-positive breast cancer. N Engl J Med. 2011 Oct 6;365(14):1273-83. [PMID: 21991949]

Swain SM, Whaley FS, Ewer MS. Congestive heart failure in patients treated with doxorubicin: a retrospective analysis of three trials. Cancer. 2003 Jun 1;97(11):2869-79. [PMID: 12767102]

Yeh ET, Tong AT, Lenihan DJ, et al. Cardiovascular complications of cancer therapy: diagnosis, pathogenesis, and management. Circulation. 2004 Jun 29;109(25):3122-31. [PMID: 15226229]

Pregnancy and Cardiovascular Disease

De Santo LS, Romano G, Della Corte A, et al. Mechanical aortic valve replacement in young women planning on pregnancy: maternal and fetal outcomes under low oral anticoagulation, a pilot observational study on a comprehensive pre-operative counseling protocol. J Am Coll Cardiol. 2012 Mar 20;59(12):1110-5. [PMID: 22421305]

European Society of Gynecology (ESG); Association for European Paediatric Cardiology (AEPC); German Society for Gender Medicine (DGesGM); Regitz-Zagrosek V, Blomstrom Lundqvist C, Borghi C, et al; ESC Committee for Practice Guidelines. ESC Guidelines on the management of cardiovascular diseases during pregnancy: the Task Force on the Management of Cardiovascular Diseases during Pregnancy of the European Society of Cardiology (ESC). Eur Heart J. 2011 Dec;32(24):3147-97. [PMID: 21873418]

Siu SC, Sermer M, Colman JM, et al; Cardiac Disease in Pregnancy (CARPREG) Investigators. Prospective multicentre study of pregnancy outcomes in women with heart disease. Circulation. 2001 Jul 31;104(5):515-21. [PMID: 11479246]

Sliwa K, Blauwet L, Tibazarwa K, et al. Evaluation of bromocriptine in the treatment of acute severe peripartum cardiomyopathy: a proof-of-concept pilot study. Circulation. 2010 Apr 6;121(13):1465-73. [PMID: 20308616]

Sliwa K, Hilfiker-Kleiner D, Petrie MC, et al; Heart Failure Association of the European Society of Cardiology Working Group on Peripartum Cardiomyopathy. Current state of knowledge on aetiology, diagnosis, management, and therapy of peripartum cardiomyopathy: a position statement from the Heart Failure Association of the European Society of Cardiology Working Group on peripartum cardiomyopathy. Eur J Heart Fail. 2010 Aug;12(8):767-78. [PMID: 20675664]

Warnes CA, Williams RG, Bashore TM, et al; American College of Cardiology; American Heart Association Task Force on Practice Guidelines (Writing Committee to Develop Guidelines on the Management of Adults With Congenital Heart Disease); American Society of Echocardiography; Heart Rhythm Society; International Society for Adult Congenital Heart Disease; Society for Cardiovascular Angiography and Interventions; Society of Thoracic Surgeons. ACC/AHA 2008 guidelines for the management of adults with congenital heart disease: a report of the American College of Cardiology/American Heart Association Task Force on Practice Guidelines (Writing Committee to Develop Guidelines on the Management of Adults With Congenital Heart Disease). Developed in Collaboration With the American Society of Echocardiography, Heart Rhythm Society, International Society for Adult Congenital Heart Disease, Society for Cardiovascular Angiography and Interventions, and Society of Thoracic Surgeons. J Am Coll Cardiol. 2008 Dec 2;52(23):e143-263. [PMID: 19038677]

Cardiovascular Medicine Self-Assessment Test

This self-assessment test contains one-best-answer multiple-choice questions. Please read these directions carefully before answering the questions. Answers, critiques, and bibliographies immediately follow these multiple-choice questions. The American College of Physicians is accredited by the Accreditation Council for Continuing Medical Education (ACCME) to provide continuing medical education for physicians.

The American College of Physicians designates MKSAP 17 **Cardiovascular Medicine** for a maximum of **21** *AMA PRA Category 1 Credits*™. Physicians should claim only the credit commensurate with the extent of their participation in the activity.

Earn "Instantaneous" CME Credits Online

Print subscribers can enter their answers online to earn Continuing Medical Education (CME) credits instantaneously. You can submit your answers using online answer sheets that are provided at mksap.acponline.org, where a record of your MKSAP 17 credits will be available. To earn CME credits, you need to answer all of the questions in a test and earn a score of at least 50% correct (number of correct answers divided by the total number of questions). Take any of the following approaches:

➢ Use the printed answer sheet at the back of this book to record your answers. Go to mksap.acponline.org, access the appropriate online answer sheet, transcribe your answers, and submit your test for instantaneous CME credits. There is no additional fee for this service.

➢ Go to mksap.acponline.org, access the appropriate online answer sheet, directly enter your answers, and submit your test for instantaneous CME credits. There is no additional fee for this service.

➢ Pay a $15 processing fee per answer sheet and submit the printed answer sheet at the back of this book by mail or fax, as instructed on the answer sheet. Make sure you calculate your score and fax the answer sheet to 215-351-2799 or mail the answer sheet to Member and Customer Service, American College of Physicians, 190 N. Independence Mall West, Philadelphia, PA 19106-1572, using the courtesy envelope provided in your MKSAP 17 slipcase. You will need your 10-digit order number and 8-digit ACP ID number, which are printed on your packing slip. Please allow 4 to 6 weeks for your score report to be emailed back to you. Be sure to include your email address for a response.

If you do not have a 10-digit order number and 8-digit ACP ID number or if you need help creating a user name and password to access the MKSAP 17 online answer sheets, go to mksap.acponline.org or email custserv@acponline.org.

CME credit is available from the publication date of July 31, 2015, until July 31, 2018. You may submit your answer sheets at any time during this period.

Directions

*Each of the numbered items is followed by lettered answers. Select the **ONE** lettered answer that is **BEST** in each case.*

Self-Assessment Test

Item 1

A 33-year-old woman is evaluated as an outpatient following an episode of atrial fibrillation. The episode resolved shortly after arriving at the emergency department. She has a history of tetralogy of Fallot with repair performed at the age of 4 years.

On physical examination, blood pressure is 110/70 mm Hg, pulse rate is 62/min and regular, and respiration rate is 18/min. BMI is 28. The estimated central venous pressure is normal. The apical impulse is normal; there is a parasternal impulse at the left sternal border. S_1 is normal. The S_2 is single, and there is a soft early systolic murmur at the second left intercostal space. A grade 2/6 decrescendo diastolic murmur that increases with inspiration is noted at the left sternal border. The remainder of the physical examination is normal.

Which of the following is the most likely diagnosis?

(A) Aortic valve regurgitation
(B) Pulmonary valve regurgitation
(C) Recurrent ventricular septal defect
(D) Tricuspid valve regurgitation

Item 2

A 58-year-old man is evaluated during a routine appointment and asks for advice on cardiac risk assessment. He does not have any current cardiac symptoms, exercises 4 days per week, and has never smoked. He has no chronic health issues and takes no medications. He has no known drug allergies. Results of the physical examination are normal.

Cardiovascular risk calculation using the Pooled Cohort Equations predicts a 6% risk of a myocardial infarction or coronary death in the next 10 years.

Which of the following tests should be performed next?

(A) Adenosine cardiac magnetic resonance (CMR) imaging
(B) Cardiac CT angiography
(C) Fractionated lipoprotein profile
(D) High-sensitivity C-reactive protein assay
(E) Stress echocardiography

Item 3

A 64-year-old woman is evaluated during a routine examination. She has no symptoms. Medical history is significant for hypertension and type 2 diabetes mellitus. Medications are amlodipine, losartan, atorvastatin, and metformin.

On physical examination, she is afebrile, blood pressure is 154/77 mm Hg and equal on both sides, pulse rate is 82/min, and respiration rate is 16/min. BMI is 28. Cardiac examination shows a grade 1/6 decrescendo diastolic murmur heard best over the apex. There are no changes with a Valsalva maneuver or change in position. Peripheral pulses are normal.

Electrocardiogram shows sinus rhythm with nonspecific ST changes.

Which of the following is the most appropriate diagnostic test to perform next?

(A) Chest CT
(B) Exercise echocardiography stress testing
(C) Transthoracic echocardiography
(D) No further testing

Item 4

A 58-year-old woman is evaluated during a routine physical examination. She has a history of atrial fibrillation and had an atrial fibrillation ablation procedure 6 months ago. Before her ablation, she had persistent atrial fibrillation with palpitations and dyspnea. Since her ablation, she has been asymptomatic with no palpitations. Ambulatory electrocardiographic monitoring at 3 and 6 months after the ablation demonstrated no atrial fibrillation. Medical history is also significant for a transient ischemic attack, hypertension, and hyperlipidemia. Her medications are warfarin, metoprolol, candesartan, and simvastatin.

On physical examination, the patient is afebrile, blood pressure is 130/80 mm Hg, pulse rate is 64/min, and respiration rate is 16/min. BMI is 30. Heart rate and rhythm are regular.

An electrocardiogram shows normal sinus rhythm.

Which of the following is the most appropriate management?

(A) Continue warfarin
(B) Continue warfarin and add aspirin
(C) Discontinue warfarin
(D) Discontinue warfarin and start aspirin
(E) Discontinue warfarin and start aspirin and clopidogrel

Item 5

A 52-year-old woman is seen in follow-up for dyspnea. Over the past 6 months, she has noticed increasing shortness of breath during her daily run, which she has had to decrease from 2 miles to 1 mile. She is able to complete other aerobic exercises, such as biking and tennis, with minimal limitation. She has experienced no chest pain or syncope. Medical history is significant for hypertension, diagnosed 10 years ago. Her only medication is hydrochlorothiazide.

On physical examination, blood pressure is 122/70 mm Hg and pulse rate is 66/min. Lungs are clear to auscultation. Cardiac examination reveals a rapid carotid upstroke and a grade 3/6 holosystolic murmur heard best at the left lower sternal border. The murmur increases during both end-expiration and squat-to-stand maneuvers.

Transthoracic echocardiogram shows left ventricular hypertrophy and dynamic left ventricular outflow tract obstruction consistent with a diagnosis of hypertrophic cardiomyopathy.

Which of the following is the most appropriate next step in treatment?

(A) Discontinue hydrochlorothiazide
(B) Dual-chamber pacemaker
(C) Initiate lisinopril
(D) Surgical myectomy

Item 6

A 71-year-old man is evaluated in the emergency department for severe pain in the chest and back that was abrupt in onset and has persisted for 3 hours. He has no abdominal pain, leg pain, or neurologic symptoms. His medical history is notable for hypertension. Medications are amlodipine and lisinopril.

On physical examination, the patient is afebrile, blood pressure is 180/100 mm Hg in both arms, pulse rate is 98/min, and respiration rate is 18/min. Oxygen saturation is 96% on ambient air. Cardiac auscultation discloses an S_4 gallop but no murmur. Pulmonary examination is normal. Pulses are symmetric and equal in all extremities.

Laboratory studies show a D-dimer level of 1.2 µg/mL (1.2 mg/L) and a serum creatinine level of 1.0 mg/dL (88.4 µmol/L). Initial serum cardiac troponin I level is not elevated.

Electrocardiogram shows left ventricular hypertrophy with repolarization abnormalities. Chest radiograph shows an enlarged cardiac silhouette. Chest CT scan with intravenous contrast demonstrates a focal penetrating ulcer in the thoracic descending aorta (shown).

Which of the following is the most appropriate immediate next step in management?

(A) Heparin followed by warfarin
(B) Endovascular stenting
(C) Intravenous β-blockade followed by intravenous sodium nitroprusside
(D) Open surgical repair

Item 7

A 52-year-old woman is evaluated for fatigue and lower extremity swelling. One year ago, she had acute idiopathic pericarditis treated with anti-inflammatory medications and colchicine. Symptoms initially improved and her medications were discontinued. However, for the past 3 months, she has had worsening symptoms of exertional fatigue and edema in both legs. She currently takes no medications.

On physical examination, she is afebrile, blood pressure is 130/78 mm Hg, pulse rate is 88/min, and respiration rate is 16/min. Pulsus paradoxus of 15 mm Hg is present. The estimated central venous pressure is 10 cm H_2O, and the jugular venous pulse contour shows diminished y descents. The lungs are clear to auscultation. Heart sounds are normal, with no rubs or gallops. Hepatomegaly is present, and peripheral edema is noted in both lower extremities up to the knees.

A 12-lead electrocardiogram is normal. Echocardiogram shows the cardiac chambers to be normal in size and function with a moderate circumferential pericardial effusion. A CT of the heart shows normal pericardial thickness.

A pericardiocentesis fails to resolve the elevated right atrial pressure documented on right heart catheterization.

Which of the following is the most likely diagnosis?

(A) Cor pulmonale
(B) Effusive constrictive pericarditis
(C) Heart failure
(D) Recurrent acute pericarditis

Item 8

A 58-year-old man is evaluated during a routine appointment. He is asymptomatic. He was diagnosed with type 2 diabetes mellitus 4 years ago and has hypertension, dyslipidemia, and obesity. His medications are enteric-coated low-dose aspirin, lisinopril, fluvastatin (20 mg/d), and metformin.

His calculated 10-year risk of atherosclerotic cardiovascular disease (ASCVD) using the Pooled Cohort Equations is 10%.

On physical examination, blood pressure is 126/78 mm Hg and pulse rate is 72/min. The remainder of the examination is normal.

Laboratory studies:

Total cholesterol	186 mg/dL (4.82 mmol/L)
LDL cholesterol	123 mg/dL (3.19 mmol/L)
HDL cholesterol	44 mg/dL (1.14 mmol/L)
Triglycerides	109 mg/dL (1.23 mmol/L)

Which of the following is the most appropriate statin management?

(A) Increase fluvastatin to 40 mg/d
(B) Switch to atorvastatin, 40 mg/d
(C) Switch to lovastatin, 20 mg/d
(D) Switch to pravastatin, 20 mg/d
(E) Switch to simvastatin, 10 mg/d

Item 9

A 34-year-old woman with idiopathic heart failure diagnosed 9 months ago is evaluated for a 3-month history of nonproductive cough. She sleeps on one pillow and has no paroxysmal nocturnal dyspnea. Medical history is otherwise unremarkable, and she has never smoked. Medications are lisinopril, carvedilol, and furosemide.

On physical examination, the patient is afebrile, blood pressure is 102/70 mm Hg, pulse rate is 64/min, and respiration rate is 16/min. Oxygen saturation on ambient air is 98%. The remainder of the examination, including heart and lung examinations, is unremarkable.

Her most recent left ventricular ejection fraction is 40%. Chest radiograph is unremarkable.

Which of the following is the most appropriate management?

(A) Discontinue lisinopril and start valsartan
(B) Echocardiography
(C) Obtain B-type natriuretic peptide level
(D) Pulmonary function testing

Item 10

A 48-year-old man with newly diagnosed hypertension is referred for an echocardiogram to assess findings of left ventricular hypertrophy noted on the electrocardiogram. He is asymptomatic, and his medical history is unremarkable other than hypertension. His only medication is chlorthalidone.

On physical examination, blood pressure is 128/70 mm Hg, pulse rate is 60/min and regular, and respiration rate is 18/min. BMI is 24. The cardiac examination is normal other than the presence of an S_4.

The transthoracic echocardiogram demonstrates normal left ventricular size, function, and mass index. An atrial septal aneurysm with a small left-to-right shunt indicative of a patent foramen ovale is noted by color-flow Doppler imaging. The right ventricular chamber size, systolic function, and estimated pressures are normal.

Which of the following is the most appropriate management based on this patient's echocardiographic findings? .

(A) Anticoagulation therapy
(B) Closure of the defect
(C) Transesophageal echocardiography
(D) No further evaluation or treatment

Item 11

A 69-year-old man is evaluated for exertional chest pain that began 2 months ago. The patient describes the chest pain as tightness in the left side of his chest that occurs after walking approximately a half-mile. This chest tightness improves with rest. Two years ago, he had a myocardial infarction. The patient's medications are low-dose aspirin, metoprolol, lisinopril, and rosuvastatin.

On physical examination, blood pressure is 124/72 mm Hg and pulse rate is 52/min. The remainder of the examination is normal.

Resting electrocardiogram (ECG) shows no evidence of left ventricular hypertrophy and no ST- or T-wave changes.

Exercise ECG is performed. The patient is able to exercise on the Bruce protocol for 10 minutes and 20 seconds; blood pressure rises appropriately, but he develops chest tightness and stops because of breathlessness. There are no ECG changes.

Which of the following is the most appropriate management?

(A) Add diltiazem
(B) Add isosorbide mononitrate
(C) Coronary angiography
(D) Pharmacologic nuclear stress test

Item 12

A 32-year-old man is evaluated during an initial office visit. He has no symptoms and no significant medical history. He takes no medications.

On physical examination, blood pressure is 120/70 mm Hg in both arms, pulse rate is 64/min, and respiration rate is 12/min. Cardiac examination reveals a grade 1/6 decrescendo diastolic murmur heard best at the left lower sternal border. Femoral pulses are equal.

Which of the following is the most likely cause of the patient's murmur?

(A) Aortic coarctation
(B) Atrial septal defect
(C) Bicuspid aortic valve
(D) Mitral stenosis

Item 13

A 69-year-old woman is evaluated for follow-up 3 months after a non–ST-elevation myocardial infarction. She was assessed to be at low risk, and she was treated medically. Since the acute event, the patient has done well. She has no chest discomfort or shortness of breath. She has hypercholesterolemia and hypertension. Medications are lisinopril, metoprolol, atorvastatin, aspirin, and clopidogrel. She has modified her diet and has begun performing physical activity 5 days a week.

On physical examination, the patient is afebrile, blood pressure is 125/80 mm Hg, pulse rate is 60/min, and respiration rate is 12/min. BMI is 26. A normal carotid upstroke without carotid bruits is noted, jugular venous pulsations are normal, and normal S_1 and S_2 heart sounds are heard without murmurs. Lung fields are clear, distal pulses are normal, and no peripheral edema is present.

Laboratory studies show adherence to her lipid therapy and are otherwise normal.

Which of the following will offer this patient the greatest reduction in her risk of future cardiovascular events?

(A) Colchicine
(B) Folic acid
(C) Influenza vaccine
(D) Vitamin E

Self-Assessment Test

Item 14

A 51-year-old woman is admitted to the hospital with community-acquired pneumonia after outpatient therapy was unsuccessful. She presented 5 days ago with cough, fever, and dyspnea, and she was found to have right lower lobe crackles on examination and a corresponding infiltrate on chest radiography. She was started on oral moxifloxacin. However, she has remained febrile with worsening shortness of breath and is now admitted to the hospital for further treatment. Medical history is significant for hypertension and depression, for which she takes carvedilol and amitriptyline. Her current medications are moxifloxacin, carvedilol, and amitriptyline.

On physical examination, temperature is 38.4 °C (101.1 °F), blood pressure is 140/90 mm Hg, pulse rate is 88/min, and respiration rate is 18/min. Oxygen saturation breathing ambient air is 89%. BMI is 25. Chest examination is consistent with right lower lobe consolidation. The remainder of the physical examination is unremarkable.

An electrocardiogram (ECG) at the time of hospital admission is shown.

Which of the following medications should be discontinued based on this patient's ECG findings?

(A) Amitriptyline
(B) Amitriptyline and carvedilol
(C) Amitriptyline and moxifloxacin
(D) Moxifloxacin

Item 15

A 74-year-old man is evaluated in the emergency department for a 7-day history of progressive exertional dyspnea associated with a dry cough, increasing orthopnea (from two to four pillows), and inability to buckle his belt. He has a 20-year history of hypertension treated with diltiazem.

On physical examination, blood pressure is 162/86 mm Hg, pulse rate is irregularly irregular at 84/min, and respiration rate is 18/min. Estimated central venous pressure is 14 cm H_2O. Cardiac examination reveals an irregularly irregular rhythm and an S_4. Bibasilar crackles are heard on auscultation of the lungs. His liver is enlarged 2 cm below the costal margin. His extremity examination reveals bilateral pitting edema.

Serum electrolyte levels and kidney function tests are normal. Serum B-type natriuretic peptide level is 2472 pg/mL (2472 ng/L).

Electrocardiogram shows atrial fibrillation. Echocardiogram shows a left ventricular ejection fraction of 60%, septal wall thickness of 1.5 cm, and posterior wall thickness of 1.4 cm. Chest radiograph shows hazy bilateral infiltrates.

Which of the following is the most appropriate next step in management?

(A) β-Blocker
(B) Cardioversion
(C) Furosemide
(D) Spironolactone

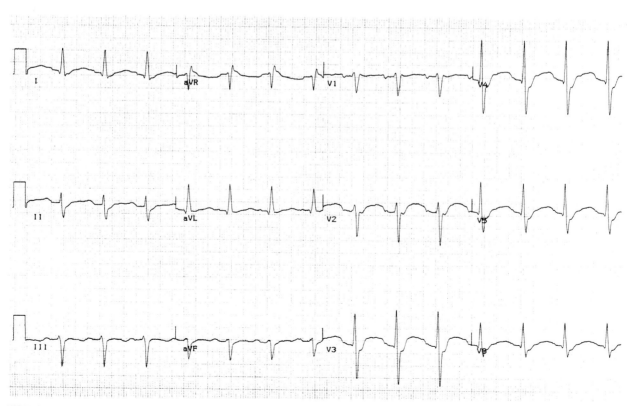

ITEM 14

Item 16

A 58-year-old man is evaluated in the hospital for weakness, fatigue, and hypotension. The patient reports a 3-week history of anorexia and 2-year history of non–small cell lung cancer with metastatic involvement in the liver treated with combination cytotoxic chemotherapy.

On physical examination, the patient appears cachectic. Blood pressure is 70/52 mm Hg and pulse rate is 110/min. The lungs are clear to auscultation. The jugular venous pulse contour is flat. Carotid upstrokes are brisk. S_1 and S_2 are distant. No rubs, gallops, or murmurs are present. No peripheral edema is noted. The remainder of the physical examination is unremarkable.

Echocardiogram shows a small left ventricular cavity with hyperdynamic function (ejection fraction, 75%). A moderately sized circumferential pericardial effusion is evident. Diastolic inversion of the right atrium and significant respiratory variation in the mitral inflow pattern are present.

The blood pressure does not change after administration of a 1-L bolus of intravenous fluid.

In addition to continued intravenous fluid, which of the following is the most appropriate next step in treatment?

(A) Intra-aortic balloon pump
(B) Pericardiocentesis
(C) Phenylephrine
(D) Window pericardiectomy

Item 17

A 54-year-old man is evaluated during a routine appointment. He has hypertension, dyslipidemia, obesity, and erectile dysfunction. He currently drinks three alcoholic beverages daily. His mother had a nonfatal myocardial infarction (MI) at age 55 years, and he is concerned about his risk of MI. Medications are hydrochlorothiazide, atorvastatin, and sildenafil as needed.

Which of the following components of this patient's medical history is associated with the greatest risk for future myocardial infarction?

(A) Alcohol consumption
(B) Dyslipidemia
(C) Hypertension
(D) Obesity

Item 18

A 63-year-old man is evaluated for follow-up of coronary artery disease that was diagnosed by exercise stress testing 3 weeks ago. For his exertional chest pain, he was started on a β-blocker and nitrate in addition to his baseline medications. He reports that his symptoms have improved, although he remains limited in his activities because of exertional chest pain. Medical history is significant for hypertension, type 2 diabetes mellitus, and hyperlipidemia. His current medications are aspirin, lisinopril, simvastatin, insulin, metoprolol, isosorbide mononitrate, and as-needed sublingual nitroglycerin.

On physical examination, he is afebrile, blood pressure is 112/72 mm Hg, pulse rate is 62/min, and respiration rate is 12/min. Cardiac examination shows a normal S_1 and S_2 without S_3, S_4, murmurs, or rubs. Lung examination is normal. He has no lower extremity edema. The remainder of the examination is normal.

Diagnostic coronary angiography reveals a 90% stenosis in the proximal left anterior descending artery; the left circumflex artery has a diffuse 70% stenosis, and the right coronary artery has a 70% ostial stenosis. Left ventriculography shows a left ventricular ejection fraction of 50% with mild anterior wall hypokinesis.

Which of the following is the most appropriate management?

(A) Change metoprolol to amlodipine
(B) Coronary artery bypass graft surgery
(C) Multivessel percutaneous coronary intervention
(D) Myocardial viability nuclear perfusion scan

Item 19

A 74-year-old woman is evaluated for a 3-week history of left shoulder pain and dyspnea on exertion. Medical history is significant for COPD, hypertension, and coronary artery disease; she underwent stenting of the mid–left anterior descending coronary artery 3 years ago. Because of her lung disease, she has limited exercise ability. Medications are lisinopril, hydrochlorothiazide, atorvastatin, aspirin, fluticasone, albuterol, and ipratropium.

On physical examination, the patient is afebrile, blood pressure is 142/88 mm Hg, pulse rate is 82/min, and respiration rate is 18/min. BMI is 29. Estimated central venous pressure is 8 cm H_2O. Cardiac examination reveals a grade 2/6 midsystolic murmur heard best at the cardiac base and late expiratory wheezing bilaterally.

Electrocardiogram shows left ventricular hypertrophy and repolarization abnormalities.

Which of the following is the most appropriate diagnostic test to perform next?

(A) Adenosine single-photon emission CT myocardial perfusion imaging
(B) Coronary catheterization
(C) Dobutamine stress echocardiogram
(D) Exercise stress echocardiogram

Item 20

A 68-year-old man is evaluated for a newly diagnosed cardiac murmur. He is active and swims and jogs regularly. Medical history is otherwise unremarkable, and he takes no medications.

On physical examination, he is afebrile, blood pressure is 140/70 mm Hg, pulse rate is 82/min, and respiration rate is 16/min. Cardiac examination reveals a late-peaking systolic murmur located at the right upper sternal border with an audible S_2.

Transthoracic echocardiogram shows normal left ventricular systolic function. Aortic valve area is 0.8 cm². The mean gradient is 44 mm Hg, with a peak gradient of 53 mm Hg.

Which of the following is the most appropriate management?

(A) Balloon aortic valvuloplasty

(B) Follow-up echocardiography in 6 to 12 months

(C) Surgical aortic valve replacement

(D) Transcatheter aortic valve replacement

Item 21

A 66-year-old woman is evaluated at the hospital for 6 hours of chest pressure and shortness of breath. Earlier this day, the patient's husband was diagnosed with lung cancer. Medical history is otherwise unremarkable.

On physical examination, temperature is 36.8 °C (98.2 °F), blood pressure is 110/62 mm Hg, and pulse rate is 98/min. BMI is 25. Cardiac examination shows a normal S_1 and S_2 without S_3, S_4, murmur, or rub. Lung examination is normal. Serum troponin T level is 2.0 ng/mL (2.0 µg/L).

Electrocardiogram is shown.

The patient is administered aspirin, clopidogrel, and unfractionated heparin. Emergency coronary angiography shows normal coronary anatomy. Diastolic (*left panel*) and systolic (*right panel*) images from left ventriculography are shown.

Which of the following is the most appropriate management?

(A) Endomyocardial biopsy

(B) Intra-aortic balloon pump

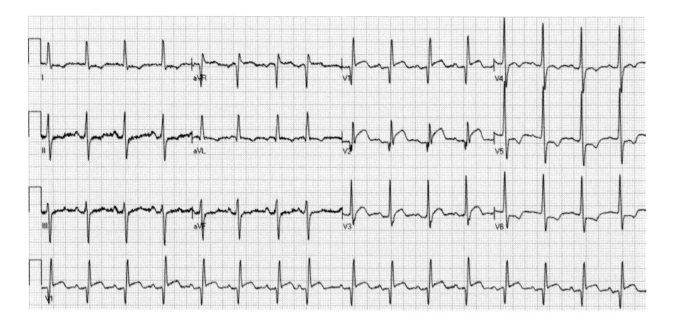

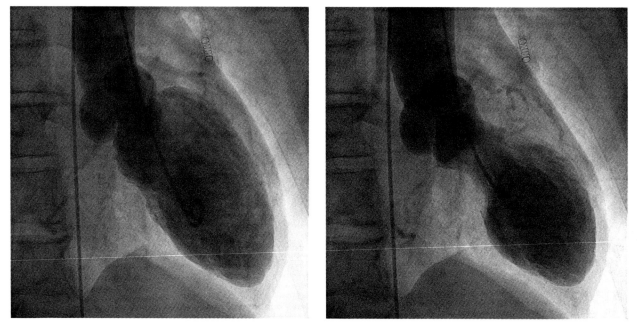

(C) Metoprolol and captopril

(D) Thrombolytic therapy

CONT.

Item 22

A 56-year-old woman is evaluated during an appointment to establish care. She has a developmental delay, and she is known to have pulmonary hypertension due to a congenital cardiac condition. There is no history of cardiac surgery. She is on low-dose aspirin and thyroid replacement therapy.

On physical examination, blood pressure is 110/70 mm Hg, pulse rate is 68/min and regular, and respiration rate is 18/min. BMI is 32. The central venous pressure is elevated with a prominent a wave. The apical impulse is normal. There is a prominent parasternal impulse at the left sternal border. The S_1 is normal; the S_2 is loud. There is a grade 1/6 holosystolic murmur at the left lower sternal border. The toes demonstrate cyanosis and digital clubbing; her hands appear normal. The remainder of the physical examination is unremarkable.

Which of the following is the most likely cause of this patient's pulmonary hypertension?

(A) Atrial septal defect

(B) Patent ductus arteriosus

(C) Tetralogy of Fallot

(D) Ventricular septal defect

Item 23

A 56-year-old man with heart failure is admitted to the hospital with a 2-week history of increasing exertional dyspnea and fatigue. He also has type 2 diabetes mellitus. Medications are metformin, lisinopril, carvedilol, furosemide, metolazone, and digoxin.

On physical examination, blood pressure is 88/60 mm Hg, pulse rate is 95/min, and respiration rate is 20/min. He is somewhat confused and inattentive. Jugular venous distention is present to the angle of the jaw while sitting. Cardiac examination reveals an S_3. There are bibasilar crackles on pulmonary examination. He has edema to the midthighs. Extremities appear mottled and are cool to the touch.

Serum creatinine level is 3.1 mg/dL (274 µmol/L); baseline value was 1.1 mg/dL (97.2 µmol/L). Serum sodium level is 133 mEq/L (133 mmol/L). Electrocardiogram shows no evidence of ischemia. Chest radiograph shows cardiomegaly and vascular congestion.

In addition to intravenous diuresis, which of the following is the most appropriate management?

(A) Dobutamine

(B) Intra-aortic balloon pump

(C) Milrinone

(D) Right heart catheterization

Item 24

A 46-year-old man is evaluated in the emergency department for severe pain in the chest and upper back that began acutely about 1 hour ago. The pain is described as "deep" and constant. He has no other associated symptoms. Medical history is significant for hypertension, and his medications are chlorthalidone and valsartan.

On physical examination, the patient is in significant pain. He is afebrile, blood pressure is 118/70 mm Hg in both upper extremities, pulse rate is 122/min, and respiration rate is 22/min. The estimated central venous pressure is 10 cm H_2O. The lungs are clear. The heart examination is notable for an early diastolic decrescendo murmur heard loudest at the right upper sternal border. The dorsalis pedis and posterior tibialis pulses are palpable and equal bilaterally.

Serum cardiac troponin T level is 0.4 ng/mL (0.4 µg/L). Electrocardiogram shows sinus tachycardia but is otherwise normal. Chest radiograph is normal. Chest CT with intravenous contrast is shown.

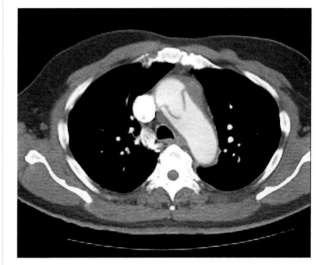

An intravenous β-blocker is started.

Which of the following is the most appropriate next step in management?

(A) Continued medical therapy alone

(B) Emergency surgical intervention

(C) Endovascular stenting

(D) Heparin

Item 25

A 46-year-old man is evaluated in the hospital prior to undergoing an elective hernia repair. Medical history is significant for a bicuspid aortic valve and a mechanical aortic valve replacement 3 years ago for severe aortic stenosis. His only medication is warfarin.

On physical examination, blood pressure is 130/75 mm Hg, pulse rate is 82/min, and respiration rate is 14/min. Cardiac examination reveals a grade 1/6 midsystolic murmur at the right upper sternal border.

Which of the following is the most appropriate management option for endocarditis prophylaxis?

(A) Amoxicillin

(B) Ceftriaxone

(C) Clindamycin

(D) No antibiotic prophylaxis

Item 26

A 48-year-old man is evaluated for tightness in his calves. His symptoms are exacerbated with walking and resolve with rest. His medical history is significant for hypertension, type 2 diabetes mellitus, and chronic kidney injury. Medications are hydrochlorothiazide, lisinopril, metformin, glyburide, and atorvastatin. He was a cigarette smoker with a 30-pack-year tobacco use history but quit 6 months ago.

On physical examination, blood pressure is 138/74 mm Hg, pulse rate is 68/min and regular, and respiration rate is 16/min. BMI is 32. No abdominal or femoral bruit is present. No skin changes are noted in the lower extremities. The remainder of the physical examination is unremarkable.

Laboratory studies are significant for a serum creatinine level of 1.9 mg/dL (168 µmol/L), normal electrolyte levels, and a hemoglobin A_{1c} value of 6.4%.

Ankle-brachial index testing:

Right systolic brachial pressure	140 mm Hg
Left systolic brachial pressure	132 mm Hg
Right posterior tibialis pressure	200 mm Hg
Left posterior tibialis pressure	130 mm Hg
Right dorsalis pedis pressure	Not detected
Left dorsalis pedis pressure	140 mm Hg

Which of the following is the most appropriate diagnostic test to perform next?

(A) Exercise ankle-brachial index

(B) Lower extremity CT angiography

(C) Lower extremity magnetic resonance angiography

(D) Toe-brachial index

Item 27

An 81-year-old man is evaluated in the office 3 days following a percutaneous coronary intervention with placement of a bare metal stent in the left anterior descending artery for angina refractory to maximal medical therapy. He indicates that he feels well except for palpitations that were not present before the procedure. Medical history is significant for hypertension and type 2 diabetes mellitus. He has no risk factors for or history of significant bleeding. Medications are aspirin, clopidogrel, lisinopril, atorvastatin, and metformin.

On physical examination, the patient is afebrile, blood pressure is 110/60 mm Hg, pulse rate is 65/min, and respiration rate is 12/min. BMI is 32. Estimated central venous pressure is not elevated. The heart has an irregularly irregular rhythm. Lungs are clear without crackles.

An electrocardiogram shows atrial fibrillation with a heart rate of 65/min and no acute ischemic changes. An echocardiogram demonstrates a left ventricular ejection fraction of 30%.

Which of the following is the most appropriate therapeutic regimen for this patient?

(A) Aspirin and clopidogrel

(B) Aspirin and dabigatran

(C) Aspirin and warfarin

(D) Aspirin, clopidogrel, and warfarin

Item 28

A 37-year-old woman is evaluated for exertional dyspnea. She noticed mild shortness of breath with significant exercise several years ago. Although she is still active, she has had to progressively decrease the amount of exercise she is able to do because of her symptoms. She has no other health problems, takes no medications, and has no known drug allergies.

On physical examination, she is afebrile, blood pressure is 120/70 mm Hg, pulse rate is 67/min, and respiration rate is 14/min. Cardiac examination demonstrates a grade 3/6 crescendo-decrescendo systolic murmur located at the right upper sternal border with delayed carotid upstrokes.

Transthoracic echocardiography demonstrates normal systolic function with a left ventricular ejection fraction of 60%, mild concentric left ventricular hypertrophy, and a bicuspid aortic valve. The aortic valve has a mean gradient of 42 mm Hg and valve area of 0.9 cm^2.

Which of the following is the most appropriate management?

(A) Balloon aortic valvuloplasty

(B) Start an ACE inhibitor

(C) Surgical aortic valve replacement

(D) Transcatheter aortic valve replacement

Item 29

A 28-year-old woman is evaluated after a 4-hour self-limited episode of palpitations. The symptoms occurred while at work yesterday. She has no history of cardiovascular disease and has no other cardiovascular symptoms. She is active without limitations. She is on no medications.

On physical examination, blood pressure is 110/70 mm Hg, pulse rate is 60/min and regular, and respiration rate is 15/min. BMI is 23. The estimated central venous pressure is elevated. The apical impulse is normal; there is a parasternal impulse present at the left sternal border, and a soft midsystolic murmur is heard at the second left intercostal space. Fixed splitting of the S_2 is noted throughout the cardiac cycle. The remainder of the physical examination is normal.

Electrocardiogram is shown (see top of next page).

Which of the following is the most likely diagnosis?

(A) Atrial septal defect

(B) Bicuspid aortic valve with aortic stenosis

(C) Congenital pulmonary valve stenosis

(D) Mitral valve prolapse with mitral regurgitation

Item 30

A 32-year-old woman is evaluated for a prepregnancy assessment. She has a heart murmur but is asymptomatic. She has no history of atrial fibrillation. Her only medication is prenatal vitamins.

On physical examination, blood pressure is 102/60 mm Hg and pulse rate is 70/min and regular. The estimated central venous pressure is elevated. The apical impulse is tapping, and there is a parasternal impulse at the left sternal border. The S_1 and S_2 are loud, and a grade

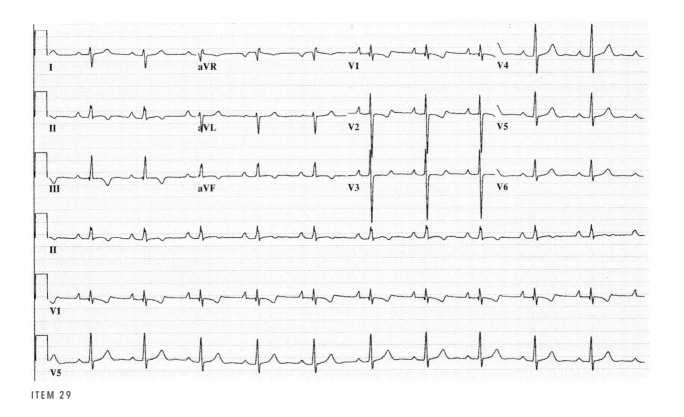

ITEM 29

2/6 diastolic decrescendo murmur is heard at the apex. No opening snap is appreciated. The lungs are clear, and there is no edema.

A transthoracic echocardiogram demonstrates normal left ventricular size and function. The mitral valve is thickened with diastolic doming. The mitral valve mean gradient is 12 mm Hg; the calculated mitral valve area is 0.9 cm². There is no mitral valve regurgitation. The estimated pulmonary artery systolic pressure is 55 mm Hg.

Which of the following is the most appropriate management at this time?

(A) Initiate an ACE inhibitor and dabigatran

(B) Obtain cardiac magnetic resonance imaging

(C) Proceed with mitral valve intervention

(D) Proceed with pregnancy without interventions or testing

Item 31

A 52-year-old woman is evaluated in the office during a routine visit. Her medical history is significant for type 2 diabetes mellitus and hypertension. Medications are aspirin, lisinopril, amlodipine, insulin glargine, insulin aspart, and rosuvastatin.

On physical examination, the patient is afebrile, blood pressure is 128/80 mm Hg, pulse rate is 73/min, and respiration rate is 18/min. BMI is 24. The lungs are clear to auscultation, and no cardiac murmurs are heard. Abdominal examination reveals a pulsatile mass in the epigastrium.

An infrarenal abdominal aortic aneurysm with maximum diameter of 5.7 cm is noted on abdominal ultrasound.

Which of the following is the most appropriate management of this patient's abdominal aortic aneurysm?

(A) Refer for aneurysm repair

(B) Repeat abdominal ultrasonography in 6 months

(C) Repeat abdominal ultrasonography in 12 months

(D) Switch amlodipine to propranolol

Item 32

A 74-year-old man is evaluated 4 months after undergoing uncomplicated bioprosthetic surgical aortic valve replacement. Within the past 2 weeks, he has developed exertional dyspnea, fatigue, and lower extremity edema. Medical history is otherwise unremarkable, and he takes no medications.

On physical examination, vital signs are normal. The estimated central venous pressure is 12 cm H₂O, and the jugular venous pulse shows prominent y descents. A pericardial knock is present. Peripheral edema is noted.

An echocardiogram reveals no evidence of pericardial effusion. The aortic and mitral valves are functioning normally. The inferior vena cava is markedly enlarged. A Doppler ultrasound shows expiratory flow reversals in the hepatic veins consistent with constrictive pericarditis.

Which of the following is the most appropriate next step in management?

(A) Ibuprofen

(B) Invasive cardiac hemodynamic evaluation

(C) Pericardiectomy

(D) Transesophageal echocardiography

Item 33

A 52-year-old man is evaluated during a follow-up visit. He was initially evaluated for severe palpitations 4 months ago. Evaluation at that time included 48-hour ambulatory electrocardiographic monitoring that was significant for frequent premature ventricular contractions (PVCs) and ventricular bigeminy. A stress echocardiogram showed no evidence of ischemia and normal left ventricular function. Cardiac magnetic resonance (CMR) imaging demonstrated no evidence of myocardial scarring. He was started on a β-blocker for treatment of PVCs at that time. He now reports continued significant palpitations despite therapy but does not have presyncope, syncope, or chest pain. He has no family history of sudden cardiac death or heart failure. His only medication is metoprolol.

On physical examination, the patient is afebrile, blood pressure is 110/60 mm Hg, pulse rate is 82/min and irregular, and respiration rate is 12/min. BMI is 34. B-type natriuretic peptide level is mildly elevated.

Electrocardiogram shows frequent monomorphic PVCs but is otherwise normal; the QRS interval on conducted sinus beats is 110 ms. Ambulatory 24-hour electrocardiographic monitoring shows frequent monomorphic PVCs (21% of all beats) and continued frequent ventricular bigeminy. An echocardiogram is significant for mild to moderate global decreased left ventricular function but without regional wall motion abnormalities; ejection fraction is estimated at 40%.

Which of the following is the most appropriate management?

(A) Amiodarone
(B) Cardiac resynchronization therapy
(C) Catheter ablation of premature ventricular contractions
(D) Implantable cardioverter-defibrillator

Item 34

A 66-year-old woman is evaluated prior to discharge. She has ischemic cardiomyopathy and was admitted to the hospital 5 days ago for worsening symptoms of heart failure. She skipped taking her diuretics during a recent business trip. Today, she feels well and is able to walk around the ward twice without any symptoms.

This was her first hospitalization in 3 years, although she has skipped her diuretics during other business trips during this time without apparent ill effect. She had an implantable cardioverter-defibrillator placed 3 years ago. An echocardiogram 1 month ago showed a left ventricular ejection fraction of 15% (stable for the past 6 years). Medications are captopril, metoprolol succinate, digoxin, furosemide, and spironolactone.

On physical examination, blood pressure is 110/72 mm Hg, pulse rate is 56/min, and respiration rate is 14/min. She has no jugular venous distention and no S_3. Lungs are clear, and she has no edema.

Electrocardiogram shows sinus rhythm, a QRS interval of 90 ms, and Q waves in V_1 through V_4. There are no changes compared with the admission electrocardiogram recorded 3 years ago.

Which of the following is the most appropriate management?

(A) Discharge and schedule follow-up within 7 days
(B) Measure B-type natriuretic peptide
(C) Obtain echocardiography prior to discharge
(D) Upgrade to biventricular implantable cardioverter-defibrillator

Item 35

A 20-year-old man is evaluated for newly noted hypertension. He is asymptomatic and his medical history is unremarkable. He takes no medications and has no family history of hypertension.

On physical examination, blood pressure is 180/80 mm Hg in both upper extremities, pulse rate is 60/min and regular, and respiration rate is 18/min. BMI is 20. The estimated central venous pressure is normal. The apical impulse is displaced and sustained. The S_1 and S_2 are normal. An S_4 is noted at the apex. A soft systolic murmur is noted over the left posterior chest. An abdominal bruit is audible. The femoral pulses are difficult to palpate, and there is a radial artery–to–femoral artery pulse delay.

The electrocardiogram is consistent with left ventricular hypertrophy.

Which of the following is the most likely diagnosis?

(A) Aortic coarctation
(B) Essential hypertension
(C) Hypertrophic cardiomyopathy
(D) Renovascular hypertension

Item 36

A 29-year-old woman who is 10 weeks pregnant is evaluated for hypertension; this is her first pregnancy. She has no symptoms and no prior cardiovascular disease. She is taking no medications. She has a family history of hypertension, and she does not recall when she last had her blood pressure checked.

On physical examination, blood pressure is 156/96 mm Hg and pulse rate is 80/min. BMI is 31. There is an apical S_4, but no murmurs are detected. Pulses are normal throughout. The remainder of the examination is unremarkable.

Serum creatinine level, plasma glucose level, and urinalysis all are normal. An ambulatory blood pressure monitor demonstrates an average blood pressure of 155/92 mm Hg.

Which of the following is the most appropriate treatment?

(A) Start labetalol
(B) Start lisinopril
(C) Start losartan
(D) No intervention is necessary

Item 37

A 28-year-old pregnant woman is evaluated for a cardiac murmur identified on examination by her obstetrician. She is asymptomatic. She is in her 24th week of pregnancy. Medical history is unremarkable, and there is no family history of heart disease. She takes prenatal vitamins and no other medications.

On physical examination, she is afebrile, blood pressure is 120/70 mm Hg, pulse rate is 86/min, and respiration rate is 18/min. Cardiac examination reveals a midsystolic ejection click followed by a grade 3/6 early peaking, crescendo-decrescendo murmur at the right upper sternal border. The murmur radiates toward the apex and decreases slightly with the Valsalva maneuver. No diastolic murmur is heard.

Which of the following is the most likely diagnosis?

(A) Bicuspid aortic valve
(B) Hypertrophic obstructive cardiomyopathy
(C) Mammary souffle
(D) Mitral valve prolapse
(E) Physiologic murmur of pregnancy

Item 38

A 64-year-old man is evaluated for chest discomfort that he has had over the past year. It does not always occur with exercise. There is no associated nausea or diaphoresis. Medical history is significant for hypertension and hyperlipidemia. Medications are metoprolol, hydrochlorothiazide, and lisinopril.

On physical examination, vital signs are normal, as is the remainder of the physical examination. Electrocardiogram is normal.

The patient is scheduled for exercise stress testing.

Which of the following should be done prior to the stress test?

(A) Stop hydrochlorothiazide
(B) Stop lisinopril
(C) Stop metoprolol
(D) Stop all medications

Item 39

A 43-year-old woman is evaluated for a 1-month history of chest discomfort. She states that she experiences a vague pressure-like sensation in her chest that occurs intermittently, with each episode lasting less than 5 minutes. She has had approximately two episodes each week, and several have seemed to be associated with exertion but also appear to have resolved after taking antacids. Her medical history is significant for hypertension. Her only medication is lisinopril. She is a current smoker with a 15-pack-year history. Family history is negative for coronary artery disease.

On physical examination, the patient is afebrile, blood pressure is 132/78 mm Hg, pulse rate is 85/min, and respiration rate is 12/min. BMI is 32. Cardiopulmonary examination is unremarkable, as is the remainder of her physical examination.

An electrocardiogram shows sinus rhythm, normal PR and QRS intervals, and no ST-segment or T-wave abnormalities or Q waves.

An exercise electrocardiographic treadmill test is performed. The patient is able to exercise for 4 minutes to a heart rate of 82% of the maximum predicted and energy expenditure of 4 metabolic equivalents until the study is discontinued because of fatigue. Testing did not reproduce her symptoms, and there were no significant electrocardiographic changes with exercise.

Which of the following is the most appropriate next step in management?

(A) Cardiac catheterization
(B) Pharmacologic stress testing
(C) Switch lisinopril to metoprolol
(D) Clinical observation

Item 40

A 72-year-old woman is evaluated for sharp chest pain that occurs randomly. She walks 3 to 4 miles daily, and her symptoms have never occurred with exertion. She has never smoked. Medical history is significant for hypertension, type 2 diabetes mellitus, and hyperlipidemia. Medications are low-dose aspirin, metformin, lisinopril, and simvastatin (10 mg/d). She has no known drug allergies.

On physical examination, blood pressure is 122/76 mm Hg, pulse rate is 76/min, and respiration rate is 12/min. Cardiac examination shows a normal S_1 and S_2; there is no S_3, S_4, murmur, or rub. The remainder of the examination is normal.

Laboratory findings include a serum total cholesterol level of 200 mg/dL (5.18 mmol/L), LDL cholesterol level of 126 mg/dL (3.26 mmol/L), and HDL cholesterol level of 50 mg/dL (1.30 mmol/L).

An exercise treadmill test is administered for 8 minutes, 40 seconds. There are no electrocardiogram changes at rest or with exercise. She does not have chest pain during exercise or recovery.

Which of the following is the most appropriate management?

(A) Increase simvastatin to 80 mg/d
(B) Continue current therapy
(C) Start atorvastatin, discontinue simvastatin
(D) Start clopidogrel

Item 41

A 57-year-old man is evaluated in follow-up 1 month after being diagnosed with peripheral arterial disease. He initially presented with left calf pain and was diagnosed by an abnormal ankle-brachial index. An exercise rehabilitation program was completed, but he continues to feel lower extremity discomfort in his left leg that limits his walking ability. He is a former smoker who quit 1 year ago. His medical history is otherwise notable for hypertension and dyslipidemia. Medications are enalapril, amlodipine, rosuvastatin, and aspirin.

On physical examination, blood pressure is 124/72 mm Hg, pulse rate is 78/min and regular, and respiration rate is 16/min. Peripheral examination reveals a left femoral bruit.

The left lower extremity is warm and without tenderness or skin changes. The remainder of the examination is unremarkable.

Which of the following is the most appropriate addition to his current therapy?

(A) β-Blocker

(B) Cilostazol

(C) Clopidogrel

(D) Warfarin

Item 42

A 75-year-old woman is evaluated in the hospital 4 hours after onset of chest pain with findings of an ST-elevation myocardial infarction. She was taken emergently to the catheterization laboratory and underwent emergency percutaneous coronary intervention for a totally occluded vessel. Her post-intervention ventriculogram demonstrated a left ventricular ejection fraction of 30%. One hour after the procedure, she developed an acute arrhythmia. Medications are aspirin, metoprolol, atorvastatin, and clopidogrel.

On physical examination, the patient is afebrile, blood pressure is 100/60 mm Hg, pulse rate is 92/min, and respiration rate is 12/min. BMI is 25. Neck examination demonstrates cannon *a* waves. Cardiac examination demonstrates regular rhythm with a variable S_1. Lungs are clear to auscultation.

Electrocardiogram is shown.

Which of the following is the most appropriate management?

(A) Amiodarone

(B) Cardioversion

(C) Implantable cardioverter-defibrillator

(D) Lidocaine

(E) No intervention

Item 43

A 68-year-old man is evaluated in the emergency department for a 24-hour history of persistent chest pain. He had a non–ST-elevation myocardial infarction 1 week ago that was managed medically with complete symptom recovery. Yesterday, he developed recurrent chest pain that differs from his previous angina pain. The pain is constant but exacerbated when leaning forward and not associated with other symptoms. Medications are low-dose aspirin, clopidogrel, metoprolol, and atorvastatin.

On physical examination, vital signs are normal. There is no jugular venous distention. The lungs are clear to auscultation. S_1 and S_2 are normal, and there is no S_3 or S_4. A two-component friction rub is present at the left lower sternal border, and a grade 2/6 holosystolic murmur is heard at the apex. The remainder of the physical examination is unremarkable.

Electrocardiogram shows diffuse, concave upward ST-segment elevations and PR-segment depression most prominent in leads V_1 through V_6.

Which of the following is the most appropriate primary treatment?

(A) High-dose aspirin

(B) Ibuprofen

(C) Nitroglycerin

(D) Prednisone

Item 44

A 56-year-old man is admitted to the coronary care unit with recent-onset substernal chest discomfort and dyspnea. Upon admission, he was given aspirin, ticagrelor, metoprolol, and enoxaparin. He has hyperlipidemia. Regular medications are low-dose aspirin and simvastatin.

On physical examination, temperature is 36.5 °C (97.7 °F), blood pressure is 134/82 mm Hg, and pulse rate is 82/min. Cardiac and pulmonary examinations are normal, as is the remainder of the examination.

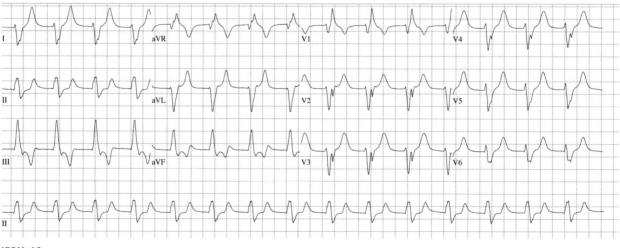

ITEM 42

Serum troponin level is elevated. Electrocardiogram shows normal sinus rhythm and heart rate of 80/min. There are nonspecific ST-T wave abnormalities but no ST-segment elevation or depression.

Cardiac catheterization is significant for preserved left ventricular systolic function and two-vessel coronary artery disease. Percutaneous coronary intervention of the mid left anterior descending artery and proximal right coronary artery is performed with placement of drug-eluting stents.

In addition to continuing aspirin, which of the following is the most appropriate management of this patient's antiplatelet regimen?

(A) Continue ticagrelor for 30 days
(B) Continue ticagrelor for 1 year
(C) Continue ticagrelor indefinitely
(D) Stop ticagrelor, start clopidogrel

Item 45

A 42-year-old woman is evaluated for a routine outpatient medical assessment. She was diagnosed with a ventricular septal defect at age 6 months. Evaluation was performed early in life and observation was recommended. She has no symptoms and is taking no medications.

On physical examination, blood pressure is 100/60 mm Hg, pulse rate is 70/min and regular, and respiration rate is 15/min. BMI is 28. The estimated central venous pressure is normal. The apical impulse is normal. There is no parasternal impulse. S_1 and S_2 are masked by a loud holosystolic murmur noted at the left lower sternal border. The rest of the examination is unremarkable.

An electrocardiogram is normal. The heart size is normal on the chest radiograph. An echocardiogram demonstrates normal left ventricular size and function with an ejection fraction of 60%. A membranous ventricular septal defect is noted with a small left-to-right shunt. The right heart chambers and valve function are normal. The estimated pulmonary artery pressure is normal.

Which of the following is the most appropriate management?

(A) Cardiac catheterization
(B) Cardiac magnetic resonance (CMR) imaging
(C) Endocarditis prophylaxis
(D) Follow-up in 3 to 5 years
(E) Stress testing to determine exercise capacity

Item 46

A 72-year-old woman is evaluated in the hospital for a 3-month history of increasing shortness of breath. Although she had previously been physically active, her ambulation is now limited to about 50 feet because of shortness of breath. Medical history is significant for rheumatic fever as a child, diverticulosis with gastrointestinal bleeding that required blood transfusions, hypertension, and hyperlipidemia. Medications are chlorthalidone and atorvastatin.

On physical examination, the patient is afebrile, blood pressure is 140/70 mm Hg, pulse rate is 83/min, and respiratory

rate is 16/min. Oxygen saturation breathing ambient air is 98%. There is no jugular venous distention. Lungs are clear. Cardiac examination reveals a regular rate and a grade 3/6 apical holosystolic murmur that radiates to the axilla. There is no lower extremity edema.

Electrocardiogram shows normal sinus rhythm and evidence of left atrial enlargement. Echocardiogram shows severe eccentric mitral regurgitation with marked calcification of the valve leaflets; left ventricular systolic function is normal.

Which of the following is the most appropriate treatment?

(A) Bioprosthetic mitral valve replacement
(B) Mechanical mitral valve replacement
(C) Oral vasodilator therapy
(D) Percutaneous mitral valvuloplasty

Item 47

A 75-year-old woman is evaluated for a 3-month history of progressive exertional dyspnea and decreased exercise tolerance. She does not have chest pain. She has a history of hypertension and COPD. She has a 55-pack-year tobacco use history but quit 3 years ago. She has no history of alcohol use. Medications are lisinopril, tiotropium, and as-needed albuterol.

On physical examination, blood pressure is 136/78 mm Hg, pulse rate is 88/min, and respiration rate is 16/min. The central venous pressure is estimated at 9 cm H_2O. There are decreased breath sounds throughout both lung fields, but no crackles are detected. An S_4 is heard on cardiac examination. There is trace bilateral lower extremity edema.

Laboratory studies, including thyroid function studies, are normal. Electrocardiogram is shown (see top of next page). A chest radiograph shows changes consistent with COPD, mild vascular congestion, and blunting of the costophrenic angles bilaterally. Echocardiogram shows a left ventricular ejection fraction of 30% and an akinetic anterior wall.

The patient is started on furosemide.

Which of the following is the most appropriate diagnostic test to perform next?

(A) Cardiac magnetic resonance (CMR) imaging
(B) Coronary artery calcium scoring
(C) Myocardial perfusion imaging stress test
(D) Endomyocardial biopsy

Item 48

A 59-year-old woman is evaluated for continued substernal chest pain. She presented with exertional chest pain 6 months ago that occurred with minimal ambulation. She was evaluated with a stress nuclear medicine myocardial perfusion study that showed no ST-segment changes but a small area of inducible ischemia in the lateral area of the left ventricle and an ejection fraction of 45%. She was initially treated medically but has continued to have chest pain with exertion despite the addition of multiple antianginal agents. Medical history is significant for hypertension, hypercholesterolemia, and type 2 diabetes mellitus. She has a 30-pack-year smoking history but quit 1 year ago.

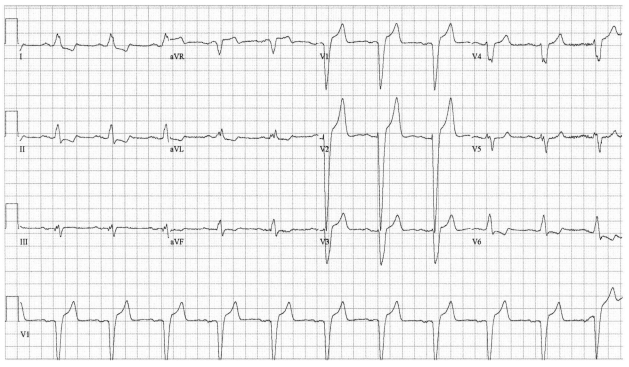

ITEM 47

Medications are aspirin, lisinopril, simvastatin, metformin, metoprolol, and long-acting nitroglycerin.

On physical examination, the patient is afebrile, blood pressure is 132/72 mm Hg, pulse rate is 68/min, and respiration rate is 16/min. BMI is 28. The remainder of her physical examination is normal.

Electrocardiogram is unchanged from the time of her stress test.

Which of the following is the most appropriate next step in management?

(A) Cardiac catheterization

(B) CT angiography

(C) Dobutamine stress echocardiography

(D) Continued medical therapy

Item 49

A 26-year-old woman is evaluated during a visit to establish care. She has noted shortness of breath for the past 18 months that is progressively worsening. She has no significant medical history. She is active and exercises regularly. She takes no medications.

On physical examination, blood pressure is 115/70 mm Hg and pulse rate is 62/min. BMI is 45. Cardiac examination reveals a midsystolic click with a grade 3/6 late systolic murmur heard over the apex and radiating toward the axilla.

Transthoracic echocardiogram (TTE) shows moderate to severe mitral regurgitation with marked prolapse of the anterior leaflet, normal left ventricular systolic function with an ejection fraction of 55%, and normal chamber sizes; the regurgitant jet is not well visualized.

Which of the following is the most appropriate management?

(A) Mitral valve repair

(B) Repeat TTE in 6 months

(C) Start lisinopril

(D) Transesophageal echocardiography

Item 50

A 35-year-old man is evaluated for a 6-month history of intermittent palpitations. His symptoms occur about once a week with no consistent pattern. He occasionally becomes lightheaded with the palpitations but has no syncope. He exercises three times weekly and does not notice symptoms during exercise. He has a history of migraine, for which he takes naproxen and sumatriptan as needed. He has no family history of sudden cardiac death.

On physical examination, the patient is afebrile, blood pressure is 138/68 mm Hg, pulse rate is 75/min, and respiration rate is 16/min. BMI is 24. Cardiac examination and the remainder of the examination are unremarkable.

Electrocardiogram is normal.

Which of the following is the most appropriate testing option?

(A) 30-Day event recorder

(B) Echocardiogram

(C) Exercise stress test

(D) 24-Hour continuous ambulatory electrocardiographic monitor

Item 51

A 76-year-old man is admitted to the hospital for recurrent palpitations and dyspnea that began 4 days ago. He has hypertension and coronary artery disease, which was treated with percutaneous intervention 8 years ago. Medications are aspirin, atorvastatin, and lisinopril.

On physical examination, temperature is 36.8 °C (98.2 °F), and blood pressure is 115/62 mm Hg. The resting heart rate is 110/min with intermittent irregularity. The estimated central venous pressure is not elevated. S_1 and S_2 are unremarkable. The lung fields are clear, and the extremities are without edema.

An electrocardiogram obtained after the physical examination is shown.

Which of the following is the most appropriate next step in treatment?

(A) Emergent cardioversion

(B) Initiate β-blocker therapy

(C) Intravenous amiodarone

(D) Intravenous procainamide

Item 52

A 74-year-old woman is evaluated during a routine examination. Her medical history is significant for hypertension and obesity. She is a former smoker, stopping 5 years ago. Medications are amlodipine, lisinopril, and aspirin.

On physical examination, she is afebrile, blood pressure is 136/78 mm Hg, pulse rate is 68/min, and respiration rate is 15/min. BMI is 32. The lungs are clear to auscultation, and no murmurs are noted. A bruit is heard over the left femoral artery.

The right ankle-brachial index is 1.2 and the left is 0.81.

Which of the following is the most appropriate management?

(A) Initiate atorvastatin

(B) Initiate cilostazol

(C) Initiate warfarin

(D) Obtain CT angiography

(E) Obtain segmental limb pressures

Item 53

A 58-year-old man is ready for hospital discharge following a non–ST-elevation myocardial infarction. He was treated with ticagrelor and underwent percutaneous coronary intervention with drug-eluting stent implantation. He has remained free of chest pain since admission to the hospital.

The patient's medical history is significant for hypertension and hyperlipidemia. Medications are low-dose aspirin, ticagrelor, metoprolol, lisinopril, atorvastatin, and sublingual nitroglycerin as needed.

On physical examination, blood pressure is 124/78 mm Hg and pulse rate is 54/min. BMI is 26. Lungs are clear to auscultation. Cardiac examination shows a normal S_1 and S_2; there is no S_3, S_4, murmur, or rub. The remainder of the examination is normal. His left ventricular systolic function is normal, as measured on transthoracic echocardiography on the day after hospital admission.

Which of the following is the most appropriate adjustment to his discharge medications?

(A) Add diltiazem

(B) Discontinue ticagrelor, start clopidogrel

(C) Increase dose of metoprolol

(D) Start eplerenone

(E) Make no changes to his medications

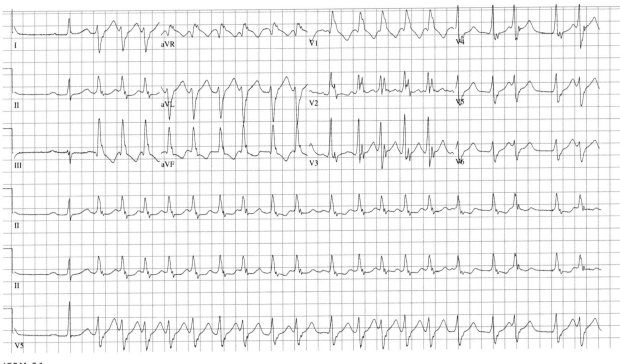

ITEM 51

Item 54

A 54-year-old man is evaluated after a recent diagnosis of systolic heart failure. He initially presented with a 4-month history of exertional dyspnea. He has not had prior regular medical care and had no known medical problems. His blood pressure was 164/96 mm Hg at the time of diagnosis. Echocardiography showed evidence of hypertensive cardiomyopathy with no regional wall motion abnormalities and a left ventricular ejection fraction of 30%. Cardiac stress testing showed no evidence of ischemia, and he exercised for 7 minutes and 10 seconds to a peak heart rate of 142/min. He was started on lisinopril and is now able to walk 6 blocks before experiencing dyspnea.

On physical examination, blood pressure is 110/72 mm Hg, pulse rate is 84/min, and respiration rate is 14/min. Estimated central venous pressure is 6 cm H_2O. The lungs are clear. Cardiac examination shows the point of maximal impulse is shifted to the left anterior axillary line. There is no lower extremity edema.

Laboratory studies, including electrolytes and kidney function, are normal.

Which of the following medications is the most appropriate addition to this patient's treatment regimen?

(A) Amlodipine
(B) Carvedilol
(C) Furosemide
(D) Spironolactone
(E) No added therapy

Item 55

A 63-year-old man is hospitalized following a recent inferior myocardial infarction. Percutaneous coronary intervention was not successful. An echocardiogram obtained following the attempted coronary intervention demonstrated a left ventricular ejection fraction of 55% with inferior wall akinesis and a dilated and dysfunctional right ventricle. On the third day after admission, the patient develops progressive oxygen desaturation and dyspnea despite oxygen therapy while upright that improves when supine.

On physical examination, his blood pressure is 90/70 mm Hg, pulse rate is 86/min and regular, and respiration rate is 25/min. Estimated central venous pressure is markedly elevated. The apical impulse is normal; there is a parasternal impulse at the left sternal border. The heart sounds are distant. There is a soft holosystolic murmur at the left sternal border that increases with inspiration. The oxygen saturation is 90% on oxygen administered by mask while the patient is sitting and improves to 94% on return to his bed. The remainder of the physical examination is normal.

Which of the following is the most likely diagnosis?

(A) Patent foramen ovale with right-to-left shunt
(B) Mitral regurgitation
(C) Severe left ventricular systolic dysfunction
(D) Ventricular septal defect

Item 56

A 77-year-old man with a 5-year history of idiopathic cardiomyopathy is evaluated for progressive exertional fatigue and dyspnea. He has recently stopped carrying groceries in from the car because of his exertional dyspnea. He had an implantable cardioverter-defibrillator placed 3 years ago. Medical history is also significant for hypertension. Medications are lisinopril, 40 mg/d; metoprolol succinate, 25 mg/d; furosemide, 40 mg/d; and spironolactone, 25 mg/d.

On physical examination, blood pressure is 94/60 mm Hg and pulse rate is 70/min. Estimated central venous pressure is 5 cm H_2O. There is no edema.

Serum electrolyte levels and kidney function are normal. Electrocardiogram shows normal sinus rhythm, a PR interval of 210 ms, QRS duration of 160 ms, and a new left bundle branch block. His left ventricular ejection fraction 3 months ago was 25%.

Which of the following is the most appropriate next step in management?

(A) Cardiac resynchronization therapy
(B) Dobutamine therapy
(C) Increase furosemide dose
(D) Left ventricular assist device placement

Item 57

A 53-year-old man is evaluated for a 6-week history of epigastric and chest discomfort. The onset of the pain has a variable relationship to stress and exercise and spicy food. The discomfort is relieved at times with antacids and with rest. He has hypertension and is a former smoker (quit 2 years ago). Medications are lisinopril and hydrochlorothiazide.

On physical examination, he is afebrile, blood pressure is 140/92 mm Hg, pulse rate is 78/min, and respiration rate is 12/min. BMI is 29. Funduscopic examination is normal. Results of the cardiac examination are normal, with no S_3 or S_4.

Electrocardiogram is shown (see top of next page).

Which of the following is the most appropriate diagnostic test to perform next?

(A) Adenosine myocardial perfusion study
(B) Cardiac magnetic resonance (CMR) imaging
(C) CT angiography
(D) Dobutamine stress echocardiography
(E) Exercise stress test

Item 58

A 58-year-old man is evaluated for a 2-week history of malaise and subjective fever. Medical history is significant for well-controlled type 2 diabetes mellitus and sinus node dysfunction. A dual-chamber pacemaker was implanted 5 years ago. He does not have dyspnea or weight loss. None of his family members have had a recent viral or febrile illness.

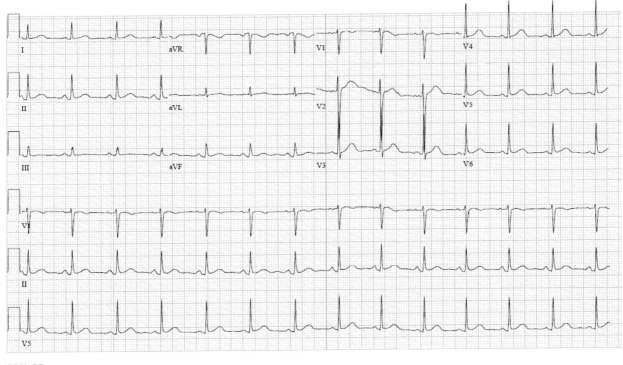

ITEM 57

On physical examination, temperature is 38.0 °C (100.4 °F), blood pressure is 132/75 mm Hg, pulse rate is 62/min, and respiration rate is 16/min. BMI is 32. His conjunctivae, oropharynx, and tympanic membranes are normal in appearance. There is no head, neck, axillary, or inguinal lymphadenopathy. The skin overlying the patient's pacemaker pocket is mildly erythematous and warm. There is no fluctuance, but there is mild tenderness to palpation. The precordial cadence is regular, and there is no evidence of cardiopulmonary congestion. Results of a complete blood count with differential and an erythrocyte sedimentation rate are pending.

Which of the following is the most appropriate management?

(A) Blood cultures

(B) Pacemaker pocket aspiration

(C) Ultrasonography of the pacemaker pocket

(D) Repeat evaluation in 1 week

Item 59

A 47-year-old man is evaluated during a routine examination. He has no symptoms. Medical history is significant for a bicuspid aortic valve. He is not taking any medications.

On physical examination, he is afebrile, blood pressure is 130/70 mm Hg, pulse rate is 56/min, and respiration rate is 15/min. Cardiac examination reveals a grade 1/6 diastolic murmur at the left lower sternal border.

Echocardiogram shows a bicuspid aortic valve with moderate aortic regurgitation, normal left ventricular systolic function, and normal left ventricular chamber size.

Which of the following is the most appropriate management?

(A) Aortic valve replacement

(B) Clinical reassessment in 1 year

(C) Endocarditis prophylaxis

(D) Start an ACE inhibitor

(E) Start a calcium channel blocker

Item 60

A 26-year-old woman with a mechanical mitral valve prosthesis visits to discuss anticoagulation management during pregnancy. Her last menstrual period was 6 weeks ago and her pregnancy was confirmed by laboratory testing in the office. Her mitral valve was replaced 5 years ago. Her medications are low-dose aspirin, metoprolol, and warfarin (4 mg/d).

On physical examination, vital signs are normal. Cardiac auscultation demonstrates a normal mechanical S_1. There are no murmurs or added sounds. Her INR is 2.6.

Which of the following anticoagulation regimens will provide the greatest protection against thromboembolism during her pregnancy?

(A) Continue warfarin and aspirin

(B) Stop warfarin and start dabigatran

(C) Stop warfarin and start subcutaneous fixed-dose unfractionated heparin

(D) Stop warfarin and start weight-based low-molecular-weight heparin

Item 61

A 72-year-old woman is evaluated in the emergency department for progressive chest pain that began 2 hours ago. She has not had recent surgery or stroke. She takes amlodipine for hypertension.

On physical examination, blood pressure is 154/88 mm Hg, and pulse rate is 88/min. Cardiac and pulmonary examinations are normal.

Initial electrocardiogram shows 2-mm ST-segment elevation in leads V_1 through V_5 with reciprocal ST-segment depression in leads II, III, and aVF. Chest radiograph shows no cardiomegaly and no evidence of pulmonary edema.

The patient is given aspirin, clopidogrel, unfractionated heparin, and a β-blocker. Because the nearest hospital with primary percutaneous coronary intervention capabilities is more than 120 minutes away, she is also given a bolus dose of tenecteplase.

Thirty minutes later, the patient's blood pressure has dropped to 85/58 mm Hg. Her chest pain persists, and she rates the pain as 8 out of 10. Pulmonary crackles are auscultated to the scapulae. Electrocardiogram shows 3-mm ST-segment elevation in leads V_1 through V_5 with reciprocal ST-segment depression in leads II, III, and aVF.

Which of the following is the most appropriate management?

(A) Continued medical therapy
(B) Glycoprotein IIb/IIIa inhibitor
(C) Repeat tenecteplase
(D) Transfer for emergency percutaneous coronary intervention

Item 62

A 56-year-old man is being evaluated after his 18-year-old son had a syncopal episode during a high school basketball game and was diagnosed with hypertrophic cardiomyopathy (HCM). The patient has had no symptoms, including with physical activity such as golfing or playing tennis. Medical history is unremarkable, and a review of family history is negative for other relatives with HCM, sudden cardiac death, or tachyarrhythmias. He takes no medications.

Findings of a comprehensive physical examination are unremarkable.

An electrocardiogram and echocardiogram are normal, with no evidence of HCM.

When should this patient next be screened for HCM?

(A) In 6 months
(B) In 1 to 2 years
(C) In 5 years
(D) No further screening is necessary

Item 63

A 73-year-old man is evaluated in the emergency department for chest pain of 2 hours' duration. He is bradycardic. He does not have dyspnea, lightheadedness, or loss of consciousness. Medical history is significant for type 2 diabetes mellitus, hypertension, and hyperlipidemia. Medications are aspirin, metformin, lisinopril, and hydrochlorothiazide.

On physical examination, the patient is afebrile, blood pressure is 120/60 mm Hg, pulse rate is 47/min, and respiration rate is 12/min. BMI is 34. He is warm and well-perfused. Trace bibasilar crackles are heard in the lungs.

The electrocardiogram is shown.

Which of the following is the most appropriate treatment?

(A) Aminophylline
(B) Low-dose dopamine
(C) Percutaneous coronary intervention
(D) Temporary pacing

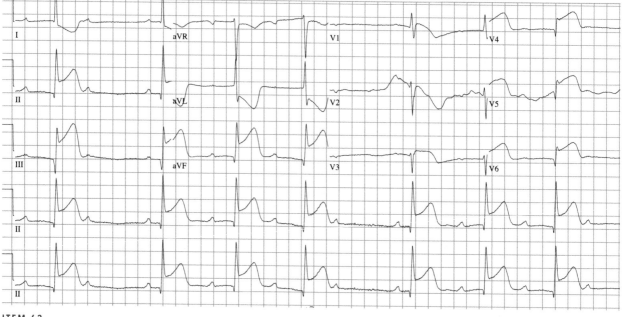

ITEM 63

Item 64

A 53-year-old woman with Eisenmenger syndrome related to a ventricular septal defect is evaluated in the emergency department for fever and chills over the past 12 hours. She has dysuria and urinary frequency. Her only outpatient medication is bosentan.

On physical examination, temperature is 38.2 °C (100.8 °F), blood pressure is 110/70 mm Hg, pulse rate is 86/min and regular, and respiration rate is 20/min. Oxygen saturation on ambient air is 85%. BMI is 24. Digital clubbing and cyanosis are evident. The estimated central venous pressure is elevated with a prominent a wave. The apical impulse is normal. A prominent parasternal impulse is present at the left sternal border. The S_1 is normal; the S_2 is loud. A soft holosystolic murmur is heard at the left lower sternal border. Mild right flank tenderness is noted.

A urinary Gram stain is positive; urine and blood culture results are pending. The hemoglobin level is 18 g/dL (180 g/L), hematocrit is 55%, and the leukocyte count is 20,000/μL (20×10^9/L).

In addition to intravenous antibiotic administration, which of the following is the most appropriate management?

(A) Air filters on intravenous lines
(B) Oxygen by close-fitting mask
(C) Phlebotomy
(D) Transthoracic echocardiogram

Item 65

A 62-year-old man is evaluated during a routine visit. He is asymptomatic and walks 1 mile most days of the week. Medical history is significant for aortic stenosis, type 2 diabetes mellitus, hypertension, and hyperlipidemia. Medications are aspirin, metformin, lisinopril, metoprolol, and rosuvastatin.

On physical examination, the patient is afebrile, blood pressure is 130/66 mm Hg, pulse rate is 68/min, and respiration rate is 14/min. BMI is 29. Cardiac examination reveals a grade 2/6 early-peaking systolic murmur at the cardiac base. Carotid upstrokes are normal. The remainder of the examination is unremarkable.

Laboratory studies demonstrate a total serum cholesterol level of 150 mg/dL (3.89 mmol/L). Electrocardiogram is within normal limits. Echocardiogram from 1 year ago shows a peak velocity of 2.0 m/s, mean transaortic gradient of 13 mm Hg, aortic valve area of 1.5 cm², and preserved ejection fraction.

Which of the following is the most appropriate management?

(A) Echocardiogram
(B) Exercise perfusion study
(C) Exercise stress test
(D) No additional testing

Item 66

A 78-year-old man is evaluated in the emergency department because of a painful right foot. He has a 1-year history of right-sided claudication. Three days ago he developed severe rest pain in the right foot that is starting to subside. He has hypertension and a 10-year history of type 2 diabetes mellitus. He has a 55-pack-year history of cigarette smoking but stopped 2 years ago. Medications are aspirin, metformin, losartan, and amlodipine.

On physical examination, vital signs are stable. The right foot is cool and pale with slow capillary refill in the nail beds. The dorsalis pedis and posterior tibialis pulses are not palpable. Arterial Doppler ultrasound signal over the dorsalis pedis is present but markedly diminished. Sensation of light touch is present but decreased over the dorsum of the right foot.

Laboratory studies are significant for normal complete blood count, electrolytes, and kidney function. Electrocardiogram demonstrates sinus rhythm.

A continuous heparin infusion is started.

Which of the following is the most appropriate next step in management?

(A) Catheter-directed thrombolytic therapy
(B) Emergent surgical amputation
(C) Initiation of warfarin
(D) Urgent angiography

Item 67

A 72-year-old man is evaluated during a routine examination. He has no symptoms or significant medical history. He is active and exercises regularly. He does not take any medications.

On physical examination, blood pressure is 135/70 mm Hg, pulse rate is 82/min, and respiration rate is 17/min. Cardiac examination reveals a grade 3/6 apical holosystolic murmur.

Echocardiogram shows severe mitral regurgitation and a left ventricular ejection fraction of 45% without evidence of regional wall motion abnormalities.

Which of the following is the most appropriate management?

(A) Vasodilator therapy
(B) Percutaneous mitral balloon valvuloplasty
(C) Repeat echocardiogram in 6 months
(D) Surgical mitral valve repair

Item 68

A 40-year-old man is evaluated in the emergency department for syncope. He was attending a baseball game when he experienced a witnessed, abrupt episode of syncope while seated. He did not experience any prodromal symptoms. He sustained some facial trauma when he struck the railing in front of him. He has experienced near-syncope on several occasions in the past. His father died suddenly at age 50 years. The patient takes no medications and has no drug allergies.

On physical examination, the patient is afebrile, blood pressure is 125/64 mm Hg, pulse rate is 64/min, and respiration rate is 16/min. BMI is 26. Estimated central venous pressure is normal. Cardiac examination shows a regular

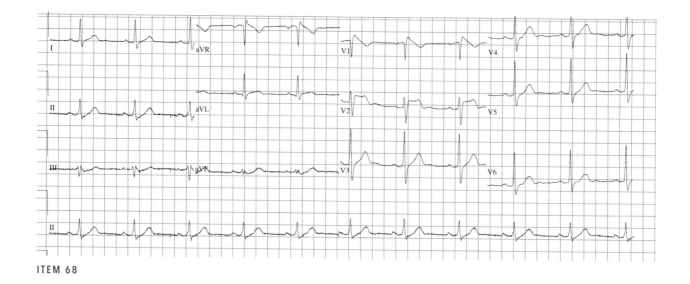

ITEM 68

rate with normal heart sounds and no murmurs. He has no peripheral edema.

Pertinent laboratory findings include a negative troponin test, a normal metabolic profile, and normal kidney function studies.

Electrocardiogram is shown. Echocardiogram demonstrates no structural heart disease and shows normal left ventricular function.

Which of the following is the most appropriate management?

(A) Cardiac magnetic resonance (CMR) imaging

(B) Exercise treadmill stress test

(C) Implantable cardioverter-defibrillator placement

(D) Tilt-table test

Item 69

A 68-year-old man is evaluated at a follow-up appointment. He has a 7-year history of heart failure secondary to ischemic cardiomyopathy. Over the past 6 months, he has had three hospitalizations for exacerbations of his heart failure. He currently has exertional dyspnea while getting dressed, and his maximal activity level is limited to riding to the store with his wife but staying in the car. Medical history is significant for disseminated prostate cancer treated with androgen deprivation therapy. Medications are aspirin, lisinopril, carvedilol, furosemide, digoxin, spironolactone, rosuvastatin, and leuprolide. He is stable on his current medications.

On physical examination, blood pressure is 92/60 mm Hg and pulse rate is 80/min. There is no jugular venous distention. An S_3 is heard on cardiac examination. The legs are cool to the touch; there is no edema.

Laboratory studies are significant for a serum sodium level of 132 mEq/L (132 mmol/L) and serum creatinine level of 1.8 mg/dL (159 μmol/L).

Which of the following is the most appropriate management?

(A) Add metolazone

(B) Cardiac transplantation evaluation

(C) Evaluation for left ventricular assist device placement

(D) Home inotropic therapy

Item 70

A 75-year-old woman is evaluated during a follow-up visit for recently diagnosed atrial fibrillation that is adequately rate controlled on medication. Medical history is significant for hypertension and end-stage kidney disease; she is on hemodialysis. Medications are metoprolol, digoxin, lisinopril, and amlodipine. She has not yet been started on stroke prevention therapy.

On physical examination, temperature is 36.8 °C (98.2 °F), blood pressure is 120/65 mm Hg, pulse rate is 72/min, and respiration rate is 16/min. BMI is 29. The precordial cadence is irregularly irregular. There is no evidence of pulmonary or peripheral congestion.

Which of the following is the most appropriate treatment?

(A) Apixaban

(B) Aspirin and clopidogrel

(C) Dabigatran

(D) Dose-adjusted warfarin

(E) Rivaroxaban

Item 71

A 62-year-old woman is evaluated in the emergency department for sudden onset of severe chest, upper abdominal, and back pain of 2 hours' duration. She has not had similar symptoms previously and notes no other symptoms. Medical history is significant for hypertension. She is a current smoker with a 55-pack-year history. Her medications are amlodipine and benazepril.

On physical examination, she is afebrile, blood pressure is 165/100 mm Hg in both arms, pulse rate is 102/min, and respiration rate is 20/min. Oxygen saturation is 98% on ambient air. Cardiac auscultation reveals an S_4 gallop but no murmurs. Pulmonary examination is normal. Pulses are symmetric and equal in all extremities. The remainder of the physical examination is unremarkable.

Laboratory studies reveal a D-dimer level of 0.8 µg/mL (0.8 mg/L) and a serum creatinine level of 2.4 mg/dL (212 µmol/L) (baseline is <1 mg/dL [88.4 µmol/L]). Initial cardiac troponin T level is 0.4 ng/mL (0.4 µg/L).

Electrocardiogram shows left ventricular hypertrophy with repolarization abnormalities. Chest radiograph demonstrates an enlarged cardiac silhouette. A magnetic resonance angiography study demonstrates aortic dissection originating distal to the left subclavian artery extending to the aortoiliac bifurcation (maximum diameter 63 mm). Bilateral renal arteries arise from the false lumen.

Treatment with analgesics, a β-blocker, and sodium nitroprusside is started.

Which of the following is the most appropriate next step in management?

(A) Aortic repair
(B) Coronary angiography
(C) Continue current medical therapy
(D) Intravenous heparin

Item 72

An 18-year-old woman with Noonan syndrome is evaluated for a heart murmur noted on a sports physical examination. She is asymptomatic and her medical history is unremarkable. She takes no medications.

On physical examination, blood pressure is 120/70 mm Hg, pulse rate is 70/min and regular, and respiration rate is 18/min. BMI is 18. The patient is of short stature and has hypertelorism, neck webbing, and a low hairline. The cen-

tral venous pressure is elevated with a prominent *a* wave. The apical impulse is normal. There is a prominent parasternal impulse at the left sternal border. The S_1 is normal; the S_2 is soft. A grade 4/6 late-peaking systolic murmur is heard at the left sternal border and second left intercostal space. An ejection click is not audible.

An echocardiogram demonstrates a dysplastic pulmonary valve with a peak instantaneous systolic gradient of 62 mm Hg and mean systolic gradient of 45 mm Hg. There is moderate pulmonary valve regurgitation. The right ventricular size and function are normal, but there is right ventricular hypertrophy. The left heart size and function are normal.

Which of the following is the most appropriate management for this patient?

(A) Endocarditis prophylaxis
(B) Exercise testing
(C) Pulmonary valve replacement
(D) Observation

Item 73

A 62-year-old man is evaluated in the emergency department (ED) for a 3-hour history of dull, substernal chest discomfort. He has type 2 diabetes mellitus, hypertension, and dyslipidemia. He does not smoke cigarettes. Medications are low-dose aspirin, lisinopril, and pravastatin. His younger sister was diagnosed with coronary artery disease at the age of 50 years.

Electrocardiogram obtained upon his arrival to the ED is shown. He is administered aspirin and sublingual nitroglycerin. His chest discomfort is relieved within 15 minutes of arrival.

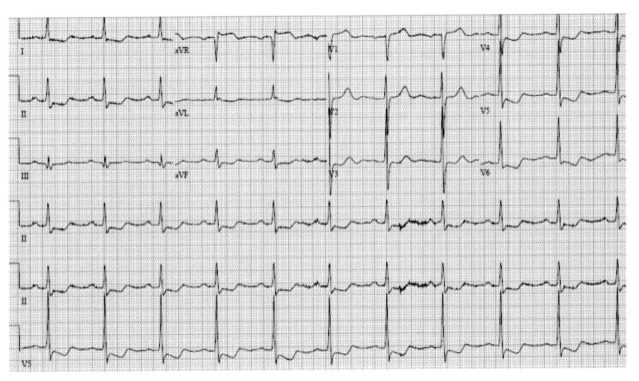

ITEM 73

On physical examination, blood pressure is 148/86 mm Hg, pulse rate is 62/min and regular, and oxygen saturation is 94% on ambient air. BMI is 28. Cardiac examination is significant only for the presence of a grade 1/6 holosystolic murmur at the left lower sternal border. The murmur does not radiate. Lungs are clear. The reminder of the examination is normal.

Initial serum troponin I concentration is 0.94 ng/mL (0.94 µg/L).

Portable chest radiograph demonstrates a normal cardiac silhouette and no evidence of pulmonary edema.

Which of the following is the most appropriate initial management?

(A) Administer clopidogrel and enoxaparin
(B) Emergent coronary angiography
(C) Exercise stress testing
(D) Monitor in the emergency department until a second set of cardiac enzyme markers is available

Item 74

A 55-year-old woman is evaluated for a 3-week history of progressive shortness of breath. She now has difficulty walking up two flights of stairs. Medical history is significant for asthma and mitral valve prolapse with moderate mitral regurgitation. Her last echocardiogram was 4 months ago and showed mild left atrial enlargement and normal left ventricular size and thickness, with an ejection fraction of 65%. Her only medication is an albuterol inhaler as needed.

On physical examination, the patient is afebrile, blood pressure is 132/56 mm Hg, pulse rate is 88/min, and respiration rate is 16/min. BMI is 27. Cardiac examination reveals a grade 3/6 holosystolic murmur radiating to the axilla. Lungs are clear to auscultation.

Electrocardiogram shows normal sinus rhythm.

Which of the following is the most appropriate diagnostic test to perform next?

(A) Exercise stress testing
(B) 24-Hour continuous ambulatory electrocardiographic monitoring
(C) Spirometry
(D) Transesophageal echocardiogram
(E) Transthoracic echocardiogram

Item 75

A 38-year-old man is evaluated for an insurance physical examination. He has a history of aortic coarctation with an end-to-end anastomosis performed at the age of 3 years. He is asymptomatic, works full time, and performs regular exercise without limitation. He takes chlorthalidone once daily for blood pressure control.

On physical examination, blood pressure is 120/80 mm Hg, pulse rate is 78/min and regular, and respiration rate is 18/min. BMI is 24. The estimated central venous pressure is normal. The apical impulse is normal. The S₁ and S₂ are normal. An ejection click is noted at the left lower sternal border. A grade 3/6 midpeaking systolic murmur is noted

at the second right intercostal space. The femoral pulses are easily palpated, and there is no radial artery–to–femoral artery pulse delay.

Which of the following is the most likely cause of the systolic murmur?

(A) Aortic valve stenosis
(B) Ascending aortic aneurysm
(C) Mitral valve regurgitation
(D) Recurrent aortic coarctation

Item 76

A 55-year-old man with a 6-month history of heart failure is evaluated during a follow-up appointment. At diagnosis, his left ventricular ejection fraction was 15%, and he had moderate mitral and tricuspid regurgitation. Cardiac catheterization at that time revealed normal coronary arteries. He was started on the appropriate medications and is now back to working at a desk job. He has dyspnea walking up a flight of stairs. Medical history is also significant for hypertension. Medications are enalapril, carvedilol (25 mg twice daily), furosemide, and spironolactone.

On physical examination, blood pressure is 100/65 mm Hg, and pulse rate is 56/min. Weight is 72 kg (159 lb). On cardiovascular examination, there is a grade 3/6 holosystolic murmur at the apex radiating to axilla and no S₃ gallop. The remainder of the examination is normal.

Serum electrolyte levels and kidney function tests are normal. Recent echocardiogram shows a left ventricular ejection fraction of 20% and moderate mitral regurgitation. Electrocardiogram demonstrates normal sinus rhythm with a QRS width of 100 ms.

Which of the following is the most appropriate management?

(A) Add an angiotensin receptor blocker
(B) Implantable cardioverter-defibrillator placement
(C) Increase carvedilol to 37.5 mg twice daily
(D) Mitral valve replacement

Item 77

A 45-year-old woman is evaluated in the emergency department for a 1-week history of dyspnea and fatigue. The patient is being treated with systemic chemotherapy for a diagnosis of breast cancer. She has received two cycles of adjuvant chemotherapy with doxorubicin (60 mg/m²) and cyclophosphamide (600 mg/m²); her first treatment occurred 3 months ago and her most recent treatment occurred 2 weeks ago. She has had no chest pain, and medical history is otherwise unremarkable. She takes no other medications.

On physical examination, blood pressure is 120/72 mm Hg and pulse rate is 88/min; BMI is 25. Carotid upstrokes are normal. The estimated central venous pressure is 10 cm H₂O. Crackles are present in both lung fields. S₁ is normal, the pulmonic component of S₂ is increased, an S₃ is present, and there is no S₄. A soft holosystolic murmur at the left lower sternal border is audible. Lower extremity edema to the midshins is present. The mastectomy site is healing well.

A chest radiograph shows infiltrates in both lung fields with a normal cardiac silhouette. Echocardiogram shows a left ventricular ejection fraction of 30%. The estimated pulmonary artery systolic pressure is 50 mm Hg. No other significant echocardiographic findings are present.

The patient is started on lisinopril and furosemide.

Which of the following is the most appropriate next step in the management of her doxorubicin chemotherapy?

(A) Continue doxorubicin
(B) Discontinue doxorubicin
(C) Reduce the dose of doxorubicin
(D) Substitute daunorubicin

Item 78

A 60-year-old man is evaluated for increasing shortness of breath. He noticed progressive exertional intolerance 1 month ago. His symptoms have worsened, and he is now short of breath with walking mild inclines. He does not have chest pain, orthopnea, paroxysmal nocturnal dyspnea, cough, wheezing, or lower extremity edema. He has a history of atrial fibrillation but remains in sinus rhythm after his second catheter ablation procedure for atrial fibrillation 1 year ago. Medical history also includes hypertension and hyperlipidemia but is negative for heart failure or left ventricular dysfunction. Medications are warfarin, metoprolol, ramipril, and atorvastatin.

On physical examination, the patient is afebrile, blood pressure is 132/78 mm Hg, pulse rate is 70/min, and respiration rate is 18/min. Pulse oximetry demonstrates 98% oxygen saturation on ambient air. BMI is 30. Cardiac rate and rhythm are regular. He has bilateral breath sounds but no wheezes, crackles, or rhonchi. There is no prolongation of the expiratory phase.

The electrocardiogram shows normal sinus rhythm. A plain chest radiograph is normal, and pulmonary function tests demonstrate no obstruction. An echocardiogram demonstrates normal left ventricular function with a left ventricular ejection fraction above 55% and evidence of mild diastolic dysfunction.

Which of the following is the most likely cause of this patient's dyspnea?

(A) Chronic thromboembolic disease
(B) Intracardiac shunting
(C) Phrenic nerve injury
(D) Pulmonary vein stenosis

Item 79

A 41-year-old man comes to the office to discuss management of hypertrophic cardiomyopathy (HCM), which was diagnosed 2 weeks ago after a murmur was detected incidentally on examination for another medical condition. HCM has since been diagnosed in his father and brother during family screening. There is no family history of sudden cardiac death. He is asymptomatic.

On physical examination, vital signs are normal. A soft holosystolic murmur is heard, which decreases during both handgrip and stand-to-squat maneuvers.

Transthoracic echocardiogram shows myocardial hypertrophy (maximal septal wall thickness, 32 mm) and mild left ventricular outflow tract obstruction at rest (gradient, 31 mm Hg). On a 24-hour ambulatory electrocardiography study, a four-beat run of nonsustained ventricular tachycardia is present.

Which of the following is the most appropriate next step in treatment?

(A) Alcohol septal ablation
(B) β-Blocker therapy
(C) Implantable cardioverter-defibrillator
(D) Surgical myectomy

Item 80

A 65-year-old man is evaluated for a routine examination. He is asymptomatic and is active, walking 2 miles on a treadmill three times a week. He has hypertension and dyslipidemia. He has a 15-pack-year smoking history but has not smoked since age 30 years. Current medications are hydrochlorothiazide, atorvastatin, and aspirin.

On physical examination, his blood pressure is 134/76 mm Hg in the right upper extremity and 146/80 mm Hg in the left. His pulse rate is 72/min. BMI is 23. He has a grade 2/6 midsystolic murmur heard loudest at his left sternal border. Abdominal examination reveals a pulsatile mass in the epigastrium.

An abdominal ultrasound reveals an aneurysm with a maximum diameter of 4.7 cm not involving the renal arteries.

Which of the following is the most appropriate management of this patient's abdominal aortic aneurysm?

(A) Refer for aneurysm repair
(B) Repeat abdominal ultrasonography in 6 to 12 months
(C) Repeat abdominal ultrasonography in 24 to 36 months
(D) No follow-up management is needed

Item 81

A 54-year-old man is evaluated in the emergency department for an episode of crushing substernal chest pain and discomfort that began 30 minutes ago. He is obese and currently smokes 1 to 2 packs of cigarettes daily. He has dyslipidemia. The patient's medications are enteric-coated low-dose aspirin and simvastatin.

On physical examination, he is afebrile, blood pressure is 146/88 Hg, pulse rate is 88/min and symmetric bilaterally, and respiration rate is 18/min. BMI is 32. Cardiac examination reveals a normal S_1 and S_2 and no S_3; there is an S_4. There are no murmurs or rubs. The remainder of the examination is normal.

Serum troponin levels are elevated. Hematocrit is 42% and platelet count is 220,000/μL (220×10^9/L). Electrocardiogram shows changes consistent with an inferior ST-elevation myocardial infarction. Portable chest radiograph shows a normal cardiac silhouette and no infiltrate.

The patient is treated with enteric-coated aspirin, nitrates, and a β-blocker. The hospital does not have capabilities to perform primary percutaneous coronary intervention (PCI), and the nearest primary PCI center is more than 2 hours away. The patient is administered intravenous tenecteplase.

Which of the following is the most appropriate treatment?

(A) Abciximab
(B) Clopidogrel
(C) Prasugrel
(D) Ticagrelor

Item 82

A 56-year-old man with Eisenmenger syndrome related to a ventricular septal defect is evaluated for recent fatigue and dyspnea. He had an elective cholecystectomy for symptomatic cholelithiasis 4 weeks ago and has had persistent fatigue and exertional dyspnea since his operation. He has no other symptoms. His current medications are sildenafil and bosentan.

On physical examination, vital signs are normal. BMI is 25. The estimated central venous pressure is elevated with a prominent *a* wave. The apical impulse is normal. There is a prominent parasternal impulse at the left sternal border. The S_1 is normal; the S_2 is loud. No murmur is appreciated. Digital clubbing and central cyanosis are noted. The abdominal wound is healing well with no evidence of infection.

Laboratory testing reveals a hemoglobin level of 11.8 g/dL (118 g/L) and hematocrit of 45%. A review of the patient's recent laboratory results shows a hemoglobin level of 18.6 g/dL (186 g/L) and hematocrit of 56% before the cholecystectomy, and a hemoglobin level of 12 g/dL (120 g/L) and hematocrit of 47% at the time of hospital discharge.

Which of the following is the most appropriate management?

(A) Erythrocyte transfusion
(B) Erythropoietin
(C) Initiate intravenous epoprostenol
(D) Initiate short-course iron therapy
(E) Refer for heart-lung transplantation

Item 83

A 55-year-old man is evaluated for cardiovascular risk assessment. He has osteoarthritis and hypertension. He is a construction worker. His brother had a myocardial infarction at the age of 53 years. The patient's medications are lisinopril and naproxen. He is a nonsmoker.

On physical examination, the patient is afebrile, blood pressure is 138/70 mm Hg, pulse rate is 78/min, and respiration rate is 14/min. BMI is 25. The remainder of the examination is unremarkable.

Laboratory studies are significant for a serum LDL cholesterol level of 135 mg/dL (3.50 mmol/L) and an HDL cholesterol level of 38 mg/dL (0.98 mmol/L).

His American College of Cardiology/American Heart Association 10-year atherosclerotic cardiovascular disease risk based on the Pooled Cohort Equations is 6%.

Which of the following is the most appropriate management?

(A) Coronary artery calcium scoring
(B) Exercise stress testing
(C) Increase dose of lisinopril
(D) Recommend antioxidant vitamin therapy

Item 84

A 61-year-old man is evaluated for a 3-month history of progressive aching pain in the left lower extremity; the pain is present during walking and is absent with rest. He has a 30-pack-year history of smoking and quit 1 year ago. His medical history is significant for New York Heart Association functional class II heart failure, hypercholesterolemia, and type 2 diabetes mellitus. Medications are aspirin, lisinopril, simvastatin, metformin, and metoprolol.

On physical examination, vital signs are stable. BMI is 25. Femoral, popliteal, and foot pulses are diminished. There is no distal ulceration or skin breakdown. The ankle-brachial index is 0.70 on the left and 0.85 on the right.

Which of the following is the most appropriate management?

(A) Initiate cilostazol
(B) Refer for endovascular repair
(C) Refer for vascular surgery
(D) Start a supervised exercise program

Item 85

A 19-year-old woman is evaluated during a routine examination. She has no symptoms or significant medical history. She takes no medications.

On physical examination, blood pressure is 130/70 mm Hg and pulse rate is 72/min. Cardiac examination reveals a grade 1/6 diastolic murmur at the base of the heart. Pulses are equal in the upper and lower extremities.

Transthoracic echocardiogram shows a bicuspid aortic valve with mild aortic regurgitation. The aortic dimension is 4.2 cm at the sinuses of Valsalva. Chest CT scan with contrast confirms the aortic root measurements, and no other pathology is noted.

Which of the following is the most appropriate management?

(A) Annual cardiac magnetic resonance (CMR) imaging
(B) Annual multidetector CT
(C) Annual transesophageal echocardiography
(D) Annual transthoracic echocardiography
(E) Reassurance and clinical observation

Item 86

A 66-year-old woman is evaluated for a 3-week history of worsening dyspnea on exertion. Medical history is significant for type 2 diabetes mellitus and hypertension.

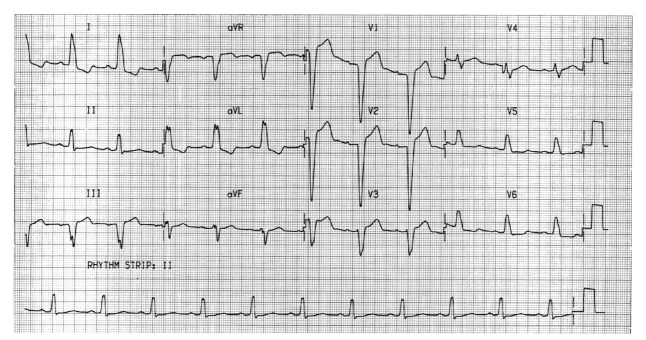

ITEM 86

Medications are metformin, lisinopril, and hydrochloro-thiazide.

On physical examination, the patient is afebrile, blood pressure is 132/78 mm Hg, pulse rate is 78/min, and respiration rate is 14/min. BMI is 28. The remainder of the examination is unremarkable.

Electrocardiogram is shown.

Which of the following is the most appropriate diagnostic test to perform next?

(A) Coronary artery calcium scoring
(B) Exercise nuclear perfusion imaging
(C) Exercise treadmill stress testing
(D) Vasodilator nuclear perfusion imaging

Item 87

A 49-year-old woman is evaluated for intermittent sharp, nonradiating, substernal chest pain for the past 2 weeks. The pain occurs more frequently in the morning and is not associated with meals or exertion but may be initiated with emotional stress. The pain does not include any pleuritic or positional components, and she states that there are no aggravating factors. The pain often lasts for 10 minutes and subsides spontaneously. She has hyperlipidemia treated with pravastatin. Her mother had a myocardial infarction and heart failure starting at the age of 52 years.

On physical examination, blood pressure is 132/82 mm Hg and pulse rate is 78/min. BMI is 28. Lungs are clear to auscultation. Cardiac examination shows a normal S_1 and S_2; there is no S_3, S_4, murmurs, rubs, or gallops. She has no lower extremity edema. The remainder of the examination is normal.

Electrocardiogram shows a heart rate of 80/min. The QRS axis is normal, and there are no ST-T wave changes.

Which of the following is the most appropriate diagnostic test to perform next?

(A) Diagnostic coronary angiography
(B) Exercise electrocardiography
(C) Exercise nuclear perfusion study
(D) Pharmacologic nuclear perfusion study

Item 88

A 48-year-old woman is evaluated during a follow-up visit. She has a 5-year history of type 2 diabetes mellitus. She has no other significant medical history. Medications are atorvastatin, metformin, and a multivitamin. She works as a mail carrier and has a walking route that takes 3 hours each day. She consumes a diet high in fruits and vegetables and does not smoke.

On physical examination, the patient is afebrile, blood pressure is 128/80 mm Hg, pulse rate is 70/min, and respiration rate is 12/min. BMI is 26. The remainder of the examination is unremarkable.

Laboratory studies are significant for a serum LDL cholesterol level of 135 mg/dL (3.50 mmol/L) and serum HDL cholesterol level of 37 mg/dL (0.96 mmol/L). Urinalysis is negative for albuminuria.

Her estimated 10-year cardiovascular risk by the Pooled Cohort Equations is 2.7%.

Which of the following is the most appropriate cardiovascular disease risk management?

(A) Aspirin
(B) Coronary artery calcium scoring
(C) Exercise stress testing
(D) Folic acid supplementation
(E) No further testing or therapy

Item 89

A 57-year-old woman is evaluated in the hospital for chronic systolic heart failure. She was admitted with progressive dyspnea of 2 weeks' duration. After 3 days of aggressive diuretic therapy with weight loss of 5 kg (11 lb), she remained very dyspneic, and right heart catheterization was performed. Medications are lisinopril, digoxin, spironolactone, and intermittent furosemide intravenously.

On physical examination, blood pressure is 96/74 mm Hg, pulse rate is 118/min, and respiration rate is 20/min. The internal jugular vein is not visible when the patient is in an upright position. Lungs are clear. An S_3 is heard on cardiac examination. There is bilateral edema to the knees. Her serum creatinine level is 1.7 mg/dL (150.3 μmol/L).

Hemodynamic measurements:

Right atrium pressure	4 mm Hg
Pulmonary capillary wedge pressure	16 mm Hg
Cardiac output	3.1 L/min (normal, 4.0-8.0 L/min)
Cardiac index	1.8 L/min/m²
Systemic vascular resistance	2050 dyne/s/cm² (normal, 800-1200 dyne/s/cm²)

Which of the following is the most appropriate change in this patient's therapy?

(A) Continuous intravenous furosemide
(B) Dopamine infusion
(C) Esmolol drip
(D) Nitroprusside

Item 90

A 47-year-old man is evaluated for a 3-month history of fatigue, abdominal fullness, and lower extremity edema. Ten years ago, the patient had acute pericarditis with cardiac tamponade; the tamponade was treated successfully with pericardiocentesis, and the pericarditis resolved following a course of an anti-inflammatory medication. He has no history of significant alcohol consumption, hepatitis, or autoimmune disease, and takes no medications.

On physical examination, the patient is icteric. Vital signs are normal; BMI is 30. The estimated central venous pressure is 12 cm H_2O, and the jugular venous pulse shows a prominent *y* descent. S_1 and S_2 are normal, and no murmurs, rubs, or gallops are heard. There is dullness to percussion at the right lung base. The remainder of the pulmonary examination is normal. Both ascites and lower extremity edema are present.

Transthoracic echocardiography is technically challenging, and limited information is obtained. Fluid obtained from abdominal paracentesis is transudative.

Which of the following is the most appropriate next step in management?

(A) Hemodynamic cardiac catheterization
(B) Liver biopsy
(C) Measurement of B-type natriuretic peptide
(D) Vigorous diuresis

Item 91

A 64-year-old woman is evaluated for a 3-month history of sharp chest discomfort that she experiences during gardening. Medical history is significant for hypertension and hyperlipidemia. The patient's father had a coronary artery bypass graft at the age of 68 years. Medications are losartan, hydrochlorothiazide, and atorvastatin, and she recently started taking low-dose aspirin daily.

On physical examination, the patient is afebrile, blood pressure is 136/84 mm Hg, pulse rate is 78/min, and respiration rate is 16/min. BMI is 26. The remainder of the physical examination is unremarkable.

Baseline electrocardiogram shows left ventricular hypertrophy with ST-segment depressions less than 0.5 mm in the lateral leads. During exercise stress testing, the patient develops 1-mm ST-segment depressions in leads II, III, and aVF. She exercised 5 minutes and 30 seconds of a Bruce protocol; her peak heart rate was 129/min (85% predicted maximum), and blood pressure was 186/76 mm Hg.

Which of the following is the most appropriate next step in the management of this patient?

(A) Add a β-blocker
(B) Cardiac catheterization
(C) Cardiac magnetic resonance (CMR) imaging
(D) Stress echocardiography

Item 92

A 66-year-old man is evaluated in the emergency department for 45 minutes of substernal chest pain that radiates to the left shoulder. The patient's medical history is significant for hypertension, type 2 diabetes mellitus, and hyperlipidemia. He has never had abnormal bleeding. Medications are low-dose aspirin, glimepiride, lisinopril, and simvastatin. He has no known drug allergies.

On physical examination, blood pressure is 174/92 mm Hg and pulse rate is 82/min. Cardiac examination shows a normal S_1 and S_2; there is no S_3, S_4, murmur, or rubs. The remainder of the physical examination is normal.

Hemoglobin concentration is 13.4 g/dL (134 g/L) and serum creatinine level is 1.0 mg/dL (88.4 μmol/L). Results of serum troponin levels are pending. Electrocardiogram is shown (see top of next page).

The patient is given aspirin, clopidogrel, unfractionated heparin, and a β-blocker. Transport to the nearest hospital with primary percutaneous coronary intervention (PCI) capabilities would take approximately 135 minutes.

Which of the following is the most appropriate management?

(A) Administer tenecteplase and transfer to a PCI-capable center
(B) Admit to the hospital and await cardiac biomarker results
(C) Initiate abciximab and transfer for urgent coronary angiography
(D) Transfer for primary percutaneous coronary intervention

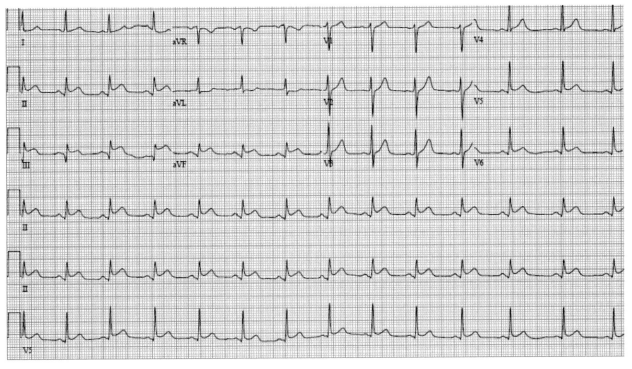

ITEM 92

Item 93

A 60-year-old man is evaluated for a murmur that was noted on a routine examination. He reports exertional dyspnea when walking up stairs. He has hypertension and takes lisinopril.

On physical examination, the patient is afebrile, blood pressure is 160/60 mm Hg, pulse rate is 90/min, and respiration rate is 16/min. Cardiac examination reveals a laterally displaced cardiac apex, soft S_1, and absent S_2. There is a grade 2/6 high-pitched blowing diastolic murmur at the left third intercostal space and a grade 1/6 rumbling mid-diastolic murmur at the apex.

Which of the following is the most likely diagnosis?

(A) Aortic regurgitation
(B) Mitral stenosis
(C) Patent ductus arteriosus
(D) Ruptured sinus of Valsalva aneurysm

Item 94

A 72-year-old woman is evaluated for cramping pain in the buttocks and thighs with standing and walking. Symptoms are exacerbated after standing at work for several hours and are relieved by sitting. Her symptoms have been present for 6 to 8 months and have been stable. Her medical history is significant for hypertension. She has a history of smoking but quit 12 years ago. Her medications are amlodipine and lisinopril.

On physical examination, vital signs are normal. BMI is 22. Deep tendon reflexes are decreased at the ankles but normal at the knees. Lower extremity muscle strength is normal. No abdominal or femoral bruit is present. No skin changes are noted in the lower extremities. Distal pulses are palpable bilaterally. The resting ankle-brachial index is 1.1 on both sides.

Which of the following is most likely to confirm the diagnosis?

(A) Exercise ankle-brachial index
(B) MRI of the lumbosacral spine
(C) Segmental limb plethysmography
(D) Toe-brachial index

Item 95

A 35-year-old woman with recently diagnosed nonischemic systolic heart failure and a left ventricular ejection fraction of 30% presents 1 week after hospital discharge with a new cough, increased exertional dyspnea, and peripheral edema. Medications are lisinopril (5 mg/d) and furosemide (40 mg/d).

On physical examination, blood pressure is 100/70 mm Hg, pulse rate is 98/min and regular, respiration rate is 13/min, and oxygen saturation on ambient air is 96%. Estimated central venous pressure is 15 cm H_2O. Her weight has increased by 2.3 kg (5 lb). Cardiac examination reveals a grade 2/6 holosystolic murmur at the apex and an S_3. Extremity examination reveals bilateral peripheral pitting edema.

Her electrocardiogram shows sinus rhythm and is unchanged from baseline. Serum electrolyte levels and kidney function tests are normal.

In addition to a low-sodium diet, which of the following is the most appropriate management?

(A) Increase furosemide
(B) Increase lisinopril
(C) Start carvedilol
(D) Start spironolactone

Item 96

A 46-year-old man is evaluated in the emergency department for an episode of left facial and left upper extremity numbness and weakness that began just over 1 hour ago. The motor symptoms have resolved fully, but some numbness persists. He has no other medical problems and takes no medications.

On physical examination, vital signs are normal. BMI is 35. There are no carotid bruits or heart murmurs. The neurologic examination is now normal, with the exception of facial numbness.

Laboratory testing and electrocardiogram are normal. Carotid ultrasonography is normal. Magnetic resonance angiography demonstrates a small right-sided ischemic stroke but no other lesions. Ultrasonography of the lower extremities is normal.

A transesophageal echocardiogram is unremarkable with the exception of a patent foramen ovale with right-to-left shunt noted with cough and Valsalva release.

Which of the following is the most appropriate treatment?

(A) Aspirin
(B) Patent foramen ovale device closure
(C) Warfarin
(D) No therapy

Item 97

A 46-year-old man is evaluated in follow-up for a bicuspid aortic valve. He exercises regularly without any activity-limiting symptoms and feels well. His medical history is otherwise negative and he takes no medications.

On physical examination, blood pressure is 138/85 mm Hg. BMI is 28. A systolic ejection click followed by a crescendo-decrescendo murmur are noted at the left sternal border. No diastolic murmur is appreciated. The lower extremity pulses are normal. The remainder of the examination is unremarkable.

Transthoracic echocardiogram shows a bicuspid aortic valve with systolic doming of the aortic valve and a valve area of 1.7 cm^2. The mean gradient across the aortic valve is 22 mm Hg. The ascending aorta is dilated at 4.5 cm; the descending thoracic aorta is incompletely visualized. Chest CT demonstrates a 4.6-cm aneurysm of the ascending aorta with no evidence of coarctation and no enlargement of the descending aorta.

Which of the following is the most appropriate next step in management?

(A) Aortic valve replacement
(B) Aortic valve replacement and ascending aortic repair
(C) Ascending aortic repair
(D) Repeat echocardiogram in 1 year

Item 98

A 42-year-old woman is evaluated for episodes of palpitations that last several seconds in duration. They occur once or twice a month and are accompanied by light-headedness and mild dyspnea. She has not experienced loss of consciousness. The episodes are not precipitated by any particular activity, including exercise. She takes no medications.

On physical examination, the patient is afebrile, blood pressure is 110/68 mm Hg, pulse rate is 72/min, and respiration rate is 16/min. BMI is 29. Cardiac examination reveals physiologic splitting of S$_2$, regular rate and rhythm, and no gallop. Estimated central venous pressure is normal. She has no edema. Serum thyroid-stimulating hormone level is normal.

A 12-lead electrocardiogram shows normal sinus rhythm.

Which of the following is the most appropriate diagnostic testing option?

(A) 30-Day wearable loop recorder
(B) Echocardiogram
(C) Exercise treadmill stress test
(D) 48-Hour ambulatory electrocardiographic monitor
(E) Implantable loop recorder

Item 99

A 56-year-old man is evaluated in the hospital for a 2-week history of fevers and malaise. Medical history is significant for a bicuspid aortic valve. The patient takes no medications.

On physical examination, temperature is 38.5 °C (101.3 °F), blood pressure is 140/50 mm Hg, pulse rate is 98/min, and respiration rate is 16/min. There is no jugular venous distention. The lungs are clear. Cardiac examination reveals a grade 1/6 diastolic murmur. There are no signs of peripheral embolic disease. No lower extremity edema is present.

Electrocardiogram shows normal sinus rhythm, a PR interval of 230 ms, and nonspecific T-wave changes. Except for the increased PR interval, there are no changes compared with a prior tracing. A transthoracic echocardiogram shows a 6-mm vegetation on the aortic valve with mild to moderate aortic regurgitation. A transesophageal echocardiogram confirms the valve findings and suggests the presence of an area of fluid around the aortic annulus posterior to the vegetation, indicative of an aortic root abscess.

Blood cultures are positive for *Staphylococcus aureus* sensitive to methicillin. Appropriate antibiotics are started.

Which of the following is the most appropriate treatment?

(A) Antibiotic therapy for 6 weeks and then reassess
(B) Antibiotic therapy for 3 months and then reassess
(C) Aortic valve replacement after 6 weeks of antibiotic therapy
(D) Urgent aortic valve replacement

Item 100

A 26-year-old woman is evaluated in the emergency department for palpitations and pounding in her neck. She often gets these episodes and they typically last several minutes; however, this episode has been going on for 30 minutes. She can usually stop the episodes by bearing down, but on this occasion this has not worked. She reports feeling a little

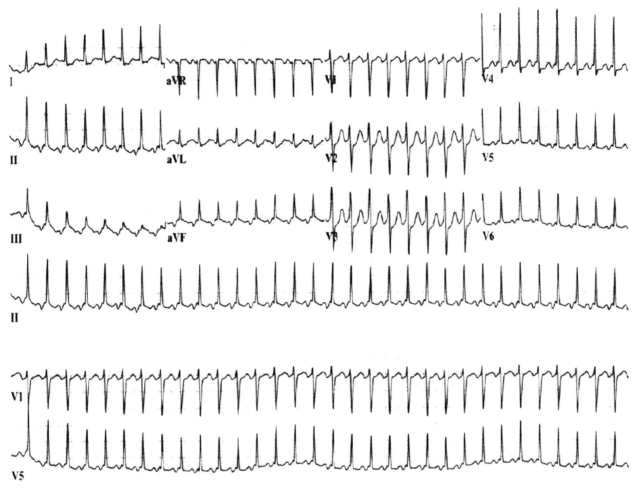

I aVR V1 V4

II aVL V2 V5

III aVF V3 V6

II

V1

V5

ITEM 100

short of breath, but she does not have chest pain or loss of consciousness. She has no other significant medical history, and her only medication is an oral contraceptive.

On physical examination, the patient is afebrile, blood pressure is 120/80 mm Hg, pulse rate is 145/min, and respiration rate is 18/min. BMI is 25. Cardiac examination shows tachycardia but regular rhythm. Lungs are clear to auscultation.

The electrocardiogram is shown.

Which of the following is the most appropriate treatment?

(A) Adenosine
(B) Amiodarone
(C) Cardioversion
(D) Ibutilide

Item 101

A 64-year-old man is evaluated before discharge from the hospital following a non–ST-elevation myocardial infarction treated with placement of a bare metal stent. He is currently pain free and tolerating his medications well. He notes no new symptoms. Medications prior to admission were aspirin, lisinopril, and atorvastatin; upon admission

to the hospital, he began receiving metoprolol, clopidogrel, and intravenous heparin.

Vital signs are normal, and his physical examination is unremarkable.

In addition to continuing aspirin indefinitely, how long should this patient's clopidogrel therapy be continued?

(A) 2 weeks
(B) 1 month
(C) 1 year
(D) Lifelong

Item 102

A 68-year-old man is evaluated for progressive shortness of breath. He underwent heart transplantation 10 years ago for ischemic cardiomyopathy and has had no limitations of his activities since then until developing dyspnea with exertion over the past 3 weeks. Medical history is otherwise significant for hypertension, hyperlipidemia, and a 45-pack-year smoking history; he stopped smoking before his transplant. Medications are aspirin, lisinopril, atorvastatin, and tacrolimus.

On physical examination, blood pressure is 140/78 mm Hg, pulse rate is 102/min, and respiration rate is 16/min.

There is no jugular venous distention. The lungs are clear, and the heart examination is unremarkable. The remainder of the examination is normal.

Electrocardiogram demonstrates sinus tachycardia, right bundle branch block, and no Q waves. Echocardiogram shows a left ventricular ejection fraction of 55%, evidence of mild diastolic dysfunction, septal wall thickness of 0.9 cm, posterior wall thickness of 1.0 cm, and moderate tricuspid regurgitation.

Which of the following is the most appropriate diagnostic test to perform next?

(A) Coronary angiography
(B) Endomyocardial biopsy
(C) Pulmonary function test
(D) Ventilation-perfusion lung scan

Item 103

A 69-year-old woman scheduled to undergo shoulder surgery is evaluated in the hospital for perioperative management of her cardiac device. She was diagnosed with heart failure 1 year ago, and a dual-chamber implantable cardioverter-defibrillator was placed. Her last device check was 3 months ago. Medical history is significant for previous myocardial infarction, coronary artery bypass graft surgery 1 year ago, ventricular tachycardia, and complete heart block. Medications are aspirin, metoprolol, lisinopril, furosemide, and spironolactone.

On physical examination, the patient is afebrile, blood pressure is 95/50 mm Hg, pulse rate is 64/min, and respiration rate is 16/min. BMI is 32. Estimated central venous pressure is normal. There is no carotid bruit. Cardiac auscultation reveals a normal rate and a fixed split S_2. Lungs are clear to auscultation. She has no edema.

An electrocardiogram shows sequential atrioventricular pacing.

Which of the following is the most appropriate preoperative device management?

(A) Disable shocking function
(B) Proceed with surgery and interrogate the device postoperatively
(C) Reprogram to asynchronous pacing and disable shocking function
(D) Advise against surgery

Item 104

A 38-year-old man is evaluated for gradually progressive exertional dyspnea. He had one episode of atrial fibrillation 1 year ago but converted spontaneously in the emergency department. No additional testing was performed at that time, and no medical therapy was initiated. He is otherwise healthy and has been active. His medical history is otherwise unremarkable. He takes no medications and has no allergies.

On physical examination, blood pressure is 120/70 mm Hg, pulse rate is 68/min and regular, and respiration rate is 16/min. BMI is 26. The estimated central venous pressure is elevated. There is a parasternal impulse at the left sternal border. Persistent splitting of the S_2 is noted. There is a soft midsystolic murmur at the second left intercostal space and a separate holosystolic murmur at the apex. The rest of the examination is normal.

The electrocardiogram is shown.

Which of the following is the most likely diagnosis?

(A) Coronary sinus atrial septal defect (ASD)
(B) Ostium primum ASD
(C) Ostium secundum ASD
(D) Patent foramen ovale
(E) Sinus venosus ASD

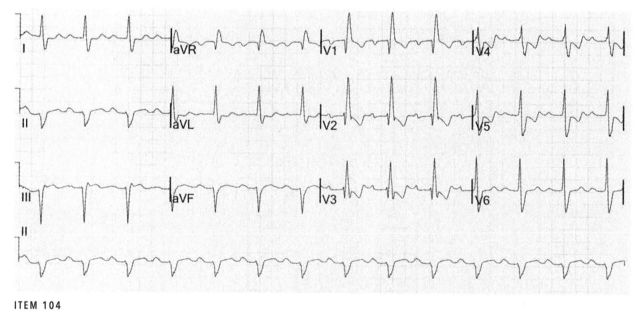

ITEM 104

Item 105

An 82-year-old man was admitted to the coronary care unit (CCU) 48 hours ago after a late presentation with anterior ST-elevation myocardial infarction. The patient underwent coronary angiography and was found to have an occluded proximal left anterior descending coronary artery but did not undergo an attempt at revascularization at the time of coronary angiography because of his late presentation and symptomatic improvement. Today, he felt faint and lost consciousness while visiting with his family in the CCU. Medications are aspirin, ticagrelor, metoprolol, lisinopril, and atorvastatin.

On physical examination, blood pressure is 72/54 mm Hg and pulse rate is 108/min. Cardiac examination shows tachycardia with a normal S_1 and S_2, new holosystolic murmur heard best at the left lower sternal border that radiates to the apex, and a right ventricular heave. Crackles are heard at the bases of both lungs, one third of the way up. He has no lower extremity edema. The remainder of the examination is normal.

Electrocardiogram shows persistent ST-segment elevation and Q waves in leads V_1 through V_4. Heart rate is 110/min. Emergency transthoracic echocardiogram shows a left ventricular ejection fraction of 35% with severe anterior-apical akinesis, a small pericardial effusion, and a color flow jet across the ventricular septum, suggestive of left-to-right flow.

Which of the following is the most appropriate management?

(A) Emergency cardiac surgery
(B) Emergency pericardiocentesis
(C) Percutaneous coronary intervention to left anterior descending artery
(D) Right heart catheterization and dopamine infusion

Item 106

A 72-year-old woman is evaluated for progressive heart failure symptoms. She has a 10-year history of nonischemic heart failure. She currently experiences exertional dyspnea with climbing one flight of stairs, which she was able to do without shortness of breath 3 months ago. Medical history is significant for hypertension, and her medications are lisinopril, carvedilol, furosemide, digoxin, and spironolactone. The patient is black.

On physical examination, blood pressure is 134/72 mm Hg and pulse rate is 66/min. BMI is 35. She has no jugular venous distention. Cardiac examination reveals a grade 1/6 holosystolic murmur but is otherwise normal. There is no lower extremity edema. The remainder of her examination is unremarkable.

Laboratory studies are significant for normal electrolyte levels and a serum creatinine level of 1.5 mg/dL (133 µmol/L).

Electrocardiogram shows normal sinus rhythm, a QRS duration of 110 ms, and nonspecific ST-T wave changes. Echocardiogram shows a left ventricular ejection fraction of 38% and trace mitral regurgitation.

Which of the following is the most appropriate treatment?

(A) Add hydralazine and isosorbide dinitrate
(B) Add losartan

(C) Add warfarin
(D) Cardiac resynchronization therapy

Item 107

A 45-year-old man being treated for infective endocarditis is seen for a follow-up examination. He was diagnosed with endocarditis 1 week ago after presenting with fatigue and fever. Initial transthoracic echocardiogram showed a bicuspid aortic valve with a small vegetation but was otherwise normal. Blood cultures were positive for methicillin-sensitive *Staphylococcus aureus*, and intravenous nafcillin was initiated. Blood cultures obtained 48 hours and 72 hours after starting antibiotic therapy showed no growth.

On physical examination, temperature is 37.8 °C (100.0 °F), blood pressure is 128/78 mm Hg, pulse rate is 88/min, and respiration rate is 16/min. BMI is 25. Physical examination reveals no cutaneous or ocular stigmata of bacterial endocarditis. Cardiac examination reveals a grade 2/6 early systolic murmur at the base of the heart, unchanged from previous examinations. The remainder of the physical examination is normal.

Electrocardiogram is unchanged from the time of diagnosis except for an increase in the PR interval from 120 to 210 ms.

Which of the following is the most appropriate next step in management?

(A) Cardiac CT
(B) Continued antibiotic therapy without additional testing
(C) Repeat transthoracic echocardiogram
(D) Transesophageal echocardiogram

Item 108

A 58-year-old man is evaluated for a 3-month history of left upper extremity symptoms and dizziness. He is left-handed and works as a carpenter. He describes an aching sensation and feeling of fatigue in his arm and occasional dizziness that occur within 2 to 3 minutes of using a hand saw; these symptoms resolve several minutes after stopping activity. He is otherwise asymptomatic. Medical history is significant for hypertension, hyperlipidemia, and type 2 diabetes mellitus. He has a 40-pack-year smoking history but quit 1 year ago. Medications are lisinopril, atorvastatin, and metformin.

On physical examination, he is afebrile, left arm blood pressure is 135/76 mm Hg, pulse rate is 68/min, and respiration rate is 16/min. BMI is 29. The carotid upstrokes are normal. The chest is clear and the cardiac examination is normal. Examination of the left upper extremity is unremarkable, with palpable distal pulses and no evidence of distal ulceration or skin breakdown. The remainder of his physical and neurologic examination is unremarkable.

Which of the following elements of the physical examination would be most helpful in establishing the diagnosis?

(A) Ankle-brachial index
(B) Bilateral blood pressure measurement
(C) Evaluation for pulsus paradoxus
(D) Thoracic outlet maneuvers

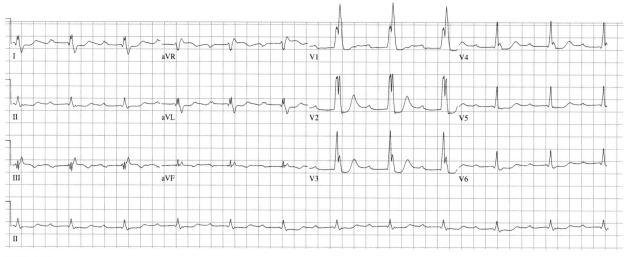

ITEM 109

Item 109

An 86-year-old man is evaluated in the emergency department after a fall. He reports tripping over a rug. He did not experience presyncope or other symptoms. He otherwise feels well and is active. Medical history is significant for hypertension. Family history is notable for pacemaker implantation in his sister. His only medication is lisinopril. A perfusion stress test 1 year ago obtained because of chest discomfort demonstrated normal left ventricular wall motion and ejection fraction.

On physical examination, temperature is 36.8 °C (98.2 °F), blood pressure is 135/80 mm Hg, pulse rate is 67/min, and respiration rate is 12/min. BMI is 24. His neck veins are flat. The point of maximal impulse is in the mid-clavicular line without heave or lift. There is mild bruising over his left hip. He has no lower extremity edema.

Plain radiographs of the left hip are negative for fracture. Laboratory evaluation demonstrates a normal metabolic profile and preserved kidney function. His 12-lead electrocardiogram is shown.

Which of the following is the most appropriate management?

(A) Adenosine nuclear stress test
(B) Dual-chamber pacemaker
(C) Single-chamber pacemaker
(D) No intervention is indicated

Item 110

A 58-year-old woman is evaluated during a routine examination. She is asymptomatic. She had a myocardial infarction 4 years ago and has hypertension and dyslipidemia. She is a former smoker and consumes one alcoholic beverage daily. She has no limitations with physical activity and is able to exercise periodically. Medications are low-dose aspirin, hydrochlorothiazide, metoprolol, and high-dose atorvastatin.

On physical examination, blood pressure is 146/94 mm, and pulse rate is 52/min. BMI is 28. The remainder of the examination is normal.

Laboratory studies:

Total cholesterol	152 mg/dL (3.94 mmol/L)
LDL cholesterol	72 mg/dL (1.86 mmol/L) (pre-treatment baseline: 150 mg/dL [3.89 mmol/L])
HDL cholesterol	46 mg/dL (1.19 mmol/L)
Triglycerides	84 mg/dL (0.95 mmol/L)

One year ago, she underwent transthoracic echocardiography that was significant for normal left ventricular systolic function and no valvular abnormalities.

Which of the following interventions offers the greatest cardiovascular risk reduction to this patient?

(A) Add fish oil
(B) Add niacin
(C) Reduce alcohol consumption
(D) Start an ACE inhibitor

Item 111

A 52-year-old man is evaluated in the hospital for progressive chest pressure over the past 3 weeks. He has a 35-pack-year history of cigarette smoking. Medical history is significant for hypertension and hyperlipidemia treated with aspirin, hydrochlorothiazide, lisinopril, and pravastatin. His brother had a myocardial infarction at age 48 years.

On physical examination, he is afebrile, blood pressure is 148/82 mm Hg, and pulse rate is 98/min. Cardiac and lung examinations are normal.

Cardiac biomarkers are elevated. Initial electrocardiogram shows 2-mm ST-segment depression in leads I, aVL, and V_4 through V_6.

He is admitted to the coronary care unit and given aspirin, metoprolol, nitroglycerin paste, and enoxaparin. Over the course of the first 12 hours, his chest pressure worsens, requiring intravenous nitroglycerin infusion. Subsequently, his chest pressure improves and he undergoes coronary angiography.

CONT.

Coronary angiography is significant for a 70% left main coronary artery stenosis, 80% mid left anterior descending stenosis, and 90% proximal right coronary artery stenosis. Left ventricular ejection fraction is 45% with mild anterior hypokinesis. Mild mitral regurgitation is noted.

He is currently hemodynamically stable and pain free.

Which of the following is the most appropriate management?

(A) Coronary artery bypass graft surgery

(B) Intra-aortic balloon pump placement

(C) Percutaneous coronary intervention

(D) Continue current therapy

Item 112

A 60-year-old woman is evaluated in the hospital for a 3-week history of worsening dyspnea and chest pain. Medical history is significant for hypertension, hyperlipidemia, and previous coronary artery bypass graft surgery. Medications are aspirin, furosemide, metoprolol, and atorvastatin.

On physical examination, she is afebrile, blood pressure is 110/70 mm Hg, pulse rate is 92/min, and respiration rate is 16/min. Estimated central venous pressure is elevated. Examination at the cardiac base demonstrates a grade 3/6 late-peaking systolic murmur and a grade 1/6 diastolic murmur. An S_2 is not heard.

Echocardiogram shows a markedly calcified bicuspid aortic valve with severe aortic stenosis and moderate aortic regurgitation.

Which of the following is the most appropriate treatment?

(A) Aortic valve repair

(B) Balloon aortic valvuloplasty

(C) Surgical aortic valve replacement

(D) Transcatheter aortic valve replacement

Item 113

A 56-year-old woman is evaluated for a 1-year history of exertional dyspnea. She also occasionally experiences light-headedness during intense aerobic activity, such as running. Symptoms are not associated with chest pain and have been relatively stable since onset. She also reports a 6.8-kg (15-lb) weight loss and intermittent fevers over the past 4 months. She had a colonoscopy and mammography 6 months ago with normal results. Medical history is otherwise unremarkable, and she takes no medications.

On physical examination, blood pressure is 120/72 mm Hg, and pulse rate is 62/min; BMI is 18. The jugular venous pulse, carotid upstroke, and lung examination findings are all normal. The precordium is quiet, and S_1 and S_2 are normal. A soft grade 2/6 diastolic rumble is heard at the apex and is preceded by an early diastolic filling sound. The remainder of the examination is unremarkable.

Echocardiogram shows a 2.5 × 2.2 cm mass in the left atrium; the mass is moderately mobile with a pedunculated stalk adherent to the fossa ovalis. Left ventricular function

and the myocardium both appear normal. No pericardial effusion or significant disease involving the cardiac valves is present.

Which of the following tumors is the most likely cause of the patient's symptoms and clinical findings?

(A) Adenocarcinoma

(B) Angiosarcoma

(C) Lipoma

(D) Myxoma

(E) Papillary fibroelastoma

Item 114

A 38-year-old woman is evaluated for a 1-week history of substernal chest pain. Symptoms are aggravated by lying in the supine position or taking a deep breath. The patient is otherwise healthy and takes no medications.

On physical examination, temperature is 37.5 °C (99.5 °F), blood pressure is 112/70 mm Hg, and pulse rate is 84/min. Systolic pressure variation with respiration is 5 mm Hg. The lungs are clear to auscultation. A loud, three-component cardiac rub is heard at the apex. S_1 and S_2 are normal. The remainder of the physical examination is unremarkable.

Laboratory studies are significant for a leukocyte count of 7000/µL (7.0×10^9/L). Echocardiogram shows normal left and right ventricles. A moderately sized circumferential pericardial effusion is noted. The inferior vena cava is normal in size. A Doppler ultrasound shows minimal change in mitral inflow with respiration.

High-dose ibuprofen, a proton pump inhibitor, and colchicine are started.

Which of the following is the most appropriate next step in management?

(A) Cardiac CT

(B) Clinical follow-up

(C) Glucocorticoid administration

(D) Inpatient monitoring

(E) Pericardiocentesis

Item 115

A 31-year-old man is evaluated for follow-up 2 days after an emergency department visit for palpitations. He reports intermittent palpitations and occasional episodes of shortness of breath. These episodes have increased in frequency and are often accompanied by light-headedness. He experienced loss of consciousness on one occasion. He does not have chest discomfort or jaw pain. His medical history is unremarkable except for a previous emergency department visit several years ago for palpitations. He has no significant family history.

On physical examination, the patient is afebrile, blood pressure is 105/68 mm Hg, pulse rate is 67/min, and respiration rate is 12/min. BMI is 24. His neck veins are flat, and the point of maximal impulse is in the midclavicular line without heave or lift. He has no lower extremity edema.

Serum thyroid-stimulating hormone level is normal.

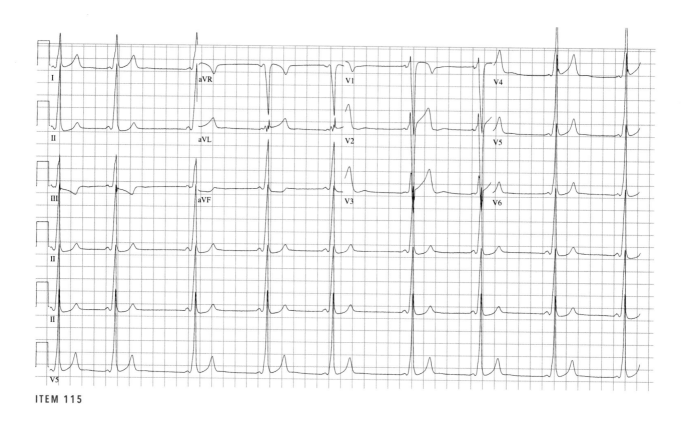

ITEM 115

Electrocardiogram is shown. Transthoracic echocardiogram shows no structural abnormalities.

Which of the following is the most appropriate next step in management?

(A) Antiarrhythmic drug therapy
(B) Diltiazem
(C) Electrophysiology study
(D) Metoprolol

Item 116

A 48-year-old woman is evaluated for a 3-week history of progressive dyspnea, palpitations, and peripheral edema. She has loose stools and a recent 2.3-kg (5-lb) weight loss. Medical history is unremarkable, and she does not use injection drugs. She does not take any medications and has no known drug allergies.

On physical examination, temperature is 37.3 °C (99.2 °F), blood pressure is 92/60 mm Hg, pulse rate is 118/min, and respiration rate is 22/min. BMI is 23. Jugular venous distention extends to the jaw. The thyroid is palpable but without identifiable nodules. The precordium is hyperdynamic, and an S₃ is heard on cardiac examination. She has severe bilateral lower extremity edema extending to the midcalf. Examination of the joints is normal, and there is no skin rash.

Leukocyte count is 6000/μL (6.0×10⁹/L) with a normal differential. Results of complete blood count are normal. Electrocardiogram shows sinus tachycardia, no Q waves or T-wave abnormalities, and no signs of left ventricular

hypertrophy. Echocardiogram shows a left ventricular ejection fraction of 10% and no valvular regurgitation.

Which of the following is the most appropriate diagnostic test to perform next?

(A) Antinuclear antibody level
(B) Endomyocardial biopsy
(C) Thyroid studies
(D) Viral titers

Item 117

A 31-year-old woman is evaluated during a follow-up examination. Marfan syndrome was diagnosed 6 months ago and was confirmed by significant family history and the presence of ectopia lentis. She has been in good health and physically active. She does not report any chest discomfort, shortness of breath, syncope, or presyncope.

On physical examination, the patient is tall and slender. Blood pressure is 100/62 mm Hg and equal in both arms. Significant findings include a high arched palate, pectus excavatum, and arachnodactyly. The jugular and carotid examinations are normal. There is a grade 1/6 blowing diastolic murmur best heard at the left sternal border. The remainder of the examination is unremarkable.

Except for pectus excavatum, a chest radiograph is unremarkable. Transthoracic echocardiography shows enlargement of the aortic root, measuring 3.9 cm with mild aortic regurgitation, unchanged from previous imaging studies. The remainder of the echocardiographic examination is unremarkable.

How frequently should this patient undergo surveillance imaging?

(A) Every 6 months
(B) Every 12 months
(C) Every 24 months
(D) Every 3 to 5 years

Item 118

A 59-year-old man is evaluated for a 3-month history of intermittent exertional chest discomfort. He has hypertension treated with lisinopril and amlodipine.

On physical examination, the patient is afebrile, blood pressure is 138/92 mm Hg, pulse rate is 82/min, and respiration rate is 14/min. BMI is 27. The remainder of the examination is unremarkable.

Exercise electrocardiographic stress testing shows 1.5-mm ST-segment depressions in leads II, III, and aVF; in addition, the patient developed chest pressure during this test. He exercised 4 minutes and stopped because of chest discomfort. Heart rate and blood pressure increased appropriately. Duke treadmill score is -11.5.

Which of the following is the most appropriate next step in management?

(A) Begin aspirin, β-blocker, and statin and re-evaluate in 2 weeks
(B) Cardiac catheterization
(C) Dobutamine stress echocardiography
(D) Exercise myocardial perfusion imaging

Item 119

A 26-year-old woman is evaluated in the emergency department for progressive dyspnea. She is 2 weeks postpartum. The pregnancy was complicated by preeclampsia but resulted in a normal delivery. The infant is healthy. She has no history of cardiovascular disease. Her only medication is prenatal vitamins.

On physical examination, the patient is afebrile. Blood pressure is 100/70 mm Hg in both arms, pulse rate is 105/min and regular, and respiration rate is 25/min. BMI is 29. The oxygen saturation on ambient air is 96%. The estimated central venous pressure is elevated. The apical impulse is diffuse. The S_1 and S_2 are soft. An S_3 and S_4 are present. A soft holosystolic murmur is heard at the apex. Crackles are heard over both lung fields. Pitting edema is noted to the knees.

An electrocardiogram is shown. An echocardiogram reveals a global reduction in contractility and left ventricular enlargement without hypertrophy.

Which of the following is the most likely diagnosis?

(A) Acute pulmonary embolism
(B) Ischemic cardiomyopathy
(C) Peripartum cardiomyopathy
(D) Stress-induced cardiomyopathy

Item 120

A 37-year-old man is evaluated for a 6-month history of exercise intolerance and shortness of breath when walking up stairs. He has no significant medical history and takes no medications.

On physical examination, blood pressure is 140/70 mm Hg, pulse rate is 62/min, and respiration rate is 16/min. Cardiac examination reveals an irregularly irregular rhythm. An opening snap is heard after S_2, followed by a grade 1/6 diastolic rumble at the apex.

Electrocardiogram shows atrial fibrillation. Transthoracic echocardiographic findings are consistent with rheumatic valve disease, showing a mildly thickened mitral valve with minimal calcification and mild restriction in leaflet motion. The subchordal apparatus is mildly thickened, and there is mild mitral regurgitation and marked left atrial enlargement. Mean gradient across the mitral valve is 13 mm Hg. Mitral valve area is 1.2 cm². Transesophageal echocardiogram shows no left atrial appendage thrombus and confirms transthoracic echocardiographic findings.

In addition to anticoagulation therapy, which of the following is the most appropriate management?

(A) Medical management; repeat echocardiogram in 6 months
(B) Mitral valve replacement
(C) Percutaneous mitral balloon valvuloplasty
(D) Surgical mitral valve repair

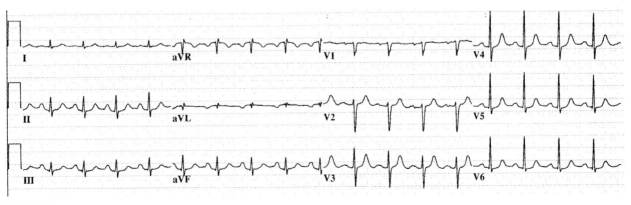

ITEM 119

Answers and Critiques

Item 1   Answer: B

Educational Objective: Diagnose pulmonary valve regurgitation as a late consequence of tetralogy of Fallot repair.

The most likely diagnosis is pulmonary valve regurgitation. Tetralogy of Fallot comprises a large subaortic ventricular septal defect, infundibular or valvular pulmonary stenosis, aortic override, and right ventricular hypertrophy. Pulmonary regurgitation is the most common structural disorder that occurs following tetralogy of Fallot repair. The clinical findings include features of right heart volume overload with a parasternal (right ventricular) lift and a soft systolic pulmonary outflow murmur. There is a single S_2 because the function of the pulmonary valve is sacrificed during repair. The diastolic murmur heard at the left sternal border that increases in intensity with inspiration is caused by pulmonary valve regurgitation.

Aortic valve regurgitation can occur late in patients following tetralogy of Fallot repair owing to progressive aortic enlargement. The aortic diastolic murmur is generally heard at the left sternal border, but it decreases in intensity with inspiration. A right ventricular prominence would not be expected in a patient with aortic regurgitation.

Recurrent ventricular septal defect also can occur in patients following tetralogy of Fallot repair. However, the physical examination findings would include a systolic murmur heard at the left sternal border, which often obliterates the S_1 and S_2. A right ventricular prominence would not be expected in a patient with a recurrent ventricular septal defect.

Tricuspid valve regurgitation may occur late in patients following tetralogy of Fallot repair owing to progressive right ventricular and annular dilatation from long-standing severe pulmonary valve regurgitation. The physical examination findings include a holosystolic murmur located at the lower left sternal border that increases with inspiration. The systolic murmur in the patient presented here is soft and heard over the pulmonary valve region.

KEY POINT

- Pulmonary regurgitation is the most common structural disorder that occurs following tetralogy of Fallot repair.

Bibliography

Ferraz Cavalcanti PE, Sá MP, Santos CA, et al. Pulmonary valve replacement after operative repair of tetralogy of Fallot: meta-analysis and meta-regression of 3,118 patients from 48 studies. J Am Coll Cardiol. 2013 Dec 10;62(23):2227-43. [PMID: 24080109]

Item 2   Answer: D

Educational Objective: Use high-sensitivity C-reactive protein level to guide treatment and cardiac risk stratification in a patient at intermediate risk of cardiovascular disease.

The most appropriate management of this patient is to obtain high-sensitivity C-reactive protein (hsCRP) levels. He has an intermediate risk of myocardial infarction and coronary death (5% to below 7.5% as defined by the Pooled Cohort Equations). The measurement of hsCRP has been proved to be useful for guiding primary prevention strategies in intermediate-risk patients, with as many as 30% of patients being reclassified as either low risk or high risk based on hsCRP measurement.

When used for this purpose, the CRP assay should be able to detect levels to at least 0.03 mg/L (high sensitivity); a single test is appropriate in patients with levels below 1.0 mg/L, but testing should be repeated in 2 weeks for values of 1.0 mg/L or higher to assess for persistent elevation. Patients with hsCRP measurement below 1.0 mg/L are considered at a low relative risk for coronary heart disease and those with levels of 3.0 mg/L or higher are considered at a high relative risk. A meta-analysis from the Emerging Risk Factors Collaboration in 2010 found that hsCRP levels have a strong linear association with both ischemic stroke and vascular mortality. Although evidence is not strong that modification of risk can occur with treatment after hsCRP measurement, the JUPITER study randomized patients with serum LDL cholesterol levels below 130 mg/dL (3.37 mmol/L) and hsCRP levels greater than or equal to 2.0 mg/L to rosuvastatin or placebo. Patients were followed for the occurrence of death, myocardial infarction, stroke, or a composite of first major cardiovascular event for 5 years. In addition to lowering serum LDL cholesterol levels from 108 to 55 mg/dL (2.80 to 1.42 mmol/L) and hsCRP from 4.2 to 2.2 mg/L, rosuvastatin significantly reduced the incidence of major cardiovascular events.

Because this patient is asymptomatic, adenosine cardiac magnetic resonance (CMR) imaging, cardiac CT angiography, and stress echocardiography are not indicated and have not been associated with reduction in cardiovascular events.

There is currently no role for the evaluation of lipid particle size and number (fractionated lipoprotein profiling). No studies to date have shown that treatment targeted to lipoprotein particle size and number affects outcomes, and the use of these tests is not addressed in current cholesterol management guidelines.

KEY POINT

- In patients with an intermediate risk of cardiovascular disease, the measurement of high-sensitivity C-reactive protein (hsCRP) has been proved to be useful for guiding primary prevention strategies, with as many as 30% of patients being reclassified as either low risk or high risk based on the hsCRP measurement.

Bibliography

Ridker PM, Danielson E, Fonseca FA, et al; JUPITER Study Group. Rosuvastatin to prevent vascular events in men and women with elevated C-reactive protein. N Engl J Med. 2008 Nov 20;359(21):2195-207. [PMID: 18997196]

Item 3   Answer: C

Educational Objective: Evaluate a patient with a diastolic murmur.

This asymptomatic patient has a diastolic murmur and should undergo transthoracic echocardiography (TTE). TTE is indicated for asymptomatic patients with a systolic murmur that is grade 3/6 or higher, a late or holosystolic murmur, or a diastolic or continuous murmur; TTE is also indicated for patients with a murmur and accompanying symptoms.

Chest CT may be helpful in the further evaluation of patients with documented aortic valve pathology (such as identification of a bicuspid valve or screening for concomitant aortopathy in a patient with a bicuspid aortic valve), but it would not be the first step in identifying the cause of this patient's murmur and would expose the patient to unnecessary radiation.

Exercise echocardiography stress testing is most commonly used to evaluate for coronary heart disease in those ineligible for electrocardiographic stress testing, although in selected patients it may be helpful in evaluating the hemodynamic significance of valvular disease. Diastolic murmurs tend not to vary with exercise; therefore, exercise echocardiography stress testing would not be an appropriate initial test to help clarify the cause of the murmur.

Although there are multiple benign causes of systolic murmurs, diastolic murmurs are virtually always considered abnormal. Therefore, further evaluation of this patient's cardiac findings is needed.

KEY POINT

- Transthoracic echocardiography is indicated for asymptomatic patients with a systolic murmur that is grade 3/6 or higher, a late or holosystolic murmur, or a diastolic or continuous murmur and for patients with a murmur and accompanying symptoms.

Bibliography
Salazar SA, Borrero JL, Harris DM. On systolic murmurs and cardiovascular physiological maneuvers. Adv Physiol Educ. 2012 Dec;36(4):251-6. [PMID: 23209004]

Item 4   Answer: A

Educational Objective: Manage thromboembolic risk following atrial fibrillation ablation.

This patient should continue taking warfarin. She has a history of symptomatic atrial fibrillation and is now symptom-free without evidence of recurrent atrial fibrillation after catheter ablation. However, patients with successful ablation and elimination of symptoms may have transient asymptomatic atrial fibrillation with continued risk for atrial fibrillation–associated thromboembolic disease. Therefore, current consensus recommendations counsel that stroke prevention therapy following atrial fibrillation ablation be based on risk factors and not rhythm status, with the preferred risk stratification tool being the CHA_2DS_2-VASc risk score, which has improved predictive ability relative to the $CHADS_2$ score. The patient is a 58-year-old woman with a prior transient ischemic attack (TIA) and hypertension. Accordingly, her CHA_2DS_2-VASc risk score is 4 (2 points for TIA, 1 point for hypertension, and 1 point for female sex). Current guidelines advocate oral anticoagulation for any patient with nonvalvular atrial fibrillation and a CHA_2DS_2-VASc score greater than 1. She has a history of a central nervous system event, and her annual risk of stroke is high (greater than 5% annually). Therefore, she should be continued on anticoagulation with warfarin.

Concomitant aspirin therapy with warfarin is reserved for patients with active coronary artery disease. This patient has risk factors for atherosclerosis, but she does not have a history of coronary artery disease or acute coronary syndromes. The addition of aspirin to warfarin significantly increases the risk of bleeding.

Discontinuation of warfarin and substitution with aspirin or dual antiplatelet therapy is not correct. Aspirin is insufficient therapy for a patient at high risk of stroke. The Atrial fibrillation Clopidogrel Trial with Irbesartan for prevention of Vascular Events (ACTIVE-W) trial compared warfarin with therapy with aspirin and clopidogrel and found that aspirin with clopidogrel was inferior to warfarin for stroke prevention with no statistically significant difference in bleeding.

Anticoagulation with a novel oral anticoagulant (such as dabigatran, rivaroxaban, or apixaban) could be considered; however, these agents have been associated with increased gastrointestinal bleeding compared with warfarin.

KEY POINT

- Stroke prevention therapy after catheter ablation of atrial fibrillation should be based upon risk stratification, not heart rhythm status.

Bibliography
Calkins H, Kuck KH, Cappato R, et al; Heart Rhythm Society Task Force on Catheter and Surgical Ablation of Atrial Fibrillation. 2012 HRS/EHRA/ECAS expert consensus statement on catheter and surgical ablation of atrial fibrillation: recommendations for patient selection, procedural techniques, patient management and follow-up, definitions, endpoints, and research trial design: a report of the Heart Rhythm Society (HRS) Task Force on Catheter and Surgical Ablation of Atrial Fibrillation. Developed in partnership with the European Heart Rhythm Association (EHRA), a registered branch of the European Society of Cardiology (ESC) and the European Cardiac Arrhythmia Society (ECAS); and in collaboration with the American College of Cardiology (ACC), American Heart Association (AHA), the Asia Pacific Heart Rhythm Society (APHRS), and the Society of Thoracic Surgeons (STS). Endorsed by the governing bodies of the American College of Cardiology Foundation, the American Heart Association, the European Cardiac Arrhythmia Society, the European Heart Rhythm Association, the Society of Thoracic Surgeons, the Asia Pacific Heart Rhythm Society, and the Heart Rhythm Society. Heart Rhythm. 2012 Apr; 9(4):632-696.e21. [PMID: 22386883]

Item 5   Answer: A

Educational Objective: Treat a patient with hypertrophic cardiomyopathy.

Hydrochlorothiazide should be discontinued in this patient. She has mild symptoms of obstructive hypertrophic cardiomyopathy (HCM). Dynamic left ventricular outflow tract (LVOT) obstruction affects 70% of patients with HCM and is exacerbated by decreases in preload (for example, from diuretic use or squat-to-stand maneuvers) and afterload (for example, from expiration or vasodilator therapy) and by increases in myocardial contractility (for example, from digoxin therapy). For patients with symptoms of HCM, the initial treatment is medical therapy that addresses the factors that predispose toward LVOT obstruction. Use of hydrochlorothiazide and other diuretics, particularly in high doses, will exacerbate the propensity towards dynamic LVOT obstruction and, therefore, should be avoided in patients with HCM. Similarly, vasodilator therapy also should not be used. Negative inotropic agents, such as β-receptor antagonists, calcium channel blockers, and disopyramide, are the cornerstone of medical therapy in these patients. This patient was previously stable on hydrochlorothiazide; however, HCM and its associated pathophysiology can manifest at any age and result in symptoms of heart failure.

Dual-chamber pacemaker implantation previously was considered to be a therapeutic option but was found to be relatively ineffective in randomized clinical trials of patients with HCM. These trials showed a significant placebo effect (40%-50%) from dual-chamber pacing without clear clinical benefit.

ACE inhibitors, such as lisinopril, reduce afterload and can exacerbate LVOT obstruction, and therefore they should be avoided in patients with HCM.

For patients with drug-refractory, severely symptomatic obstructive HCM, septal reduction therapy with surgical myectomy or alcohol septal ablation may be considered. Neither myectomy nor alcohol ablation is recommended for patients with the minimal symptoms that this patient has or for those without an adequate trial of appropriate pharmacotherapy.

KEY POINT

- Diuretics, particularly in high doses, will exacerbate the propensity towards dynamic left ventricular outflow tract obstruction and, therefore, should be avoided in patients with hypertrophic cardiomyopathy.

Bibliography

Gersh BJ, Maron, BJ, Bonow, RO, et al; American College of Cardiology Foundation/American Heart Association Task Force on Practice Guidelines. 2011 ACCF/AHA Guideline for the Diagnosis and Treatment of Hypertrophic Cardiomyopathy: a report of the American College of Cardiology Foundation/ American Heart Association Task Force on Practice Guidelines. Developed in collaboration with the American Association for Thoracic Surgery, American Society of Echocardiography, American Society of Nuclear Cardiology, Heart Failure Society of America, Heart Rhythm Society, Society for Cardiovascular Angiography and Interventions, and Society of Thoracic Surgeons. J Am Coll Cardiol. 2011 Dec 13;58(25):e212-60. [PMID: 22075469]

Item 6   Answer: C

Educational Objective: Treat a penetrating atherosclerotic ulcer in the descending aorta.

The most appropriate management for this patient is intravenous β-blockade followed by intravenous sodium nitroprusside. The CT scan (shown, see top of next column) reveals a focal penetrating atherosclerotic ulcer (PAU) in the proximal descending aorta (*arrow*), a type B acute aortic syndrome. PAU is a focal defect or lesion occurring at the site of an intimal atherosclerotic plaque. Patients tend to be older and with greater cardiovascular comorbidity. PAU occurs most

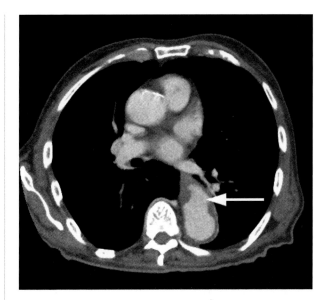

commonly in the descending aorta, which may reflect a greater burden of atheromatous disease at this site. Elevation of the D-dimer level frequently accompanies acute aortic syndromes. Uncomplicated type B acute aortic injury is best treated medically, initially with β-blockade to decrease the heart rate to below 60/min followed by a parenteral arterial vasodilator as needed to control blood pressure.

Chest pain is a common presenting symptom in the emergency department, and three potentially lethal causes must be rapidly excluded: acute myocardial infarction, pulmonary embolism, and an acute aortic syndrome. Anticoagulation therapy would be considered standard of care if an acute coronary syndrome were suspected. In this patient, although a non–ST-elevation myocardial infarction cannot be excluded based on the electrocardiogram, it is less likely given his normal troponin I level; the troponin level would likely be elevated after 3 hours of ongoing cardiac ischemia. The patient also has a low pretest probability of pulmonary embolism by Wells scoring. Given his clinical and radiographic presentation, neither alternative diagnosis to an acute aortic syndrome is likely, and anticoagulation is not indicated in acute aortic syndrome.

Malperfusion syndromes are uncommon with an aortic penetrating atherosclerotic ulcer but could occur with transformation to classic dissection. In such cases, emergency endovascular stenting with or without fenestration may be necessary. This patient shows no evidence of lower limb or visceral malperfusion, and catheterization with endovascular repair is not indicated. Emergency open surgery is rarely indicated in this setting with the advent of endovascular therapies.

KEY POINT

- Uncomplicated type B acute aortic injury is best treated medically, initially with β-blockade followed by a parenteral arterial vasodilator to control blood pressure.

Bibliography

Nienaber CA, Powell JT. Management of acute aortic syndromes. Eur Heart J. 2012 Jan;33(1):26-35b. [PMID: 21810861]

Item 7   Answer: B

Educational Objective: Diagnose effusive constrictive pericarditis.

The most likely diagnosis in this patient is effusive constrictive pericarditis. Effusive constrictive pericarditis is a clinical entity in which patients who have a pericardial effusion, with or without cardiac tamponade, experience persistent symptoms and hemodynamic derangements after treatment and relief of the pericardial effusion. In some patients with constrictive pericarditis, pericardial inflammation results in an effusion, which is placed under pressure by the inelastic pericardium. Symptoms of low cardiac output, systemic congestion, and an elevated jugular venous pulse are seen, as in constrictive pericarditis; however, in patients with effusive constrictive pericarditis, a pericardial knock is absent and the y descent of the jugular venous pulse may be less prominent. Additionally, pulsus paradoxus may be present, which is not a typical finding of constrictive pericarditis. This disorder is caused by pericarditis involving the visceral layer of the pericardium. Thickening of the visceral layer of the pericardium can be difficult to detect with CT and other noninvasive imaging, and a high index of clinical suspicion is necessary to establish the diagnosis. In this patient, effusive constrictive pericarditis is suggested by the persistently elevated right atrial pressure following pericardiocentesis.

Similar findings in the jugular venous pulse can occur in patients with cor pulmonale or heart failure. With cor pulmonale, however, evidence of right ventricular dysfunction or chamber enlargement is usually seen on imaging. The clear lungs on auscultation do not support the presence of heart failure.

The presence of a normal electrocardiogram and the absence of the typical symptom of chest pain argue against recurrent acute pericarditis as a diagnosis. Additionally, acute pericarditis cannot explain this patient's pulsus paradoxus and elevated jugular venous pulse.

KEY POINT

- Effusive constrictive pericarditis is a clinical entity in which patients who have a pericardial effusion experience persistent symptoms and hemodynamic derangements after relief of the pericardial effusion.

Bibliography

Syed FF, Ntsekhe M, Mayosi BM, Oh JK. Effusive-constrictive pericarditis. Heart Fail Rev. 2013 May;18(3):277-87. [PMID: 22422296]

Item 8   Answer: B

Educational Objective: Manage high LDL cholesterol level in a patient with diabetes mellitus and an elevated risk for coronary artery disease.

The most appropriate management in this patient with a coronary heart disease (CHD) risk equivalent is to switch to atorvastatin, 40 mg/d. Current guidelines recommend that statin therapy be initiated in patients at high risk for CHD. The intensity of the statin therapy should be tailored to the CHD risk. Candidates for high-intensity statin therapy include:

- Patients with known atherosclerotic disease (clinical CHD, cerebrovascular disease, or peripheral arterial disease)
- Patients with an LDL cholesterol level 190 mg/dL (4.92 mmol/L) or greater
- Patients with diabetes mellitus, an LDL cholesterol level below 190 mg/dL (4.92 mmol/L), and calculated 10-year CHD risk of 7.5% or higher
- Some patients without diabetes with an LDL cholesterol level below 190 mg/dL (4.92 mmol/L) and calculated 10-year CHD risk of 7.5% or higher

Moderate-intensity statin therapy can be considered for:

- Patients with diabetes who are not receiving high-intensity therapy
- Most patients without diabetes with an LDL cholesterol level below 190 mg/dL (4.92 mmol/L) and calculated 10-year CHD risk of 7.5% or higher
- Some patients without diabetes with an LDL cholesterol level below 190 mg/dL (4.92 mmol/L) and calculated 10-year CHD risk of 5% or higher but lower than 7.5%

This patient has diabetes, an LDL cholesterol level less than 190 mg/dL (4.92 mmol/L), and a calculated 10-year CHD of 10%, and, therefore, should be considered for high-intensity statin therapy. Drugs and doses that constitute high-intensity statin therapy include atorvastatin, 40 to 80 mg/d; rosuvastatin, 20 to 40 mg/d; and simvastatin, 80 mg/d. (The FDA has issued a warning regarding the incidence of muscle injury with products that contain 80 mg of simvastatin and recommends that patients be switched to a different statin rather than increasing the dosage of simvastatin to 80 mg/d.)

Fluvastatin, 40 mg/d; lovastatin, 20 mg/d; pravastatin, 10 mg/d; and simvastatin, 10 mg/d, are all classified as low-intensity dosing and are inadequate to reduce this patient's CHD risk.

KEY POINT

- Patients with diabetes mellitus should receive moderate- or high-intensity statin therapy to reduce their risk of coronary heart disease.

Bibliography

Stone NJ, Robinson JG, Lichtenstein AH, et al; American College of Cardiology/American Heart Association Task Force on Practice Guidelines. 2013 ACC/AHA guideline on the treatment of blood cholesterol to reduce atherosclerotic cardiovascular risk in adults: a report of the American College of Cardiology/American Heart Association Task Force on Practice Guidelines. Circulation. 2014 Jun 24;129(25 Suppl 2):S1-45. Erratum in: Circulation. 2014 Jun 24;129(25 Suppl 2):S46-8. [PMID: 24222016]

Item 9   Answer: A

Educational Objective: Manage ACE inhibitor side effects in a patient with heart failure.

The most appropriate treatment for this patient is to switch from her ACE inhibitor (lisinopril) to an angiotensin receptor blocker (ARB), such as valsartan, and observe her closely for several weeks to see if her cough resolves. For patients with heart failure, the two most common causes of a nonproductive cough are volume overload and ACE inhibitors. An ACE inhibitor–induced cough may occur at any time after an ACE inhibitor has been initiated, and it would not be surprising that she could develop an ACE inhibitor cough after 9 months of therapy. The most appropriate course of therapy, therefore, would be to switch to an ARB. Although data regarding mortality outcomes in patients with heart failure taking ARBs are limited, results thus far demonstrate equivalent mortality outcomes and fewer medication-related adverse events in this setting.

An echocardiogram evaluates left ventricular function and valvular abnormalities. It would not be helpful in a patient with diagnosed heart failure to assess for volume overload. Indications for repeating echocardiograms in patients with heart failure include a decline in functional status and to reassess function after uptitrating medications. Additionally, in patients followed over time, repeating an echocardiogram every 2 to 3 years is indicated to assess for further left ventricular dilation and evaluate left ventricular ejection fraction for further decline. It is unlikely to be helpful in this patient, who has no evidence of volume overload on examination and no pulmonary edema on chest radiograph.

B-type natriuretic peptide (BNP) level is useful for the assessment of acute dyspnea. Studies have shown that levels of BNP are elevated in patients with heart failure. Additionally, higher levels are associated with an increase in mortality. BNP has not been demonstrated to be useful to guide diuresis in patients with heart failure. In a patient with a history of heart failure, a random BNP level would not help in the assessment of fluid overload being the cause of a cough.

Pulmonary function testing is useful primarily in the evaluation of dyspnea or to assess for the presence of underlying lung disease that might contribute to cough, such as cough-variant asthma. However, this patient has no clinical history or increased risk for lung disease, is a never-smoker, and has a normal lung examination. Therefore, pulmonary function testing would not be appropriate prior to a trial of medication adjustment.

KEY POINT

- An ACE inhibitor–induced cough may occur at any time after an ACE inhibitor has been initiated; the best course of therapy is to switch to an angiotensin receptor blocker.

Bibliography

Heran BS, Musini VM, Bassett K, Taylor RS, Wright JM. Angiotensin receptor blockers for heart failure. Cochrane Database Syst Rev. 2012 Apr 18;4:CD003040. [PMID: 22513909]

Item 10   Answer: D

Educational Objective: Manage incidental finding of atrial septal aneurysm with patent foramen ovale.

No further evaluation or treatment is the appropriate management approach for this patient with an incidentally discovered atrial septal aneurysm. Atrial septal aneurysm is redundant atrial septal tissue that is often associated with a patent foramen ovale. When atrial septal aneurysm is identified incidentally, no medical treatment or intervention is needed. Antiplatelet therapy is recommended for patients with cryptogenic stroke and an isolated atrial septal aneurysm.

In patients with an atrial septal aneurysm and recurrent stroke while taking antiplatelet therapy, anticoagulant therapy is recommended if no other cause of stroke is identified.

Rarely, surgical excision of an atrial septal aneurysm and defect closure is considered in patients in whom antiplatelet or warfarin therapy fails to prevent stroke recurrence or in patients with a large left-to-right shunt causing right heart enlargement. Percutaneous device closure is rarely performed in patients with atrial septal aneurysms, because a large device is required to plicate the atrial septal aneurysm and close multiple fenestrations.

Atrial septal aneurysms are most commonly detected by transesophageal echocardiogram. However, when an incidental atrial septal aneurysm is well visualized by transthoracic echocardiogram, additional imaging with a transesophageal echocardiogram is not needed.

KEY POINT

- When an atrial septal aneurysm is identified incidentally, no further evaluation, medical treatment, or intervention is needed.

Bibliography

Burger AJ, Sherman HB, Charlamb MJ. Low incidence of embolic strokes with atrial septal aneurysms: A prospective, long-term study. Am Heart J. 2000 Jan; 139(1 Pt 1):149-52. [PMID: 10618576]

Item 11   Answer: B

Educational Objective: Manage a patient with stable angina pectoris and a low-risk stress test result.

In this patient with ongoing stable angina pectoris and a low-risk exercise stress test result (that is, a Duke treadmill score of +6), initiation of a long-acting nitrate such as isosorbide mononitrate is recommended by current guidelines. β-Blockers and nitrates improve functional capacity, delay onset of exercise-induced myocardial ischemia, and decrease the frequency and severity of anginal episodes. Most patients with stable angina will require combination therapy with these two classes of drugs to achieve effective control of anginal symptoms. Although this patient is at low risk, initiation of medical therapy is also appropriate in patients who are at intermediate risk and high risk based on clinical risk factors, symptom burden, and/or stress testing results. Those patients with intermediate-risk stress test findings (Duke treadmill score of -10 to +4) and high-risk stress testing findings (Duke treadmill score of less than -11) have a 1% to 3% cardiovascular mortality per year and a 3% or higher cardiovascular mortality rate per year, respectively.

Calcium channel blockers, such as diltiazem, are second-line therapy in patients with stable angina pectoris who are intolerant of β-blockers or who have continued symptoms on β-blockers and nitrates. This patient is tolerating his β-blocker well and is not yet taking a nitrate for his angina. Therefore, diltiazem is not indicated at this time.

Because of the invasive nature of coronary angiography and the inherent risks of vascular complications, it should be reserved for patients with lifestyle-limiting angina despite optimal medical therapy or high-risk criteria on noninvasive stress testing such as significant ST-segment depression at a low work load, ST-segment elevation, or hypotension.

Pharmacologic nuclear stress testing is not indicated in this patient owing to the presence of stable symptoms, lack of optimal medical therapy, and low-risk findings on exercise stress testing.

KEY POINT

- First-line antianginal therapy for patients with stable angina pectoris is β-blockers and nitrates.

Bibliography

Qaseem A, Fihn SD, Dallas P, Williams S, Owens DK, Shekelle P; Clinical Guidelines Committee of the American College of Physicians. Management of stable ischemic heart disease: summary of a clinical practice guideline from the American College of Physicians/American College of Cardiology Foundation/American Heart Association/American Association for Thoracic Surgery/Preventive Cardiovascular Nurses Association/Society of Thoracic Surgeons. Ann Intern Med. 2012 Nov 20;157(10):735-43. [PMID: 23165665]

Item 12   Answer: C

Educational Objective: Diagnose bicuspid aortic valve.

This patient most likely has a bicuspid aortic valve. Bicuspid aortic valve is the most common congenital heart lesion, occurring in approximately 0.5% to 2% of the general population. It is the second most common cause of aortic stenosis after calcific degeneration of a tricuspid aortic valve and the second most common cause of aortic regurgitation after aortic root dilation. Many patients with a bicuspid aortic valve are asymptomatic, with the diagnosis being suggested based on incidentally noted auscultatory findings. The presenting murmur depends on the degree of valve dysfunction, with a systolic ejection murmur that varies in intensity, ranging from minimal flow disturbance to findings consistent with the murmur of aortic stenosis as the degree of outflow obstruction increases. A diastolic murmur may occur if aortic valve incompetence with regurgitation is present, as in this patient. Bicuspid aortic valve has an increased prevalence associated with congenital lesions such as aortic coarctation, interrupted aortic arch, and Turner syndrome. More than 70% of patients with a bicuspid aortic valve will require surgical intervention for a stenotic or regurgitant valve or aortic pathology over the course of a lifetime. The presence of a bicuspid aortic valve increases the risk for aortic stenosis or regurgitation, and stenosis proceeds at a faster rate when the aortic valve is bicuspid. The risk for infective endocarditis also is increased in these patients. In addition, bicuspid aortic valve is associated with aortopathy and a predisposition to aneurysm formation and thoracic aortic dissection.

Adults with previously undiagnosed aortic coarctation may present with hypertension or a murmur. Palpation of reduced femoral pulses and measurement of discrepant blood pressures during routine examination are helpful in raising suspicion for the diagnosis. The murmur associated with coarctation may be nonspecific but is usually a systolic murmur in the left infraclavicular area and under the left scapula.

The murmur associated with an atrial septal defect is a midsystolic flow murmur caused by the ejection of increased right-sided volume, owing to the left-to-right shunt that occurs initially with this defect. This murmur is best heard over the pulmonic area of the chest and may radiate toward the back, as with the murmur of pulmonary stenosis. The most characteristic finding on auscultation in patients with an atrial septal defect is a fixed split S_2.

The murmur of mitral stenosis is a diastolic low-pitched decrescendo murmur heard best in the left lateral decubitus position. With mitral stenosis, S_1 has increased intensity and S_2 is normal. The opening snap, which is due to forceful opening of the mitral valve, occurs when the pressure in the left atrium is greater than the pressure in the left ventricle. As the severity of the mitral stenosis increases, the pressure in the left atrium increases, and the mitral valve opens earlier in ventricular diastole.

KEY POINT

- A bicuspid aortic valve is often discovered incidentally; the murmur depends on the degree of valve dysfunction, with a systolic ejection murmur that may range from a minimal flow disturbance to findings consistent with the murmur of aortic stenosis as the degree of outflow obstruction increases.

Bibliography

Siu SC, Silversides CK. Bicuspid aortic valve disease. J Am Coll Cardiol. 2010 Jun 22;55(25):2789-800. [PMID: 20579534]

Item 13   Answer: C

Educational Objective: Recommend influenza vaccination for the secondary prevention of ischemic heart disease.

Providing this patient with an annual influenza vaccination would significantly reduce her risk of future cardiovascular events. A meta-analysis of randomized trials demonstrated that use of the influenza vaccine was associated with a 36%

lower risk of major adverse cardiovascular events compared with nonimmunized patients. Based on these data, the American Heart Association and American College of Cardiology recommend influenza vaccination for the secondary prevention of ischemic heart disease. In addition to influenza vaccination as a preventive measure for cardiovascular disease, this patient also qualifies for influenza vaccination according to Advisory Committee on Immunization Practices (ACIP) guidelines that recommend all persons aged 6 months or older receive the influenza vaccination.

Colchicine has anti-inflammatory properties, and observational studies of patients taking colchicine for gout or familial Mediterranean fever suggest a decreased risk of cardiovascular disease associated with treatment. However, its use for secondary prevention of cardiovascular disease has not been established.

Folic acid lowers homocysteine levels, which have been associated with increased cardiovascular disease in observational studies. However, clinical trials examining the effectiveness of lowering homocysteine levels by folic acid supplementation have failed to show a reduction in adverse cardiovascular events. Folic acid supplementation for this purpose is therefore not recommended as secondary prevention.

Because inflammation and oxidative stress are involved in atherosclerosis, the use of antioxidant agents, including vitamins E and C and β-carotene, has been proposed as both a primary and secondary preventive intervention for cardiovascular disease. Although supported by some basic science and observational data, several large, randomized controlled trials have failed to document benefit of antioxidant therapy for either purpose. Therefore, the use of vitamin E supplementation would not be appropriate in this patient.

KEY POINT

- Influenza vaccine should be administered to patients with established cardiovascular disease to reduce the risk of future cardiovascular events.

Bibliography
Udell JA, Zawi R, Bhatt DL, et al. Association between influenza vaccination and cardiovascular outcomes in high-risk patients: a meta-analysis. JAMA. 2013 Oct 23;310(16):1711-20. [PMID: 24150467]

Item 14   Answer: C

Educational Objective: Treat acquired QT-interval prolongation.

Both amitriptyline and moxifloxacin should be discontinued in this patient. Her electrocardiogram (ECG) demonstrates QT-interval prolongation. Many medications may prolong the QT interval, including amitriptyline and moxifloxacin; QT prolongation may be markedly increased in patients taking more than one medication with this effect.

The corrected QT interval (QTc) is most often determined using the Bazett formula (QT interval / $\sqrt{R}$-R interval). This patient's ECG at the time of admission shows a QTc

interval of 630 ms; a normal QTc is defined as 460 ms or less in women and 440 ms or less in men. A QTc greater than 500 ms is associated with increased risk of torsades de pointes.

The cause of this patient's QT prolongation is likely her pharmacotherapy. Many drugs have been implicated in QT-interval prolongation, including antiarrhythmic agents, antibiotics (including some macrolides and fluoroquinolones), antipsychotic drugs, and antidepressants. A list of QT-prolonging drugs is available at http://crediblemeds.org/. The large degree of QTc prolongation in this patient may be caused by either the presence of two QT-prolonging medications or an underlying ion channel variant that is only evident in the setting of a QT-prolonging medication.

Although both medications may lead to her ECG findings, discontinuing either the moxifloxacin or amitriptyline in isolation is insufficient treatment given the significant degree of QT prolongation on this patient's ECG.

Carvedilol does not prolong the QT interval directly, although it may increase the risk of bradycardia-related arrhythmias in patients with acquired QT-interval prolongation by slowing the heart rate. However, the most important intervention in this patient is to reduce the risk of torsades de pointes by discontinuing the offending QT-prolonging agents.

KEY POINT

- A corrected QT interval greater than 500 ms is associated with increased risk of torsades de pointes; patients with this degree of QT-interval prolongation should discontinue any potentially QT-interval prolonging drugs.

Bibliography
Isbister GK, Page CB. Drug induced QT prolongation: the measurement and assessment of the QT interval in clinical practice. Br J Clin Pharmacol. 2013 Jul;76(1):48-57. [PMID: 23167578]

Item 15   Answer: C

Educational Objective: Manage heart failure with preserved ejection fraction with diuretics.

This patient should be admitted to the hospital and given intravenous furosemide. His presentation is characteristic for heart failure with preserved ejection fraction (HFpEF). He has volume overload manifested by increasing abdominal girth, increased exertional dyspnea, and progressive orthopnea. His left ventricular ejection fraction is normal, but he has mild left ventricular hypertrophy and a long history of hypertension. Additionally, he has a markedly elevated B-type natriuretic peptide level. The etiology of his acute exacerbation into heart failure is most likely acute atrial fibrillation, but because he is already on diltiazem and has a normal heart rate, he may have been in atrial fibrillation for some time and not noticed it.

In contrast to patients with a reduced ejection fraction, no drugs have been shown to reduce mortality rates in patients with HFpEF. Instead, guidelines emphasize controlling blood pressure and volume. Patients with HFpEF are

CONT.

often volume sensitive, and careful use of diuretics to maintain euvolemia is important. This patient is not already taking a diuretic, and starting with a low dose of furosemide is a reasonable approach. If the patient were already on an oral diuretic, giving at least the equivalent dose intravenously would be suggested. Patients with HFpEF should be encouraged to monitor their weight closely, as small differences in volume can quickly cause volume overload and subsequent hospital admissions.

β-Blocker therapy is relatively contraindicated in this patient with acute decompensated heart failure as it may exacerbate his heart failure. Once his heart failure is successfully treated with diuretics, this patient may benefit from β-blocker therapy to help manage his heart rate and blood pressure, but this should be avoided in the setting of acute volume overload, whenever possible.

Despite the fact that the patient is currently in atrial fibrillation, cardioversion at this point is incorrect. Because he is hemodynamically stable with good rate control, there is no indication for immediate cardioversion. In addition, because it is unclear how long he has been in atrial fibrillation, cardioversion without a transesophageal echocardiogram to rule out thrombus or initiation of prophylactic anticoagulation would place the patient at risk for embolization at the time of the procedure.

Several small trials have suggested that aldosterone antagonists may improve diastolic function in patients with HFpEF. However, a recent trial comparing spironolactone with placebo showed a reduction in heart failure hospitalizations but no difference in mortality rates or all-cause hospitalizations in patients with HFpEF, and spironolactone was associated with significant increases in serum creatinine and potassium levels. Given this minimal benefit but substantial increase in risk of adverse effects, the addition of spironolactone for his current symptoms is not appropriate in this patient with HFpEF.

KEY POINT

- Patients with heart failure with preserved ejection fraction are often volume sensitive, and careful use of diuretics to maintain euvolemia is important.

Bibliography

Heart Failure Society of America; Lindenfeld J, Albert NM, Boehmer JP, et al. HFSA 2010 Comprehensive Heart Failure Practice Guideline. J Card Fail. 2010 Jun;16(6):e1-e194. [PMID: 20610207]

Item 16   Answer: B

Educational Objective: Treat low-pressure cardiac tamponade.

This patient should undergo pericardiocentesis. He has low-pressure cardiac tamponade, which is tamponade occurring in the setting of clinical dehydration. Evidence of cardiac tamponade on echocardiography includes diastolic inversion of the right-sided chambers and respiratory variation in the mitral inflow pattern; a ventricular septal shift and plethora of the inferior vena cava also may be present. However, because

of volume contraction, the intracardiac filling pressures are low, and tamponade does not result in an elevation of estimated central venous pressure. Therefore, several physical examination findings usually associated with pericardial tamponade, such as jugular venous distention and pulsus paradoxus, may not be evident in many patients. Low-pressure cardiac tamponade may be caused by malignancy, tuberculosis, or other severe chronic illnesses that result in both dehydration and pericardial effusions, with metastatic involvement of the pericardium likely present in this patient with known disseminated cancer.

In cardiac tamponade, the pericardial effusion causes intrapericardial pressure to exceed ventricular diastolic pressures, which leads to impairment in ventricular filling and stroke volume. Sinus tachycardia, as evident in this patient, is a compensatory response to maintain forward cardiac output. Treatment should consist of acute intravenous hydration to augment ventricular preload and stroke volume and, most importantly, procedures to relieve the tamponade, specifically pericardiocentesis.

An intra-aortic balloon pump is used in patients with hemodynamic instability, usually as a bridging device until definitive treatment can be undertaken. Because removal of pericardial fluid in this patient would be expected to markedly improve his hemodynamic status, pericardiocentesis is indicated prior to pursuing additional supportive therapy.

Phenylephrine is a potent vasoconstrictor. Although phenylephrine may improve this patient's blood pressure by increasing his systemic vascular resistance, the increase in resistance will reduce stroke volume, which is already significantly impaired by tamponade and hypovolemia. Phenylephrine, therefore, would not be an appropriate intervention prior to treating the tamponade and ensuring adequate volume expansion.

A window pericardiectomy procedure is performed in the operating room either as an open procedure or using video-assisted thoracoscopy by cardiac surgery and would be indicated only if this patient's tamponade was unresponsive to pericardiocentesis, a less invasive bedside procedure.

KEY POINT

- Treatment of low-pressure cardiac tamponade should include acute intravenous hydration to augment ventricular preload and stroke volume and pericardiocentesis to relieve the tamponade.

Bibliography

Sagristà-Sauleda J, Angel J, Sambola A, Alguersuari J, Permanyer-Miralda G, Soler-Soler J. Low-pressure cardiac tamponade: clinical and hemodynamic profile. Circulation. 2006 Aug 29;114(9):945-52. [PMID: 16923755]

Item 17   Answer: B

Educational Objective: Identify the importance of individual risk factors in the risk of myocardial infarction.

The presence of dyslipidemia places this patient at highest risk for future myocardial infarction (MI), accounting for approximately 50% of the risk of developing acute MI. The INTERHEART study assessed the prevalence of nine potentially modifiable risk factors in more than 15,000 patients with first acute MI and almost 15,000 asymptomatic age- and sex-matched controls. Nine risk factors were strongly associated with acute MI in the 52 countries included in the trial. In descending order, these are: dyslipidemia, smoking, psychosocial stressors, diabetes mellitus, hypertension, obesity, alcohol consumption, physical inactivity, and diet low in fruits and vegetables. Results of the INTERHEART study suggest that these modifiable risk factors account for more than 90% of the risk for acute MI.

KEY POINT

- Nine modifiable risk factors account for more than 90% of the risk for acute myocardial infarction; in descending order, these are: dyslipidemia, smoking, psychosocial stressors, diabetes mellitus, hypertension, obesity, alcohol consumption, physical inactivity, and diet low in fruits and vegetables.

Bibliography

Yusuf S, Hawken S, Ounpuu S, et al; INTERHEART Study Investigators. Effect of potentially modifiable risk factors associated with myocardial infarction in 52 countries (the INTERHEART Study): case-control study. Lancet. 2004 Sep 11-17;364(9438):937-52. [PMID: 15364185]

Item 18   Answer: B

Educational Objective: Manage a patient with diabetes mellitus and three-vessel coronary artery disease.

The appropriate management of this patient is coronary artery bypass grafting (CABG). He has type 2 diabetes mellitus and multivessel coronary artery disease (CAD) with moderate to severe symptoms despite optimal medical therapy. In multiple observational studies and randomized controlled trials, performing CABG compared with percutaneous coronary intervention (PCI) as the initial revascularization strategy in patients with a clear indication was associated with improved outcomes, including reduced rates of death, myocardial infarction (MI), and stroke. The FREEDOM trial evaluating management of multivessel CAD in patients with diabetes showed that the composite endpoint of death, MI, and stroke was significantly lower in patients treated with CABG versus PCI. This difference was driven by a statistically significant reduction in the occurrence of death and MI in CABG patients, although stroke rates were higher in the CABG group than the PCI group. CABG is recommended for patients who remain symptomatic despite optimal medical therapy and have specific angiographic findings (either left main disease or multivessel disease with involvement of the proximal left anterior descending artery), concomitant reduced systolic function, or diabetes mellitus.

β-Blockers are first-line antianginal agents because of their ability to reduce heart rate, myocardial contractility, and blood pressure, resulting in reduced myocardial oxygen demand. Calcium channel blockers are reasonable second-line therapy in patients who are intolerant of β-blockers or who have continued symptoms on β-blockers and nitrates. However, it would not be appropriate to switch to a calcium channel blocker, such as amlodipine, in this patient who currently tolerates an effective dose of a β-blocker.

Myocardial viability testing is performed with a radionuclide radiotracer that is taken up by viable myocardial tissue. Viability testing may demonstrate hypoperfused regions of the heart that might show functional improvement if revascularization is performed. However, information from a substudy of the Surgical Treatment of Ischemic Heart Failure (STICH) trial demonstrated no relationship between the results of viability imaging and the effectiveness of bypass surgery. Therefore, in this patient who remains symptomatic despite optimal medical therapy and is a reasonable surgical candidate, revascularization is indicated, and myocardial perfusion testing would not contribute significant information regarding medical decision making. Myocardial perfusion testing is typically limited to use in patients at high risk for revascularization surgery in whom assessing the degree of viable myocardium present may influence the risk-benefit ratio of surgical treatment.

KEY POINT

- Coronary artery bypass grafting is recommended for patients who remain symptomatic with optimal medical therapy and have specific angiographic findings (either left main disease or multivessel disease with involvement of the proximal left anterior descending artery), concomitant reduced systolic function, or diabetes mellitus.

Bibliography

Farkouh ME, Domanski M, Sleeper LA, et al; FREEDOM Trial Investigators. Strategies for multivessel revascularization in patients with diabetes. N Engl J Med. 2012 Dec 20;367(25):2375-84. [PMID: 23121323]

Item 19   Answer: C

Educational Objective: Evaluate coronary artery disease in a patient with COPD.

This patient should undergo dobutamine stress echocardiography. She has a history of coronary artery disease (CAD) with new atypical, but exertional, symptoms suggestive of cardiac ischemia. Because she has baseline electrocardiogram abnormalities (left ventricular hypertrophy with repolarization abnormalities) that will make interpretation of ST-segment changes difficult, she should undergo stress testing with imaging, with either stress echocardiography with dobutamine or myocardial perfusion imaging with a vasodilator.

With stress echocardiography, regional myocardial function is assessed in real time. Stress images are obtained at peak or immediately after stress, before cardiac function returns to baseline. Wall motion abnormalities indicate either infarction (seen on stress and rest images) or ischemia (seen on stress images only). For patients who cannot exercise, such as this patient, pharmacologic stressors such as dobutamine in combination with imaging can be used in place of exercise and imaging.

Because of her COPD with active wheezing on examination, pharmacologic testing with vasodilators should be avoided. Pharmacologic vasodilators, such as dipyridamole, adenosine, and regadenoson, can cause bronchospasm and are therefore contraindicated in a patient who is actively wheezing. These agents can be used with caution in a patient with a history of bronchospastic airways disease, but the presence of active wheezing in this patient precludes the use of a vasodilator. Therefore, stress testing with dobutamine is the correct choice.

This patient has no symptoms to indicate an acute coronary syndrome that would prompt cardiac catheterization as the initial diagnostic test. Evaluation of the extent and severity of disease would be the first step in deciding management in this patient. If she has a small perfusion defect, she could be treated medically with more intensive antianginal therapies.

KEY POINT

- Pharmacologic vasodilators, such as dipyridamole, adenosine, and regadenoson, can cause bronchospasm during cardiac stress testing; these agents can be used with caution in a patient with a history of COPD but are contraindicated in a patient who is actively wheezing.

Bibliography
Qaseem A, Fihn SD, Williams S, Dallas P, Owens DK, Shekelle P; Clinical Guidelines Committee of the American College of Physicians. Diagnosis of stable ischemic heart disease: summary of a clinical practice guideline from the American College of Physicians/American College of Cardiology Foundation/American Heart Association/American Association for Thoracic Surgery/Preventive Cardiovascular Nurses Association/Society of Thoracic Surgeons. Ann Intern Med. 2012 Nov 20;157(10):729-34. [PMID: 23165664]

Item 20   Answer: B

Educational Objective: Manage asymptomatic severe aortic stenosis.

Although this patient has severe aortic stenosis based on quantitative echocardiographic findings, he is asymptomatic with normal left ventricular (LV) systolic function; therefore, follow-up echocardiography in 6 to 12 months is the most appropriate management. Appropriate follow-up in patients with asymptomatic severe aortic stenosis includes a clinical evaluation and echocardiography every 6 to 12 months. Patients should also be educated to identify and report possible aortic stenosis–related symptoms, such as dyspnea, reduced exercise tolerance, exertional chest pain, lightheadedness, and syncope, before scheduled follow-up.

Balloon valvuloplasty, although important in the treatment of the pediatric patient with severe aortic stenosis, has a more limited role in adults owing primarily to its limited efficacy and the high rate of complications

associated with the procedure. Additionally, this patient is asymptomatic, so there is no indication for intervention at present.

Surgical aortic valve replacement is indicated for symptomatic patients with severe aortic stenosis, asymptomatic patients with severe aortic stenosis and LV systolic dysfunction (LV ejection fraction <50%), and patients with severe aortic stenosis who are undergoing coronary artery bypass graft or surgery on the aorta or other heart valves. This patient is asymptomatic with normal LV systolic function, and he does not have any other cardiac procedures planned.

Transcatheter aortic valve replacement (TAVR) is indicated for patients with symptomatic severe aortic stenosis who are considered unsuitable for conventional surgery because of severe comorbidities. Currently, TAVR should not be performed in patients with intermediate or low surgical risk, and no therapeutic intervention is currently indicated in this asymptomatic patient.

KEY POINT

- In patients with asymptomatic severe aortic stenosis, close clinical follow-up with echocardiography every 6 to 12 months is appropriate.

Bibliography
Manning WJ. Asymptomatic aortic stenosis in the elderly: a clinical review. JAMA. 2013 Oct 9;310(14):1490-7. [PMID: 24104373]

Item 21   Answer: C   H

Educational Objective: Diagnose stress cardiomyopathy (takotsubo cardiomyopathy).

This patient's clinical history and presentation are consistent with stress cardiomyopathy (takotsubo cardiomyopathy). The absence of coronary artery stenosis and the presence of hypokinesis of the mid and apical left ventricle on ventriculography confirm this diagnosis. This patient with takotsubo cardiomyopathy without evidence of cardiogenic shock should be administered metoprolol and captopril. The treatment of stress cardiomyopathy is supportive, including the use of β-blockers and ACE inhibitors, and most patients have resolution of symptoms and recovery of left ventricular function within 7 days.

Takotsubo cardiomyopathy often mimics non–ST-elevation myocardial infarction (NSTEMI) or ST-elevation myocardial infarction (STEMI). Patients present with chest pain or shortness of breath, electrocardiographic changes consistent with anterior and/or lateral ST-segment elevation, and elevated cardiac biomarkers. Although not required for diagnosis, many patients develop symptoms following a stressful or emotional event. The diagnosis of stress cardiomyopathy requires (1) ST-segment elevation on electrocardiography, (2) transient wall motion abnormalities of the mid and apical left ventricle, (3) the absence of significant obstructive coronary artery disease, and (4) the absence of other causes of transient left ventricular dysfunction, such as myocarditis.

Endomyocardial biopsy is generally not indicated for the initial evaluation of heart failure unless a specific diagnosis that would influence management or prognosis is suspected based on clinical data or noninvasive testing. This patient's presentation, with acute onset following a stressful event, ST-segment elevation, and hypokinesis of the cardiac apex, is characteristic of takotsubo cardiomyopathy, and an endomyocardial biopsy is not indicated as an initial diagnostic test. Myocarditis has a variable presentation, but focal ST-segment changes and apical hypokinesis are not typical.

More than 95% of patients with stress cardiomyopathy recover ventricular function with conservative supportive care (β-blockers and ACE inhibitors). This patient does not have evidence of hemodynamic compromise, and intra-aortic balloon pump implantation is not indicated.

In this patient, the lack of coronary artery obstructive disease in the presence of ST-segment elevation and elevated cardiac biomarkers eliminates STEMI or NSTEMI as possible etiologies for this presentation. Therefore, thrombolytic therapy is not indicated.

KEY POINT

- Stress cardiomyopathy presents similarly to myocardial infarction, with ST-segment elevation and, often, elevated cardiac biomarkers; however, coronary angiography demonstrates an absence of significant obstructive coronary artery disease.

Bibliography

Prasad A, Lerman A, Rihal CS. Apical ballooning syndrome (Tako-Tsubo or stress cardiomyopathy): a mimic of acute myocardial infarction. Am Heart J. 2008 Mar;155(3):408-17. [PMID: 18294473]

Item 22   Answer: B

Educational Objective: Diagnose Eisenmenger syndrome due to a patent ductus arteriosus.

The patient has a patent ductus arteriosus (PDA) with secondary pulmonary hypertension (Eisenmenger syndrome). Clinical features of an Eisenmenger PDA include clubbing and oxygen desaturation affecting the lower body. This differential cyanosis and clubbing are caused by desaturated blood reaching the lower part of the body preferentially.

Pulmonary hypertension occurs infrequently in patients with unrepaired atrial septal defects owing to the relatively small shunt size. Clinical features of unrepaired atrial septal defect with pulmonary hypertension include cyanosis and clubbing that affects the hands and feet equally. The clinical findings are otherwise similar to findings in patients with idiopathic pulmonary arterial hypertension, with a parasternal lift and increased S_2.

Unrepaired tetralogy of Fallot consists of right ventricular outflow tract obstruction and a large ventricular septal defect with secondary features of right ventricular hypertrophy and aortic override. Clinical features include cyanosis and clubbing that affect the hands and

feet equally and a loud early systolic murmur heard at the left sternal border related to the right ventricular outflow tract obstruction. The pulmonic component of the S_2 is generally soft or absent depending on the degree of pulmonary valve stenosis. Right ventricular hypertension but not pulmonary hypertension is present; the pulmonary vasculature is protected by the presence of pulmonary valve stenosis.

A ventricular septal defect can cause pulmonary hypertension if it remains open beyond age 2 years. Clinical features include cyanosis and clubbing that affect the hands and feet equally, a parasternal lift, and increased S_2. Differential clubbing and cyanosis would not occur in a patient with pulmonary hypertension related to a ventricular septal defect.

KEY POINT

- A patent ductus arteriosus with Eisenmenger syndrome is characterized by differential cyanosis and clubbing affecting the lower body.

Bibliography

Srinivas SK, Manjunath CN. Differential clubbing and cyanosis: classic signs of patent ductus arteriosus with Eisenmenger syndrome. Mayo Clin Proc. 2013 Sep;88(9):e105-6. [PMID: 24001503]

Item 23   Answer: A

Educational Objective: Treat a patient with acute decompensated heart failure and evidence of low cardiac output.

This patient should be started on dobutamine for probable cardiogenic shock. Cardiogenic shock is present when there is systemic hypotension and evidence for end-organ hypoperfusion, primarily due to inadequate cardiac output. Cardiogenic shock usually requires treatment with intravenous vasoactive medications and, in severe cases, device-based hemodynamic support. Manifestations of end-organ hypoperfusion may include acute kidney failure, elevated serum aminotransferase levels or hyperbilirubinemia, cool extremities, and decreased mental status. In this patient, initiating inotropic therapy is reasonable. Both dobutamine and milrinone are used to increase cardiac output; however, in the setting of kidney dysfunction, dobutamine would be the appropriate choice because milrinone is metabolized by the kidneys. Also, milrinone is a vasodilator, which could exacerbate his hypotension.

Mechanical therapy for cardiogenic shock should be considered in patients with end-organ dysfunction that does not rapidly show signs of improvement (within the first 12-24 hours) with intravenous vasoactive medications and correction of volume overload. Options for mechanical therapy include placement of an intra-aortic balloon pump and percutaneous or surgically implanted ventricular assist devices (VADs). An intra-aortic balloon pump is timed to inflate during diastole, augmenting coronary and systemic perfusion, and deflate during systole, reducing left ventricular afterload. It is premature to consider mechanical therapy for this patient.

Right heart catheterization can be helpful to guide therapy if volume status or cardiac output is uncertain. However, it has not been shown to improve outcomes in patients hospitalized with heart failure. This patient has clinical evidence of volume overload, including jugular venous distention, pulmonary crackles, edema to the mid thighs, pulmonary edema on chest radiography, and an S_3. Additionally, he has evidence of low cardiac output (narrow pulse pressure, hypotension, acute kidney injury, mottled and cool extremities). Placement of a right heart catheter is not necessary prior to initiating inotropic therapy.

KEY POINT

- Cardiogenic shock usually requires treatment with intravenous vasoactive medications and, in severe cases, device-based hemodynamic support.

Bibliography

Nativi-Nicolau J, Selzman CH, Fang JC, Stehlik J. Pharmacologic therapies for acute cardiogenic shock. Curr Opin Cardiol. 2014 May;29(3):250-7. [PMID: 24686400]

Item 24   Answer: B

Educational Objective: Manage type A aortic dissection.

The most appropriate management for this patient with an acute type A aortic dissection is emergency surgical intervention. The abrupt onset of severe chest and back pain is typical of an acute aortic syndrome. A diastolic murmur consistent with aortic valvular insufficiency increases the clinical suspicion for a proximal (type A) aortic dissection that has disrupted normal valve leaflet coaptation. Acute aortic dissection is the most common life-threatening disorder affecting the aorta. In the Stanford classification, type A dissections involve the ascending aorta, and type B dissections are those that do not involve the ascending aorta. Type A dissections require emergency surgical repair, whereas medical therapy, consisting of a β-blocker to decrease the heart rate to below 60/min plus additional medications as needed to control hypertension, is usually the initial strategy for acute type B dissections. Therefore, pursuing medical management alone would not be appropriate in this patient. The immediate mortality rate in aortic dissection is as high as 1% per hour over the first several hours, making early diagnosis and treatment critical for survival.

Although most patients with dissection have underlying hypertension, only a tiny fraction of all persons with hypertension ever have a dissection. Syncope occurs in approximately 10% of patients with an acute aortic dissection and is more commonly associated with proximal dissection. Pulse deficits occur in less than 20% of type A dissections. Abnormal aortic contour or widening of the aortic silhouette may be an important clue to the diagnosis of aortic dissection. However, a normal chest radiograph is seen in nearly 15% of patients with acute aortic dissection. The 10-year survival rate of patients with acute dissection who survive initial hospitalization is reported to be 30% to 60%.

Endovascular treatment of dissection is used as an alternative to open surgery primarily in complicated type B dissections. Although endovascular procedures for type A dissections have shown some promise, they are not routinely used, particularly in patients with valve dysfunction requiring surgical repair.

Although heparin is commonly used in the initial treatment of acute coronary syndromes and pulmonary embolism, heparin is not indicated in the setting of an acute type A aortic dissection. The use of heparin in this setting can be complicated by major bleeding and cardiac tamponade. Moreover, heparin can increase the risk of life-threatening major bleeding when used in patients with very elevated blood pressures (commonly seen during a dissection).

KEY POINT

- A dissection involving the ascending aorta (Stanford type A) is a surgical emergency.

Bibliography

Braverman AC. Aortic dissection: prompt diagnosis and emergency treatment are critical. Cleve Clin J Med. 2011 Oct;78(10):685-96. [PMID: 21968475]

Item 25   Answer: D

Educational Objective: Manage antibiotic prophylaxis in a patient with a mechanical aortic valve prosthesis.

For this patient with a mechanical valve preparing for hernia repair surgery, antibiotic prophylaxis to prevent bacterial endocarditis is not indicated. Prophylaxis to prevent bacterial endocarditis is appropriate before certain dental procedures for patients with specific indications placing them at high risk for an adverse outcome from infective endocarditis (class IIa recommendation). These indications include previous endocarditis, a history of cardiac transplantation, a prosthetic valve, and specific forms of complex congenital heart disease. However, prophylaxis is not recommended for nondental procedures, including transesophageal echocardiography and genitourinary or gastrointestinal procedures (such as upper endoscopy, colonoscopy, or hernia repair), in the absence of active infection (class III recommendation). Dental procedures for which antibiotic prophylaxis is reasonable include those that involve manipulation of gingival tissue or the periapical region of teeth or perforation of the oral mucosa. Prophylaxis is not recommended for routine dental procedures, including radiographs and orthodontics.

When antibiotic prophylaxis is indicated, it should be given as a single dose 30 to 60 minutes before the dental procedure. If the prophylactic medication is inadvertently not administered, it may be given up to 2 hours after the procedure. Options include amoxicillin, 2 g orally, or ampicillin, 2 g intravenously. For patients allergic to penicillin or amoxicillin, alternatives include clindamycin, 600 mg orally;

azithromycin, 500 mg orally; or cefazolin/ceftriaxone, 1 g intramuscularly or intravenously.

CONT.

KEY POINT

- Antibiotic prophylaxis to prevent bacterial endocarditis is not recommended for nondental procedures, including transesophageal echocardiography and genitourinary or gastrointestinal procedures, in the absence of active infection.

Bibliography

Bonow RO, Carabello BA, Chatterjee K, et al; American College of Cardiology/American Heart Association Task Force on Practice Guidelines. 2008 focused update incorporated into the ACC/AHA 2006 guidelines for the management of patients with valvular heart disease: a report of the American College of Cardiology/American Heart Association Task Force on Practice Guidelines (Writing Committee to revise the 1998 guidelines for the management of patients with valvular heart disease). Endorsed by the Society of Cardiovascular Anesthesiologists, Society for Cardiovascular Angiography and Interventions, and Society of Thoracic Surgeons. J Am Coll Cardiol. 2008 Sep 23;52(13):e1-142. [PMID: 18848134]

Item 26   Answer: D

Educational Objective: Diagnose peripheral arterial disease in a patient with uninterpretable ankle-brachial index testing.

The most appropriate diagnostic test to perform next in this patient is a toe-brachial index. The ankle-brachial index (ABI) is obtained by measuring the systolic pressures in the dorsalis pedis and posterior tibialis arteries on both sides. The ABI for each leg is the highest ankle pressure for that side divided by the highest brachial pressure (regardless of side). An ABI of 0.90 or lower establishes a diagnosis of peripheral arterial disease (PAD). In this patient, the right ABI is greater than 1.40. An ABI above 1.40 suggests noncompressible vessels, which may reflect medial calcification but is not diagnostic of flow-limiting atherosclerotic disease. An ABI greater than 1.40 is associated with worse cardiovascular outcomes than a normal ABI. In such patients, an appropriate next step is to either measure great toe pressure or calculate a toe-brachial index (systolic great toe pressure divided by systolic brachial pressure). Vessels within the great toe rarely become noncompressible, and a great toe systolic pressure below 40 mm Hg or a toe-brachial index of less than 0.70 is consistent with PAD.

An ABI obtained immediately following symptom-limited exercise is useful when a high clinical suspicion for PAD remains despite a normal (1.00-1.40) or borderline resting ABI. A decrease of the ABI by 20% compared with the resting ABI is consistent with significant PAD. This patient's resting ABI is above the normal range; therefore, exercise ABI would not help to establish the diagnosis.

In patients with an established diagnosis of PAD and indications for revascularization, further vascular anatomic data can be obtained noninvasively using gadolinium-enhanced magnetic resonance angiography or contrast-enhanced multi-detector CT angiography. However, these tests should be reserved for planning intervention in patients who have not benefited from medical therapy; they should not be used for the diagnosis of PAD. Moreover, this patient has chronic kidney injury, and use of contrast for either study should be avoided if possible.

KEY POINT

- In a patient with suspected peripheral arterial disease, an ankle-brachial index above 1.40 is uninterpretable; measurement of the great toe systolic pressure can establish the diagnosis.

Bibliography

Aboyans V, Criqui MH, Abraham P, et al; American Heart Association Council on Peripheral Vascular Disease; Council on Epidemiology and Prevention; Council on Clinical Cardiology; Council on Cardiovascular Nursing; Council on Cardiovascular Radiology and Intervention, and Council on Cardiovascular Surgery and Anesthesia. Measurement and interpretation of the ankle-brachial index: a scientific statement from the American Heart Association. Circulation. 2012 Dec 11;126(24):2890-909. Erratum in: Circulation. 2013 Jan 1;127(1):e264. [PMID: 23159553]

Item 27   Answer: D

Educational Objective: Manage atrial fibrillation in a patient following percutaneous coronary intervention for treatment of refractory angina.

This patient should be treated with aspirin, clopidogrel, and warfarin ("triple therapy"). He has new-onset atrial fibrillation in the setting of recent bare metal stent placement for medically refractory angina. Patients with a bare metal stent should be treated with dual antiplatelet therapy for at least 1 month to allow endothelialization of the stent; with drug-eluting stents, the requirement for dual antiplatelet therapy is longer and depends upon the type of stent implanted. This patient is also at high risk of thromboembolic disease associated with atrial fibrillation. He has a CHA_2DS_2-VASc score of 5 (2 points for age >75 years, 1 point each for diabetes mellitus, hypertension, and vascular disease). Therefore, oral anticoagulant therapy is also indicated. Although triple therapy with two antiplatelet agents and systemic anticoagulation is associated with a significant increase in bleeding risk, this regimen is appropriate treatment in this patient for at least 1 month until stent endothelialization can be assured, at which time he can be transitioned to only aspirin and an oral anticoagulant to decrease bleeding risk but provide adequate thromboembolic prophylaxis. If warfarin is used as an anticoagulant during triple therapy, careful maintenance of the INR within the recommended range of 2.0 to 2.5 in patients without mechanical valves may reduce the overall bleeding risk.

Aspirin and clopidogrel are inferior to oral anticoagulation for the prevention of stroke in patients with an indication for anticoagulation for thromboembolism prophylaxis in atrial fibrillation.

Treatment with aspirin and dabigatran is not optimal for two reasons. First, in the Randomized Evaluation of Long Term Anticoagulant Therapy (RE-LY) trial, there was a numeric excess of myocardial infarctions observed with dabigatran. More importantly, no data are available regarding the efficacy of aspirin and dabigatran for the prevention of stent thrombosis following an acute coronary syndrome.

CONT.

Treatment with dual antiplatelet therapy is indicated in all patients with a coronary stent, with the recommended duration based on the underlying condition and type of stent placed. Therefore, treatment with aspirin and warfarin does not optimally prevent acute stent occlusion in a patient with stent placement.

KEY POINT

- Patients with atrial fibrillation and recent stent placement should be treated with appropriate systemic anticoagulation and antiplatelet therapy as determined by risk scoring and the type of stent placed.

Bibliography

Lip GY, Huber K, Andreotti F, et al; Consensus Document of European Society of Cardiology Working Group on Thrombosis. Antithrombotic management of atrial fibrillation patients presenting with acute coronary syndrome and/or undergoing coronary stenting: executive summary—a Consensus Document of the European Society of Cardiology Working Group on Thrombosis, endorsed by the European Heart Rhythm Association (EHRA) and the European Association of Percutaneous Cardiovascular Interventions (EAPCI). Eur Heart J. 2010 Jun;31(11):1311-8. [PMID: 20447945]

Item 28   Answer: C

Educational Objective: Manage symptomatic severe aortic stenosis.

The patient should be referred for surgical aortic valve replacement. She has symptomatic severe aortic stenosis, a class I indication for valve replacement. Surgical aortic valve replacement is the treatment of choice for most patients with symptomatic severe aortic stenosis and is associated with low mortality rates (1%-3%) in patients younger than 70 years.

Balloon valvuloplasty of the aortic valve has an extremely limited role in treating aortic stenosis owing to the high risk of complications associated with the procedure (10%-20%), a short-lived clinical benefit, and poor long-term outcomes. It would not be an appropriate treatment option in this patient.

Medical therapy for aortic stenosis is limited. Multiple agents have been evaluated for treatment of aortic stenosis, including ACE inhibitors, angiotensin receptor blockers, digoxin, diuretics, and statins. None have been shown to alter the progression of disease and valve replacement remains the indicated therapy. These agents are appropriate if there are other indications for their use, none of which are present in this patient.

Transcatheter aortic valve replacement (TAVR) is an option for patients with an indication for aortic valve replacement but who are not operative candidates or are at high risk for death or major morbidity with open aortic valve replacement. However, TAVR is not currently approved in patients with a bicuspid aortic valve, and given this patient's age and significant lack of comorbidities, she would appear to be a good candidate for surgical replacement.

KEY POINT

- Surgical aortic valve replacement is the treatment of choice for most patients with symptomatic severe aortic stenosis.

Bibliography

Joint Task Force on the Management of Valvular Heart Disease of the European Society of Cardiology (ESC); European Association for Cardio-Thoracic Surgery (EACTS), Vahanian A, Alfieri O, Andreotti F, et al. Guidelines on the management of valvular heart disease (version 2012). Eur Heart J. 2012 Oct;33(19):2451-96. [PMID: 22922415]

Item 29   Answer: A

Educational Objective: Diagnose atrial septal defect.

This patient has features of an ostium secundum atrial septal defect. Adults with atrial septal defects often present with atrial arrhythmias. The characteristic physical examination findings in atrial septal defect are fixed splitting of the S_2 and a right ventricular heave. A pulmonary midsystolic flow murmur and a tricuspid diastolic flow rumble caused by increased flow through the right-sided valves from a large left-to-right shunt may be heard. In ostium secundum atrial septal defect, the electrocardiogram (ECG) demonstrates right axis deviation and incomplete right bundle branch block. Ostium primum atrial septal defects are nearly always associated with anomalies of the atrioventricular valves, particularly a cleft in the anterior mitral valve leaflet or defects of the ventricular septum. The ECG in ostium primum atrial septal defect characteristically demonstrates first-degree atrioventricular block, left axis deviation, and right bundle branch block.

Bicuspid aortic valve with aortic stenosis causes a systolic murmur at the second right intercostal space. The central venous pressure is normal in aortic stenosis, and a right ventricular impulse would not be expected. Fixed splitting of the S_2 is not heard in patients with bicuspid aortic valve with aortic stenosis. The ECG typically demonstrates a normal axis and features of left ventricular hypertrophy.

Patients with pulmonary valve stenosis may demonstrate jugular venous pressure elevation with prominence of the a wave and a parasternal impulse from increased right ventricular pressure. The ejection murmur of pulmonary valve stenosis is heard at the second left intercostal space, and the timing of the peak of the murmur is related to stenosis severity. An ejection click is often heard; the proximity of the click to the S_2 varies depending on the severity of stenosis. Splitting of the S_2 results from prolonged ejection delay in the pulmonary valve component and may become fixed in severe pulmonary valve stenosis. The ECG typically demonstrates right axis deviation and features of right ventricular hypertrophy.

Mitral valve prolapse with mitral regurgitation may cause symptoms of palpitations. The murmur of mitral regurgitation is generally heard best at the apex. The central venous pressure is generally normal, and a right ventricular impulse would not be expected. Fixed splitting of the S_2 is not heard in patients with mitral valve prolapse. The ECG is typically normal.

> **KEY POINT**
>
> • Fixed splitting of the S_2 throughout the cardiac cycle and a right ventricular heave are characteristic clinical features of atrial septal defect.

Bibliography

Baumgartner H, Bonhoeffer P, De Groot NM, et al; Task Force on the Management of Grown-up Congenital Heart Disease of the European Society of Cardiology (ESC); Association for European Paediatric Cardiology (AEPC); ESC Committee for Practice Guidelines (CPG). ESC Guidelines for the management of grown-up congenital heart disease (new version 2010). Eur Heart J. 2010 Dec;31(23):2915-57. [PMID: 20801927]

Item 30   Answer: C

Educational Objective: Manage a patient with mitral valve stenosis considering pregnancy.

This patient has clinical and echocardiographic features of severe mitral valve stenosis as indicated by mitral valve mean gradient, valve area, and pulmonary artery systolic pressure greater than 50 mm Hg. Planned pregnancy is a class I indication for intervention in patients with severe mitral stenosis despite the absence of baseline symptoms. Most young patients will be candidates for mitral balloon valvuloplasty.

In severe mitral valve stenosis, negative chronotropic drugs such as β-blockers allow increased diastolic filling time of the left ventricle and may improve symptoms. If atrial fibrillation develops (even if paroxysmal), chronic anticoagulation therapy with warfarin is indicated to reduce the risk of thromboembolism, which is much higher than in nonvalvular atrial fibrillation. ACE inhibitors provide no particular benefit to patients with mitral stenosis and are contraindicated in pregnant patients. Dabigatran is approved for prevention of systemic embolism in adults with nonvalvular atrial fibrillation; however, its effectiveness in preventing embolism in patients with valvular heart disease is unknown, and it is not recommended in this setting.

Cardiac magnetic resonance imaging will not add incremental information to determine therapeutic strategy for this patient with rheumatic mitral stenosis considering pregnancy.

Pregnancy is associated with a marked increase in blood volume and cardiac output. Patients with severe mitral stenosis and moderate pulmonary hypertension often develop symptoms during pregnancy and should receive intervention prior to pregnancy.

> **KEY POINT**
>
> • Planned pregnancy is a class I indication for mitral valve intervention in patients with severe mitral valve stenosis despite the absence of baseline symptoms.

Bibliography

European Society of Gynecology (ESG); Association for European Paediatric Cardiology (AEPC); German Society for Gender Medicine (DGesGM), Regitz-Zagrosek V, Blomstrom Lundqvist C, Borghi C, et al; ESC Committee for Practice Guidelines. ESC Guidelines on the management of cardiovascular diseases during pregnancy: the Task Force on the Management of Cardiovascular Diseases during Pregnancy of the European Society of Cardiology (ESC). Eur Heart J. 2011 Dec;32(24):3147-97. [PMID: 21873418]

Item 31   Answer: A

Educational Objective: Manage abdominal aortic aneurysm with referral for repair.

The most appropriate management is to refer this patient for abdominal aortic aneurysm (AAA) repair. AAA is a common and potentially life-threatening condition, and management of detected aneurysms is based on size or rate of expansion. Elective repair to prevent rupture in asymptomatic patients is optimal management in those meeting criteria for intervention. Once an aneurysm reaches 5.5 cm in men and 5.0 cm in women, repair is generally warranted. Repair may be performed by an open approach or an endovascular approach, if the anatomy of the aneurysm is amenable; the mode of therapy should be decided by the surgeon, the internist, and the patient after a comprehensive discussion of risks and long-term benefits. Randomized trials show that endovascular aneurysm repair (EVAR) is associated with lower perioperative morbidity and mortality compared with open AAA repair, but EVAR does not completely eliminate the future risk of AAA rupture. Open repair is associated with higher perioperative morbidity and mortality than EVAR, but it provides a more definitive repair.

The optimal surveillance schedule for patients once an AAA has been identified has not been clearly defined. Annual surveillance is recommended, but larger aneurysms expand faster than small ones and may require more frequent surveillance. Aneurysm diameter is the most important factor predisposing to rupture, with risk increasing markedly at aneurysm diameters greater than 5.5 cm. For asymptomatic patients, the risk of AAA rupture generally exceeds the risk associated with elective AAA repair when aneurysm diameter exceeds 5.0 cm in a woman and 5.5 cm in a man. This patient's AAA is 5.7 cm in diameter; therefore, she should be referred for repair, rather than continuing surveillance.

Although controlling risk factors for cardiovascular disease is essential in patients with AAA, there is little compelling evidence for treating hypertension in these patients with a specific agent, including β-blockers, to prevent aneurysm expansion. As this patient's blood pressure is well controlled, no change in antihypertensive therapy is indicated.

> **KEY POINT**
>
> • An abdominal aortic aneurysm larger than 5.5 cm in men and 5.0 cm in women is an indication for referral for repair.

Bibliography

Buck DB, van Herwaarden JA, Schermerhorn ML, Moll FL. Endovascular treatment of abdominal aortic aneurysms. Nat Rev Cardiol. 2014 Feb;11(2):112-23. Erratum in: Nat Rev Cardiol. 2014 Feb;11(2):i. [PMID: 24343568]

Item 32   Answer: A

Educational Objective: Treat a patient with potentially transient constrictive pericarditis.

This patient has evidence of constrictive pericarditis and should be treated with an anti-inflammatory medication, such as a high-dose NSAID or prednisone. Supportive findings are symptoms and signs of right heart failure and congestion, with hemodynamic evidence of constriction on echocardiography. In some patients with constrictive pericarditis, the constriction can be transient and either spontaneously resolve or respond to medical therapy. This subtype of constrictive pericarditis more frequently has idiopathic, viral, or postsurgical causes. Although a minority of patients will have this transient constrictive pericarditis, a trial of medical therapy with an anti-inflammatory medication is reasonable. If medical therapy is successful, then surgical pericardiectomy can be avoided. Anti-inflammatory medication regimens for potentially transient constrictive pericarditis are similar to those for acute pericarditis, with relatively high doses of NSAIDs used (for example, ibuprofen, 800 mg three times daily; indomethacin, 50 mg three times daily; aspirin, 650 mg three times daily), with a slow taper over 2 to 3 weeks.

Cardiac catheterization for hemodynamic assessment of possible constriction is only indicated when diagnostic information cannot be obtained with echocardiography, which is not the case in this patient.

Pericardiectomy is inappropriate before a 2- to 3-month trial of anti-inflammatory medication in this patient. Although pericardiectomy is the definitive treatment for relief of heart failure in patients with constrictive pericarditis, it is a complex, invasive procedure that should not be used in patients with transient constriction.

Transesophageal echocardiography is only indicated when data from other noninvasive imaging studies (such as transthoracic echocardiography) are inconclusive.

KEY POINT

- In some patients with constrictive pericarditis, the constriction may be transient and either spontaneously resolve or respond to medical therapy, which obviates the need for surgical pericardiectomy.

Bibliography

Haley JH, Tajik AJ, Danielson GK, Schaff HV, Mulvagh SL, Oh JK. Transient constrictive pericarditis: causes and natural history. J Am Coll Cardiol. 2004 Jan 21;43(2):271-5. [PMID: 14736448]

Item 33   Answer: C

Educational Objective: Manage symptomatic premature ventricular contractions.

This patient has frequent, symptomatic premature ventricular contractions (PVCs) with decline in his left ventricular function despite treatment with β-blocker therapy. As there is no clear underlying myocardial process, it is likely that his PVCs may represent a reversible cause of his cardiomyopathy. He

should be referred to a cardiac electrophysiologist for catheter ablation of his PVCs.

PVCs are common and are usually benign. However, symptomatic or frequent PVCs (>10,000 PVCs/24 hours or >10% of all beats) require treatment. Up to one third of patients with frequent PVCs develop PVC-induced cardiomyopathy and progressive left ventricular dysfunction. First-line therapy for symptomatic or frequent PVCs is β-blocker or calcium channel blocker therapy. Patients with medically refractory frequent PVCs or who develop left ventricular dysfunction should undergo catheter ablation of the PVCs. Catheter ablation leads to resolution of PVC-induced cardiomyopathy in most patients.

Amiodarone could be used for PVC suppression; however, it has many long-term risks, including thyroid, liver, pulmonary, and neurologic toxicity. Given this patient's relatively young age, amiodarone would not be the most appropriate therapy, particularly if long-term control is needed.

Cardiac resynchronization therapy involves the simultaneous pacing of both ventricles in patients with advanced heart failure and evidence of intraventricular conduction delay (QRS interval ≥150 ms) to reduce dyssynchrony to improve pump performance. This patient does not have severe heart failure or evidence of dyssynchrony. As his symptoms are related more to his ventricular ectopy, cardiac resynchronization therapy would not be appropriate.

An implantable cardioverter-defibrillator (ICD) is indicated in patients at risk for ventricular tachycardia or ventricular fibrillation to prevent sudden cardiac death. Although this patient has very frequent PVCs, including bigeminy, he does not have sustained tachyarrhythmias of potential hemodynamic significance. Therefore, ICD placement would not be appropriate in this patient.

KEY POINT

- Patients with frequent premature ventricular contractions and subsequent cardiomyopathy should be treated with catheter ablation.

Bibliography

Yokokawa M, Good E, Crawford T, et al. Recovery from left ventricular dysfunction after ablation of frequent premature ventricular complexes. Heart Rhythm. 2013 Feb;10(2):172-5. [PMID: 23099051]

Item 34   Answer: A   H

Educational Objective: Manage discharge of a patient with heart failure to prevent readmission.

This patient should be discharged home, with a follow-up appointment scheduled within 7 days. She has had one heart failure hospitalization in the past 3 years and her nonadherence with her diuretic medication was the most likely cause of the admission. With any heart failure hospitalization, it is important to reassess several factors before discharge. First, patients must be adequately diuresed prior to discharge. It is important to know that measuring a serum B-type natriuretic peptide level will not help with that assessment. Patients should be examined for flat neck veins, resolution of peripheral or abdominal edema (if possible), and resolution of the signs and symptoms of acute heart failure (S₃, exertional dyspnea and fatigue, orthopnea, paroxysmal nocturnal dyspnea). Second, patients should be on appropriate medical therapy for their stage of heart failure. For this patient, appropriate medications include an ACE inhibitor or angiotensin receptor blocker, β-blocker, aldosterone antagonist, and an adequate dosage of diuretic to prevent readmission. Third, it has been demonstrated that a patient being seen within 1 week after discharge is associated with a reduction of future heart failure hospitalizations. This patient is adequately diuresed and is on appropriate medications. Reducing her risk of readmission requires a follow-up visit within 7 days of discharge and appropriate patient education.

An echocardiogram performed 1 month ago demonstrated that the patient's left ventricular function is stable. There is no suggestion of ischemia or change in valvular function as a precipitant of this hospitalization. If this patient had not had an echocardiogram in at least 6 months, it would be reasonable to repeat the echocardiogram during the hospitalization; otherwise unless there is a suspicion of a change, there is no reason to do so.

Patients are candidates for a biventricular pacemaker if they have all of the following indications: on guideline-directed medical therapy, a reduced ejection fraction (≤35%), a wide QRS interval (≥150 ms) or a left bundle branch block, and New York Heart Association functional class III or IV symptoms. This patient has a narrow QRS interval and therefore would not be a candidate for upgrading to a biventricular implantable cardioverter-defibrillator.

KEY POINT

- Patients hospitalized for heart failure who are scheduled for a follow-up appointment within 1 week after discharge have a reduced risk of future heart failure hospitalization.

Bibliography

Fleming LM, Kociol RD. Interventions for heart failure readmissions: successes and failures. Curr Heart Fail Rep. 2014 Jun;11(2):178-87. [PMID: 24578234]

Item 35   Answer: A

Educational Objective: Diagnose aortic coarctation in an adult.

This patient presents with newly diagnosed hypertension and clinical features of aortic coarctation, which include upper extremity hypertension and a radial artery-to-femoral artery pulse delay suggesting a mechanical obstruction between the radial and femoral arteries; lower extremity blood pressure determinations may be low or difficult to obtain. A systolic murmur over the left posterior chest is common in patients with severe aortic coarctation; these murmurs can arise from the obstruction or the collateral blood flow. The chest radiograph (shown) demonstrates "rib notching" affecting several of the posterior ribs; rib notching results from exaggerated collateral blood flow diverting blood around the area of obstruction. Also present on the chest radiograph is the "figure 3 sign" caused by dilatation of the aorta above and below the area of coarctation.

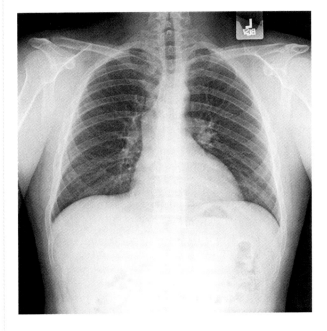

Essential hypertension is the most common cause of hypertension in adults. A family history of hypertension is common. The physical examination in a patient with severe essential hypertension often includes an S₄, but a pulse and blood pressure differential between the upper and lower extremities is not expected.

Patients with hypertrophic cardiomyopathy do not usually present with hypertension. The systolic murmurs in hypertrophic cardiomyopathy characteristically include an ejection quality murmur at the left sternal border related to outflow obstruction and a late systolic murmur at the apex related to mitral valve regurgitation.

Renovascular hypertension is a common cause of hypertension occurring primarily in patients with diffuse atherosclerosis. An epigastric bruit may be audible. The rest of the physical examination in a patient with renovascular hypertension is usually normal. A pulse and blood pressure differential between an upper and a lower extremity is not expected.

KEY POINT

- Aortic coarctation is characterized clinically by upper extremity hypertension and a radial artery–to–femoral artery pulse delay.

Bibliography

Tanous D, Benson LN, Horlick EM. Coarctation of the aorta: evaluation and management. Curr Opin Cardiol. 2009 Nov;24(6):509-15. [PMID: 19667980]

Item 36   Answer: A

Educational Objective: Treat hypertension during pregnancy.

The most appropriate treatment for this patient is labetalol. When hypertension is noted before the 20th week of gestation, it is most consistent with a new diagnosis of chronic hypertension. There is no evidence that tight control of hypertension during pregnancy will prevent preeclampsia; instead, antihypertensive therapy is warranted only to limit maternal end-organ damage in those with severe hypertension. Hypertension of the magnitude demonstrated by this patient (systolic blood pressure >150 mm Hg) is a class I indication for pharmacologic treatment during pregnancy.

If treatment is necessary, it is important to note that all antihypertensive agents cross the placenta. Methyldopa and labetalol appear to be the safest choices, whereas ACE inhibitors, angiotensin receptor blockers (ARBs), and likely renin inhibitors are not safe.

ACE inhibitors (such as lisinopril), ARBs (such as losartan), and direct renin inhibitors (aliskiren) are contraindicated during pregnancy owing to fetal toxicity. Fetal exposure to these agents during the first trimester can cause central nervous system and cardiovascular malformations, and exposure during the second trimester can cause urogenital and renal developmental malformations.

Diet and weight loss should be used in conjunction with pharmacologic therapy in this patient, but nonpharmacologic strategies alone are not sufficient in a patient with this magnitude of hypertension.

Not treating this patient's chronic hypertension may result in maternal end-organ damage and is not an acceptable option.

KEY POINT

- Labetalol has been demonstrated to be safe and effective for the treatment of hypertension during pregnancy and is the preferred β-blocker for use during pregnancy.

Bibliography

European Society of Gynecology (ESG); Association for European Paediatric Cardiology (AEPC); German Society for Gender Medicine (DGesGM), Regitz-Zagrosek V, Blomstrom Lundqvist C, Borghi C, et al; ESC Committee for Practice Guidelines. ESC Guidelines on the management of cardiovascular diseases during pregnancy: the Task Force on the Management of Cardiovascular Diseases during Pregnancy of the European Society of Cardiology (ESC). Eur Heart J. 2011 Dec;32(24):3147-97. [PMID: 21873418]

Item 37   Answer: A

Educational Objective: Diagnose a murmur heard in a pregnant woman.

The most likely cause of this woman's murmur is a bicuspid aortic valve, the most common congenital heart abnormality. The characteristic finding of a bicuspid aortic valve is an aortic ejection sound associated with either a systolic or diastolic murmur. While the murmur associated with aortic stenosis usually radiates to the carotid arteries, the murmur

of a nonstenotic bicuspid aortic valve may radiate to the apex. Fetal echocardiography is indicated if there is maternal cardiac structural disease because of the increased risk of fetal cardiac abnormalities, which is estimated to be in the range of 3% to 7%.

The altered hemodynamics of pregnancy may bring out murmurs not previously heard or may bring the pregnant patient to medical attention for the first time owing to the increase in systemic blood volume and cardiac output. Systolic murmurs are common during pregnancy. Most often these are ejection murmurs caused by increased flow through the right and left ventricular outflow tracts. The murmurs tend to be grade 1/6 or 2/6 midsystolic murmurs that do not radiate. Diastolic murmurs are not common.

The systolic murmur associated with hypertrophic obstructive cardiomyopathy generally increases with maneuvers that decrease preload, such as the Valsalva maneuver or change in position from squatting to standing.

A mammary souffle is a continuous murmur with a soft, humming quality. It is typically heard over the breast during late pregnancy and lactation and is thought to result from increased blood flow to the breast.

While the murmur of mitral valve prolapse is often late systolic and can be associated with a click, this click would not be described as an ejection click. The click associated with mitral valve prolapse is mid- to late systolic and is related to tensing of the chordae tendineae or valve leaflets. The click is responsive to changes in ventricular volume induced by posture or pharmacologic agents.

Functional murmurs, or physiologic murmurs, can occur in the absence of valvular pathology. An increase in cardiac output, as occurs in pregnancy, can result in physiologic ejection murmurs.

Given the findings on examination, it would be appropriate to obtain transthoracic echocardiography for this patient to identify the etiology of the murmur and the potential need for adjuvant screening to evaluate for associated aortopathy.

KEY POINT

- The characteristic finding of a bicuspid aortic valve is an aortic ejection sound associated with either a systolic or diastolic murmur.

Bibliography

Franklin WJ, Gandhi M. Congenital heart disease in pregnancy. Cardiol Clin. 2012 Aug;30(3):383-94. [PMID: 22813364]

Item 38   Answer: C

Educational Objective: Manage medication use prior to stress testing.

This patient's metoprolol should be withheld for 48 hours before stress testing. In this intermediate-probability patient with a normal electrocardiogram, exercise stress testing is appropriate. Exercise stress is preferred to pharmacologic stressors because it provides a gauge of functional capacity and a contextual understanding of symptoms, and it records hemodynamic response to exercise. The sensitivity of the study to detect obstructive coronary artery disease (CAD) is lowered, however, if patients are taking certain medications. β-Blockers and nondihydropyridine calcium channel blockers can blunt the maximal heart rate that can be achieved with exercise and may limit a patient's ability to reach 85% of the maximal predicted heart rate. However, dihydropyridine calcium channel blockers do not need to be withheld prior to testing. Similarly, digoxin can limit the maximal heart rate and should be withheld. Nitrates are effective antianginal agents but may minimize the ischemic response on stress testing; therefore, they should also be withheld. If, however, a patient has known CAD and the goal of testing is to determine whether symptoms are related to ischemia or to assess adequacy of antianginal therapy, there is no need to stop any of the medications.

There is no evidence that ACE inhibitors, such as lisinopril, or angiotensin receptor blockers alter the sensitivity of exercise stress testing in the diagnosis of CAD, and these agents do not need to be discontinued before testing. For this patient on several medications for hypertension, an appropriate strategy would be to continue hydrochlorothiazide and lisinopril and discontinue metoprolol.

KEY POINT

- In patients undergoing stress testing to diagnose coronary artery disease, β-blockers should be withheld for 24 to 48 hours before testing.

Bibliography

Fihn SD, Gardin JM, Abrams J, et al; American College of Cardiology Foundation; American Heart Association Task Force on Practice Guidelines; American College of Physicians; American Association for Thoracic Surgery; Preventive Cardiovascular Nurses Association; Society for Cardiovascular Angiography and Interventions; Society of Thoracic Surgeons. 2012 CCF/AHA/ACP/AATS/PCNA/SCAI/STS Guideline for the diagnosis and management of patients with stable ischemic heart disease: a report of the American College of Cardiology Foundation/American Heart Association Task Force on Practice Guidelines, and the American College of Physicians, American Association for Thoracic Surgery, Preventive Cardiovascular Nurses Association, Society for Cardiovascular Angiography and Interventions, and Society of Thoracic Surgeons. J Am Coll Cardiol. 2012 Dec 18;60(24):e44-e164. [PMID: 23182125]

Item 39   Answer: B

Educational Objective: Manage a patient with new-onset exertional angina pectoris.

This patient with an intermediate risk of ischemic heart disease and an inadequate exercise electrocardiographic (ECG) stress test should undergo pharmacologic stress testing. Although exercise ECG stress testing is the preferred diagnostic study in patients with an indication for testing who have an interpretable resting ECG and are able to exercise, in patients who are unable to meet the minimal criteria for adequacy on this study (achievement of at least 85% of the age-predicted maximal heart rate and maximal metabolic demand), additional testing is indicated to appropriately evaluate for ischemic heart disease. Dobutamine stress echocardiography or a vasodilator nuclear medicine stress test would be appropriate

studies in this clinical setting and would allow for further stratification of this patient's risk for ischemic heart disease.

Proceeding directly to cardiac catheterization may be appropriate in patients at very high risk for ischemic heart disease in whom noninvasive testing would not be expected to significantly change the pretest probability of disease. However, in this patient with an intermediate risk of disease, adequate noninvasive testing would be helpful in evaluating for the presence of ischemic heart disease, and coronary angiography would not be indicated as a next diagnostic test.

Switching the patient's antihypertensive medication to an agent with antianginal properties would not be indicated without establishing the presence of ischemic heart disease, particularly with adequate control of her blood pressure on her current regimen.

Because an inadequate exercise ECG exercise test is unable to assess for the presence of ischemic heart disease in this patient at intermediate risk, clinical observation without further evaluation would not be appropriate.

KEY POINT

- Exercise stress testing is recommended as the initial test of choice for patients with intermediate risk of ischemic heart disease who are capable of exercising and have a normal resting electrocardiogram, although advanced imaging is indicated if the exercise stress test is inadequate or indeterminate.

Bibliography

Fihn SD, Gardin JM, Abrams J, et al; American College of Cardiology Foundation/American Heart Association Task Force. 2012 ACCF/AHA/ACP/AATS/PCNA/SCAI/STS guideline for the diagnosis and management of patients with stable ischemic heart disease: a report of the American College of Cardiology Foundation/American Heart Association task force on practice guidelines, and the American College of Physicians, American Association for Thoracic Surgery, Preventive Cardiovascular Nurses Association, Society for Cardiovascular Angiography and Interventions, and Society of Thoracic Surgeons. Circulation. 2012 Dec 18;126(25):e354-471. Erratum in: Circulation. 2014 Apr 22;129(16):e463. [PMID: 23166211]

Item 40   Answer: C

Educational Objective: Manage cardiovascular risk in an older woman with diabetes mellitus.

This patient should start atorvastatin, discontinue simvastatin, and continue her other medications. The most recent cholesterol guidelines recommend a moderate- or high-intensity statin, such as atorvastatin, in patients aged 40 to 75 years with diabetes mellitus who have a 10-year cardiovascular risk greater than or equal to 7.5%. This patient's 10-year cardiovascular risk is above 10%. A cardiovascular risk calculator based on the Pooled Cohort Equations for the purpose of managing cholesterol levels is available at http://my.americanheart.org/professional/Statements-Guidelines/PreventionGuidelines/Prevention-Guidelines_UCM_457698_SubHomePage.jsp. In patients with diabetes in this age group with a 10-year risk below 7.5%, a moderate-intensity statin (such as simvastatin 20-40 mg/d) would be recommended. While there are multiple options for a high-intensity statin, the fact that atorvastatin has a generic alternative makes it a more attractive choice.

Increasing simvastatin from 10 mg/d to 80 mg/d is incorrect, as the FDA issued a black box warning against the use of simvastatin 80 mg/d because of a heightened risk of muscle adverse effects.

Continuing the patient's current medications is incorrect because this patient's cardiovascular risk warrants change to a moderate- or high-intensity statin.

The addition of clopidogrel to this patient's drug regimen is incorrect because dual antiplatelet therapy (such as aspirin plus clopidogrel) increases the risk of bleeding and is not routinely recommended for patients for primary prevention of cardiovascular events.

Despite a negative exercise stress test, aspirin therapy would be recommended in this woman who has several risk factors for cardiovascular events and stroke, including hypertension, type 2 diabetes mellitus, hyperlipidemia, and her age. In the Women's Health Study of 40,000 healthy women, 100 mg/d of aspirin decreased the risk of stroke, myocardial infarction, and cardiovascular death in patients older than 65 years.

KEY POINT

- A moderate- or high-intensity statin is recommended for patients aged 40 to 75 years with diabetes mellitus who have a 10-year cardiovascular risk greater than or equal to 7.5%.

Bibliography
Stone NJ, Robinson JG, Lichtenstein AH, et al; American College of Cardiology/American Heart Association Task Force on Practice Guidelines. 2013 ACC/AHA guideline on the treatment of blood cholesterol to reduce atherosclerotic cardiovascular risk in adults: a report of the American College of Cardiology/American Heart Association Task Force on Practice Guidelines. J Am Coll Cardiol. 2014 Jul 1;63(25 Pt B):2889-934. Erratum in: J Am Coll Cardiol. 2014 Jul 1;63(25 Pt B):3024-3025. [PMID: 24239923]

Item 41   Answer: B

Educational Objective: Manage claudication with pharmacologic therapy in a patient with peripheral arterial disease.

The most appropriate treatment is the addition of cilostazol. Cilostazol is an oral phosphodiesterase-3 inhibitor that has demonstrated increases in pain-free walking and overall walking distance in patients with claudication in randomized clinical trials. Cilostazol is contraindicated in patients with heart failure or a left ventricular ejection fraction below 40%. This contraindication exists because cilostazol has a similar pharmacologic action to the inotropic drugs milrinone and amrinone, which demonstrated increased mortality rates with long-term use in patients with heart failure. In the absence of heart failure, a therapeutic trial of cilostazol should be considered in all patients with lifestyle-limiting claudication.

Antihypertensive therapy is recommended for reduction of cardiovascular events in patients with peripheral arterial disease (PAD). Although concern has been raised in the past regarding use of β-blockers for treatment of hyper-

tension in patients with PAD because of the possibility of loss of β-receptor–mediated vasodilation causing worsening claudication, this has not been supported by study data. Therefore, β-blockers may be used in patients with PAD for blood pressure control. However, this patient's hypertension is well controlled, and β-blockade is not indicated as therapy for claudication symptoms.

Clopidogrel or another thienopyridine should be added to aspirin therapy in all patients following an acute coronary syndrome and in those undergoing coronary stent placement. However, there is no benefit in adding clopidogrel to aspirin in patients with PAD for treatment of the vascular occlusion or reducing the risk of cardiovascular events.

In the Warfarin Antiplatelet Vascular Evaluation (WAVE) trial among patients with PAD, the combination of an oral anticoagulant and antiplatelet therapy was not more effective than antiplatelet therapy alone in preventing major cardiovascular complications and was associated with an increase in life-threatening bleeding.

KEY POINT

- Cilostazol has been shown to be effective at improving pain-free walking and overall walking distance in patients with claudication.

Bibliography
Pande RL, Hiatt WR, Zhang P, Hittel N, Creager MA. A pooled analysis of the durability and predictors of treatment response of cilostazol in patients with intermittent claudication. Vasc Med. 2010 Jun;15(3):181-8. [PMID: 20385711]

Item 42   Answer: E

Educational Objective: Manage an accelerated idioventricular rhythm following myocardial infarction.

This patient requires no further intervention at this time. She developed a wide complex rhythm shortly after percutaneous coronary intervention and reperfusion of her infarct-related artery. The electrocardiogram (ECG) shows a regular wide complex rhythm at 92/min with no clearly discernible atrial activity, findings consistent with accelerated idioventricular rhythm (AIVR). AIVR is postulated to result from abnormal automaticity in the subendocardial Purkinje fibers. It is observed in up to 15% of patients who undergo reperfusion of an infarct-related artery. The rate is almost always less than 120/min and usually less than 100/min. Most studies have shown that it is a benign rhythm when it occurs within 24 hours of reperfusion. This patient is tolerating the rhythm well and is already on a β-blocker for post–myocardial infarction care; therefore, no intervention is required.

Neither amiodarone nor lidocaine is indicated because AIVR is a benign ventricular arrhythmia and usually does not recur. Studies of prophylactic lidocaine after acute coronary syndromes have demonstrated potential harm, and amiodarone has been associated with decreased survival after myocardial infarction.

Cardioversion is not indicated because AIVR is a transient rhythm and, in this patient, it is well-tolerated.

CONT.

AIVR usually indicates successful (or at least partial) reperfusion and is considered a reversible arrhythmia. Implantable cardioverter-defibrillator (ICD) placement is not indicated at this time given the patient's recent revascularization and nature of the arrhythmia. If the left ventricular ejection fraction remains low despite medical therapy, ICD placement might be indicated in the future.

KEY POINT

- Accelerated idioventricular rhythm is a common complication following coronary reperfusion and does not require intervention when it occurs within 24 hours of reperfusion.

Bibliography

Bonnemeier H, Ortak J, Wiegand UK, et al. Accelerated idioventricular rhythm in the post-thrombolytic era: incidence, prognostic implications, and modulating mechanisms after direct percutaneous coronary intervention. Ann Noninvasive Electrocardiol. 2005 Apr;10(2):179-87. [PMID: 15842430]

Item 43   Answer: A

Educational Objective: Treat a patient with acute pericarditis with high-dose aspirin.

This patient should receive high-dose aspirin. He has acute pericarditis in the setting of a recent myocardial infarction. The typical chest pain, physical examination findings, and abnormal electrocardiogram (ECG) are all consistent with this diagnosis, especially the findings of concave upward ST-segment elevation and PR-segment depression in all leads, except aVR, on the ECG. Anti-inflammatory therapy with aspirin or other NSAIDs, such as ibuprofen, is indicated in patients with acute pericarditis. In those whose pericarditis is associated with myocardial infarction, such as this patient, only aspirin should be used because ibuprofen and other NSAIDs can impair myocardial healing and increase the risk of mechanical complications. The anti-inflammatory medication should be given in relatively high doses to achieve an anti-inflammatory effect and then tapered slowly over 2 to 4 weeks to reduce the risk of recurrent pericarditis. Colchicine (0.5-1.2 mg/d) also has been shown to be effective as adjunctive therapy to anti-inflammatory agents in patients with acute pericarditis, further reducing the risk of recurrent pericarditis and treatment failure. Colchicine is not recommended for patients with post-infarction pericarditis. Colchicine may be associated with gastrointestinal side effects, liver toxicity, and bone marrow suppression but is generally well tolerated.

Nitroglycerin is an effective therapy for chest pain caused by myocardial ischemia but is not effective for symptoms caused by pericarditis.

Glucocorticoids, such as prednisone, are reserved for patients with contraindications to NSAIDs or those with refractory acute pericarditis, primarily because there is evidence that their use is associated with an increased risk of recurrent pericarditis. As this patient has no apparent contraindication to aspirin use, treatment with glucocorticoids is not indicated.

KEY POINT

- Anti-inflammatory therapy with aspirin or other NSAIDs, such as ibuprofen, is indicated in patients with acute pericarditis; when the pericarditis is associated with myocardial infarction, only aspirin should be used because other NSAIDs can impair myocardial healing and increase the risk of mechanical complications.

Bibliography

Lotrionte M, Biondi-Zoccai G, Imazio M, et al. International collaborative systematic review of controlled clinical trials on pharmacologic treatments for acute pericarditis and its recurrences. Am Heart J. 2010 Oct;160(4):662-70. [PMID: 20934560]

Item 44   Answer: B

Educational Objective: Manage dual antiplatelet therapy after drug-eluting stent placement following non–ST-elevation myocardial infarction.

This patient, who has undergone drug-eluting stent placement following a non–ST-elevation myocardial infarction, should continue taking ticagrelor for 1 year. He also should continue taking aspirin indefinitely. The American College of Cardiology/American Heart Association percutaneous coronary intervention (PCI) guidelines recommend at least 1 year of dual antiplatelet therapy for patients undergoing PCI with a drug-eluting stent (DES).

Antiplatelet drugs indicated for patients who have received a drug-eluting stent following an acute coronary syndrome are clopidogrel, ticagrelor, and prasugrel. In the PLATelet inhibition and patient Outcomes (PLATO) trial, ticagrelor was found to be superior to clopidogrel in reducing the incidence of cardiovascular death, myocardial infarction, and stroke following an acute coronary syndrome.

Dual antiplatelet therapy for patients who have undergone placement of a bare metal stent following an acute coronary syndrome is indicated for at least 4 weeks and up to 1 year. Following placement of a DES, however, a 30-day duration of ticagrelor is insufficient.

Despite numerous studies about the risk of very late stent thrombosis, defined as the occurrence of stent thrombosis greater than 1 year after placement, there is no recommendation for lifelong dual antiplatelet therapy in current treatment guidelines.

Stopping ticagrelor and starting clopidogrel is incorrect because there is no indication to stop ticagrelor, an agent that appears to be superior to clopidogrel in improving cardiovascular outcomes following an acute coronary syndrome. Cost and adverse events (including bleeding, dyspnea, and bradycardia) are the most common reasons for discontinuation of ticagrelor.

KEY POINT

- At least 1 year of dual antiplatelet therapy is recommended for patients undergoing percutaneous coronary intervention with a drug-eluting stent (DES); therapeutic options for agents to be taken with aspirin are clopidogrel, ticagrelor, and prasugrel.

Bibliography

Wallentin L, Becker RC, Budaj A, et al. Ticagrelor versus clopidogrel in patients with acute coronary syndromes. N Engl J Med. 2009 Sep 10;361(11):1045-57. [PMID: 19717846]

Item 45   Answer: D

Educational Objective: Manage a patient with ventricular septal defect.

The most appropriate management for this patient with a small uncomplicated ventricular septal defect (VSD) is follow-up in 3 to 5 years. She has clinical features of a small membranous VSD without associated volume overload of the left heart, pulmonary hypertension, or valve regurgitation.

Cardiac catheterization is not indicated for this patient because the echocardiogram does not demonstrate left heart enlargement or features that suggest pulmonary hypertension.

Cardiac magnetic resonance (CMR) imaging will usually demonstrate a membranous VSD and can quantitate the impact of the VSD on the left heart; however, it is not indicated in this patient because the clinical assessment and echocardiogram suggest that observation is appropriate. CMR imaging would be a reasonable test if the transthoracic echocardiogram images were not diagnostic.

Endocarditis prophylaxis is recommended for patients with congenital heart disease characterized by unrepaired cyanotic congenital heart disease, including palliative shunts and conduits; a completely repaired congenital heart defect with prosthetic material or device during the first 6 months after the procedure; and repaired congenital heart disease with residual defects. Patients with uncomplicated VSDs without a prior history of endocarditis do not require endocarditis prophylaxis.

Functional aerobic capacity measured by stress testing is not used to determine management in patients with small VSDs. A small VSD does not impact exercise capacity and thus assessment of exercise capacity will not change management in this patient.

KEY POINT

- A small membranous ventricular septal defect without left heart enlargement, pulmonary hypertension, recurrent endocarditis, or valve regurgitation can be observed clinically.

Bibliography

Penny DJ, Vick GW 3rd. Ventricular septal defect. Lancet. 2011 Mar 26;377(9771):1103-12. [PMID: 21349577]

Item 46   Answer: A

Educational Objective: Treat mitral regurgitation with bioprosthetic mitral valve replacement.

The most appropriate treatment for this patient is mitral valve replacement (MVR) with a bioprosthetic valve. She has a history of rheumatic fever and extensive degeneration of the mitral valve with severe mitral regurgitation on

echocardiogram, consistent with rheumatic heart disease. Indications for mitral valve surgery include symptomatic severe mitral regurgitation with left ventricular (LV) ejection fraction greater than 30% and asymptomatic severe mitral regurgitation with mild to moderate LV dysfunction (ejection fraction of 30%-60% and/or LV end-systolic diameter ≥40 mm). Although surgical valve repair is generally preferred to valve replacement, it may not be possible with extensive calcification of the valve leaflet or annulus, prolapse of more than one third of the leaflet tissue, or extensive destruction of the chordal apparatus. The choice of valve intervention and prosthetic valve type should be a shared decision-making process. When valve replacement is indicated, as in this patient, a bioprosthesis is preferred in patients of any age for whom anticoagulant therapy is contraindicated, cannot be managed appropriately, or is not desired. In addition, a bioprosthesis is a reasonable choice for patients older than 70 years. This patient's history of gastrointestinal bleeding and her advanced age make a bioprosthetic valve the more reasonable choice.

Intravenous vasodilator therapy improves forward blood flow and symptoms acutely in patients with severe mitral regurgitation. However, there is little evidence that long-term oral vasodilator therapy is beneficial for symptomatic mitral regurgitation, and it is used primarily in patients unable to undergo surgical correction. Because this patient has no clear contraindication to surgical therapy, medical therapy alone would not be appropriate.

Percutaneous mitral valve repair procedures include percutaneous valvuloplasty or implantation of a clip to reduce regurgitant flow. However, these procedures are either under investigation or their use is limited to a small group of patients.

KEY POINT

- When valve replacement is indicated, a bioprosthesis is preferred in patients of any age for whom anticoagulant therapy is contraindicated, cannot be managed appropriately, or is not desired.

Bibliography

Nishimura RA, Otto CM, Bonow RO, et al; American College of Cardiology/American Heart Association Task Force on Practice Guidelines. 2014 AHA/ACC guideline for the management of patients with valvular heart disease: executive summary: a report of the American College of Cardiology/American Heart Association Task Force on Practice Guidelines. J Am Coll Cardiol. 2014 Jun 10;63(22):2438-88. Erratum in: J Am Coll Cardiol. 2014 Jun 10;63(22):2489. [PMID: 24603192]

Item 47   Answer: C

Educational Objective: Evaluate a patient with new-onset heart failure who has evidence of coronary artery disease.

The most appropriate diagnostic test to perform next in this patient is myocardial perfusion imaging stress testing. This patient has evidence of new-onset heart failure as evidenced by her clinical presentation (decreased exercise tolerance, jugular venous distention, crackles on lung examination, and lower extremity edema). A diagnosis of new-onset heart failure should be confirmed by echocardiography, which has both high sensitivity and specificity for heart failure and may be useful in evaluating for specific possible causes of heart failure, such as valve dysfunction. Treatable causes of heart failure include coronary artery disease (CAD), thyroid disease, alcohol abuse, and some valvular diseases (such as aortic stenosis, if repaired early) and should be looked for during the initial evaluation.

As many as two thirds of cases of heart failure are caused by CAD. This patient has several risk factors for cardiovascular disease, including hypertension and a history of smoking. Her electrocardiogram (ECG) demonstrates left bundle branch block and her echocardiogram demonstrates an akinetic left wall, both of which suggest CAD. Patients with heart failure and multiple risk factors or symptoms of CAD should be evaluated by either a stress test or cardiac catheterization. The reason to evaluate for CAD is that revascularization by either percutaneous coronary intervention (PCI) or coronary artery bypass graft surgery may improve her left ventricular ejection fraction and reduce her symptoms of heart failure. Noninvasive exercise testing is often performed initially to provide information about the possible presence of ischemic heart disease but also to assist in risk stratification and prognosis. Cardiac catheterization may be helpful in patients with suggestive findings on non-invasive testing or may be an appropriate initial study in selected patients.

Cardiac magnetic resonance (CMR) imaging is not part of the routine evaluation of new-onset heart failure but may be used if an infiltrative or an inflammatory process is suspected, such as myocarditis, hemochromatosis, Wilson disease, or sarcoidosis. If the patient's evaluation for CAD as a cause of her heart failure is normal and myocarditis is a consideration, CMR imaging may be a reasonable test.

Coronary artery calcium scoring is a method of measuring vascular calcification in the coronary arteries, with increased levels of calcium being associated with an increased burden of atherosclerotic plaque and cardiac events. Its optimal use may be in providing additional information for making therapeutic decisions in asymptomatic patients at intermediate risk for atherosclerotic cardiovascular disease. However, its role in evaluating patients with heart failure believed to be caused by CAD has not been established.

Endomyocardial biopsy is indicated in patients with heart failure that progresses despite medical therapy and those with malignant arrhythmias to evaluate for giant cell myocarditis, as well as in those in whom amyloidosis or hemochromatosis is suspected. Endomyocardial biopsy is not indicated in this patient with evidence of heart failure in whom CAD has not been evaluated.

KEY POINT

- Patients with new-onset heart failure with multiple risk factors or symptoms of coronary artery disease should be evaluated by either a stress test or cardiac catheterization.

Bibliography

Hunt SA, Abraham WT, Chin MH, et al; American College of Cardiology Foundation; American Heart Association. 2009 Focused update incorporated into the ACC/AHA 2005 Guidelines for the Diagnosis and Management of Heart Failure in Adults. A Report of the American College of Cardiology Foundation/American Heart Association Task Force on Practice Guidelines Developed in Collaboration With the International Society for Heart and Lung Transplantation. J Am Coll Cardiol. 2009 Apr 14;53(15):e1-e90. Erratum in: J Am Coll Cardiol. 2009 Dec 15;54(25):2464. [PMID: 19358937]

Item 48   Answer: A

Educational Objective: Manage a patient with diabetes mellitus presenting with stable angina pectoris not controlled with optimal medical therapy.

This patient with stable angina pectoris with symptoms that are not adequately controlled on optimal medical therapy should undergo left heart catheterization for further evaluation and potential revascularization. Her myocardial perfusion imaging results are consistent with ischemic coronary artery disease (CAD); however, these findings alone would not be an indication for left heart catheterization. In patients with stable angina pectoris, coronary revascularization has not been shown to improve morbidity or mortality, and thus is not indicated in patients whose symptoms are able to be controlled with optimal medical therapy. However, in patients with coronary ischemia who fail to respond to adequate antianginal therapy, such as this patient, coronary angiography is indicated to evaluate for possible revascularization to control her angina symptoms. Catheterization may allow for percutaneous intervention to address a coronary occlusion leading to her angina symptoms, or assessment for the need for surgical revascularization if extensive or complex CAD is present.

CT angiography is an emerging technology for the non-invasive evaluation of the coronary arteries. Although it may be able to confirm the diagnosis of CAD in this patient, it would not allow the opportunity for percutaneous coronary intervention, if possible. The use of CT angiography to estimate the need or benefit of coronary artery bypass grafting also has not been established. Therefore, this study would not be indicated in this clinical setting.

Dobutamine stress echocardiography is typically used to evaluate for ischemic CAD in patients who are unable to exercise. However, in this patient with documented coronary ischemia established by a nuclear medicine myocardial perfusion study, there would be no benefit to performing this alternative diagnostic study for ischemia.

Because this patient remains symptomatic with restrictions on her quality of life, continuing her current medical therapy without additional intervention would not be appropriate.

KEY POINT

- Patients with stable angina not adequately controlled with optimal medical therapy should undergo coronary angiography to evaluate for possible revascularization.

Bibliography

Fihn SD, Gardin JM, Abrams J, et al; American College of Cardiology Foundation/American Heart Association Task Force. 2012 ACCF/AHA/ACP/AATS/PCNA/SCAI/STS guideline for the diagnosis and management of patients with stable ischemic heart disease: a report of the American College of Cardiology Foundation/American Heart Association task force on practice guidelines, and the American College of Physicians, American Association for Thoracic Surgery, Preventive Cardiovascular Nurses Association, Society for Cardiovascular Angiography and Interventions, and Society of Thoracic Surgeons. Circulation. 2012 Dec 18;126(25):e354-471. Erratum in: Circulation. 2014 Apr 22;129(16):e463. [PMID: 23166211]

Item 49   Answer: D

Educational Objective: Use appropriate imaging to evaluate mitral regurgitation.

Transesophageal echocardiography (TEE) would be the most appropriate next step in management of this patient. Evaluating the degree of mitral regurgitation and assessing the causative valve abnormalities provides essential information for guiding therapy, particularly whether surgical repair is possible or indicated. Although this information is usually obtained with transthoracic echocardiography, in situations in which full evaluation of the valve and degree of mitral regurgitation is not possible, such as in this very obese patient in whom accurate Doppler parameters cannot be obtained, TEE is indicated. Because the transducer in TEE is able to be closely approximated to the left atrium and mitral valve, structural details, including integrity of the valve leaflets and chordae, and the regurgitant jet, are almost always well visualized, allowing assessment of valvular abnormalities and accurate measurement of Doppler parameters. Chest CT angiography and cardiac magnetic resonance imaging may also be useful adjuvants, allowing assessment of coronary anatomy, valve structure, and coexisting structural heart disease. Three-dimensional echocardiography, both transthoracic and transesophageal, can further help identify leaflet and scallop involvement, likelihood of operative repair, and additional quantification of mitral regurgitation severity.

The decision to proceed with mitral valve surgery, including mitral valve repair, would be premature in this patient without adequate knowledge of the severity of mitral regurgitation and better definition of the underlying valvular abnormalities.

Although clinical follow-up with serial echocardiography may be appropriate for this patient, the appropriateness of this management strategy depends upon adequate initial evaluation of her mitral valve disease.

Medical therapy for patients with asymptomatic mitral regurgitation is limited. To date, no studies have shown benefit of ACE inhibitors, angiotensin receptor blockers, or diuretics in the absence of another specific indication, such as hypertension, left ventricular systolic dysfunction, or evidence of volume overload. This patient has none of those features.

- In patients with mitral regurgitation, transthoracic echocardiography (TTE) is used to evaluate the degree of mitral regurgitation and assess the causative valve abnormalities, thereby providing essential information for guiding therapy; if visualization is inadequate with TTE, transesophageal echocardiography is indicated.

Bibliography

Solis J, Piro V, Vazquez de Prada JA, Loughlin G. Echocardiographic assessment of mitral regurgitation: general considerations. Cardiol Clin. 2013 May;31(2):165-8. [PMID: 23743069]

Item 50   Answer: A

Educational Objective: Evaluate infrequent palpitations in a patient without syncope.

An event recorder would be appropriate to evaluate this patient's episodic symptoms of palpitations and lightheadedness. The evaluation and identification of arrhythmias can be challenging because of their intermittent nature; the modality used depends on the frequency and nature of the symptoms. In patients with infrequent symptoms, event recorders are the most effective means of obtaining rhythm information around the time of the symptoms. Event recorders record electrocardiographic (ECG) tracings only when activated by the patient and are more useful for infrequent symptoms. Two types of event recorders are used. A patient-triggered recorder is an external device without leads that is held to the chest and triggered by the patient when symptoms occur. The advantage of this device is the lack of electrode leads, making it more comfortable and convenient; however, no preceding rhythm is saved when the device is triggered. When the patient activates a looping event recorder, a permanent recording is created that includes several seconds of the presymptom rhythm, which is useful in patients with syncope.

In patients in whom pathologic structural heart disease is suspected, transthoracic echocardiography provides noninvasive, quantitative evaluation of cardiac size and function, valve morphology and function, pericardial disease, pulmonary artery pressures, and proximal great vessels. Physical examination findings in patients with structural disease include signs of heart failure and abnormal cardiac auscultation. In this patient, there is no evidence of structural heart disease by either history or examination, so an echocardiogram is not warranted.

Exercise ECG stress testing allows diagnosis of exercise-related arrhythmias, as well as assessment of the impact of the arrhythmia on blood pressure. The patient does not describe exercise-related symptoms, and an exercise stress test is not indicated.

Ambulatory ECG monitors record continuous rhythms and can be useful when patients have frequent, usually daily, symptoms. Monitors are usually worn for 24 or 48 hours.

Patients are encouraged to perform their normal activities while wearing the monitor. Patients keep a symptom diary or trigger a marker on the continuous reading that correlates with symptoms. Ambulatory ECG monitors can also be useful to detect asymptomatic arrhythmias, such as asymptomatic atrial fibrillation. This patient's symptoms occur about once a week, and a 24- or 48-hour ambulatory monitoring period is likely to miss the symptomatic episodes.

KEY POINT

- In patients with infrequent symptoms, cardiac event recorders are the most effective means of obtaining rhythm information around the time of the symptoms.

Bibliography

Zimetbaum P, Goldman A. Ambulatory arrhythmia monitoring: choosing the right device. Circulation. 2010 Oct 19;122(16):1629-36. [PMID: 20956237]

Item 51   Answer: B

Educational Objective: Treat wide-complex tachycardia due to atrial fibrillation with aberrant conduction.

The most appropriate next step in treatment of this patient is to initiate β-blocker therapy. He has paroxysmal atrial fibrillation with aberrant conduction, resulting in a wide-complex tachycardia. The electrocardiogram demonstrates a normal sinus beat followed by a run of atrial fibrillation with right bundle branch block. Note the irregularly irregular nature of the tachycardia and the QRS morphology consistent with typical right bundle branch block. Given his rapid ventricular response and his symptoms of palpitations and dyspnea, the atrial fibrillation requires treatment. β-Blocker therapy is the preferred atrioventricular nodal blocking agent given the patient's history of coronary artery disease.

Assessment of the need for anticoagulation therapy is also indicated in this patient with atrial fibrillation. Current guidelines recommend the use of the CHA_2DS_2-VASc score for this purpose, replacing the $CHADS_2$ score because of its ability to more clearly discriminate stroke risk. This patient has a CHA_2DS_2-VASc score of 4 (1 point for hypertension, 2 points for age, and 1 point for coronary artery disease), placing him at moderate risk for stroke. Therefore, initiation of oral anticoagulation also is appropriate.

Emergent cardioversion is not necessary because the patient is hemodynamically stable and appears to be having self-terminating paroxysms of tachycardia. If the patient had a sustained arrhythmia accompanied by hemodynamic instability, emergent cardioversion would be indicated regardless of the specific etiology of the arrhythmia (that is, supraventricular versus ventricular).

Intravenous amiodarone would be an appropriate treatment for recurrent ventricular tachycardia. The electrocardiogram appearance is consistent with right bundle branch block. There is an rSR pattern in lead V_1 and a terminal S wave in leads I and V_6. Right axis deviation is present (QRS axis 123 degrees); however, there is also evidence of left posterior fascicular block (small r waves and deep S waves in leads I and aVL; qR complexes in leads II, III, and aVF). Thus, these features are most consistent with aberrant conduction in the setting of atrial fibrillation rather than ventricular tachycardia.

Intravenous procainamide would be the agent of choice if this tachycardia were pre-excited (Wolff-Parkinson-White syndrome). Pre-excitation is evidenced by the presence of a delta wave. This patient's electrocardiogram does not demonstrate pre-excitation in either the sinus beat or the tachycardia.

KEY POINT

- Paroxysms of an irregularly irregular rhythm with a typical right bundle branch block appearance on electrocardiogram most likely represent atrial fibrillation with aberrant conduction.

Bibliography

Goldberger ZD, Rho RW, Page RL. Approach to the diagnosis and initial management of the stable adult patient with a wide complex tachycardia. Am J Cardiol. 2008 May 15;101(10):1456-66. Erratum in: Am J Cardiol. 2008 Aug 1;102(3):374. [PMID: 18471458]

Item 52   Answer: A

Educational Objective: Manage cardiovascular risk reduction in a patient with peripheral arterial disease.

The most appropriate management is to start a moderate- or high-intensity statin. Peripheral arterial disease (PAD) is strongly associated with smoking, diabetes mellitus, and aging. PAD is defined noninvasively by calculation of the ankle-brachial index (ABI). An ABI of 0.90 or below is diagnostic of PAD. Most patients with PAD are asymptomatic; approximately 25% have symptoms referable to circulatory compromise. PAD is considered a coronary artery disease risk equivalent and statin therapy has been demonstrated to lower cardiovascular events in patients with PAD.

Exercise and cilostazol are effective therapies for patients with stable symptomatic PAD. Cilostazol significantly increases pain-free walking time and maximal walking time, although the gains with structured exercise are two- to three-fold greater than with cilostazol alone. Since this patient is asymptomatic, cilostazol is not indicated.

Antiplatelet therapy is indicated for all patients with symptomatic PAD, previous lower extremity revascularization, or amputation due to PAD. Antiplatelet therapy is reasonable in patients with asymptomatic PAD, particularly if they have evidence of atherosclerosis elsewhere (coronary or cerebral arteries). Combination treatment with an antiplatelet agent and warfarin, and warfarin monotherapy (adjusted to an INR of 2.0-3.0), is no more effective than antiplatelet therapy alone and carries a higher risk of life-threatening bleeding.

Noninvasive angiography is performed for anatomic delineation of PAD in patients requiring surgical or endovascular intervention. CT angiography (CTA) is rapid and easily available but requires the administration of intravenous contrast dye. While CTA compares favorably with digital subtraction (invasive) angiography for the detection of occlusive arterial disease, imaging is not needed at this time because the patient does not require surgical intervention.

Lower extremity segmental pressure measurement can help determine the level and extent of PAD. Using specialized equipment in the vascular laboratory, blood pressures are obtained at successive levels of the extremity, localizing the level of disease. Many vascular laboratories use air plethysmography to measure volume changes within the limb, in conjunction with segmental limb pressure measurement. Lower extremity segmental pressure measurement is not needed at this time because localization of disease is not needed to guide therapy, such as would be required if surgical intervention were being planned.

KEY POINT

- Patients with peripheral arterial disease should be treated with a moderate- or high-intensity statin.

Bibliography
Berger JS, Hiatt WR. Medical therapy in peripheral artery disease. Circulation. 2012 Jul 24;126(4):491-500. [PMID: 22825411]

Item 53   Answer: E

Educational Objective: Choose appropriate antiplatelet agents following acute coronary syndrome and percutaneous coronary intervention.

No changes should be made to this patient's medications at the time of hospital discharge.

Calcium channel blockers, with the exception of nifedipine, can be used in patients with contraindications to β-blockers and in those with continued angina despite optimal doses of β-blockers and nitrates. This patient has no indications for a calcium channel blocker such as diltiazem.

There is no evidence to support a change from ticagrelor to clopidogrel after percutaneous coronary intervention (PCI) for acute coronary syndrome. In the PLATO (PLATelet inhibition and patient Outcomes) trial, the use of ticagrelor was associated with a 1.9% absolute risk reduction in the occurrence of cardiovascular death, myocardial infarction, and stroke when compared with clopidogrel. A $P2Y_{12}$ inhibitor (clopidogrel, prasugrel, ticagrelor) should be continued for at least 1 year for patients undergoing PCI with stent placement.

Oral β-blockers should be given to all patients with acute coronary syndrome without a contraindication (decompensated heart failure, advanced atrioventricular block, or severe reactive airways disease) and continued indefinitely. This patient is already bradycardic, and an increase in the dosage of metoprolol may be associated with symptomatic bradycardia.

In this patient with an acute coronary syndrome and preserved left ventricular function, there is no evidence to support the use of an aldosterone antagonist such as eplerenone. Based on the EPHESUS (Eplerenone Post-AMI Heart Failure Efficacy and Survival) trial, the 2007 American College of Cardiology/American Heart Association guidelines recommend the administration of an aldosterone antagonist to all patients following a non–ST-elevation myocardial infarction (NSTEMI) who are receiving an ACE inhibitor, have a left ventricular ejection fraction of 40% or below, and have either heart failure symptoms or diabetes mellitus.

ACE inhibitors inhibit postinfarction remodeling, helping to preserve ventricular function. ACE inhibitors should be continued indefinitely.

KEY POINT

- Long-term therapy following myocardial infarction includes aspirin, a β-blocker, an ACE inhibitor, and a statin; a $P2Y_{12}$ inhibitor (clopidogrel, prasugrel, ticagrelor) should be continued for at least 1 year for patients undergoing coronary percutaneous intervention with stent placement.

Bibliography
Makki N, Brennan TM, Girotra S. Acute coronary syndrome. J Intensive Care Med. 2013 Sep 18. [PMID: 24047692]

Item 54   Answer: B

Educational Objective: Treat heart failure with reduced ejection fraction with a β-blocker.

This patient with a recent diagnosis of heart failure with reduced ejection fraction (HFrEF) should be started on a β-blocker, such as carvedilol. Standard therapy for patients with HFrEF includes an ACE inhibitor and a β-blocker. This patient is already on an ACE inhibitor for treatment of his blood pressure and for afterload reduction for his heart failure. ACE inhibitors are typically started first in patients with heart failure because of their positive hemodynamic effects. An angiotensin receptor blocker (ARB) would be another treatment option, particularly if an ACE inhibitor were not tolerated. A β-blocker should then be started in stable, euvolemic patients with heart failure, either at the time of diagnosis or after acute decompensation is treated. β-Blockers have several beneficial effects and have been shown to prolong overall and event-free survival.

The β-blockers that have been shown to provide benefit in patients with HFrEF are metoprolol succinate, carvedilol, and bisoprolol. The β-blocker dosage should be increased slowly—at 1- to 2-week intervals—to the maximal dose. Like ACE inhibitors, there are data that suggest improved outcomes on higher doses of β-blockers (increased ejection fraction, reduced symptoms, lower mortality rates); therefore, attempting to up-titrate to maximally tolerated doses is important.

Although dihydropyridine calcium channel blockers, such as amlodipine, are effective antihypertensive and antianginal medications, they do not provide the same benefits as ACE inhibitors, ARBs, or β-blockers, and would not be appropriate add-on therapy in this patient who is not currently on a β-blocker and has controlled blood pressure without angina.

This patient has clear lungs, no significant jugular venous distention, and no peripheral edema. He has no evidence of volume overload and therefore does not need a diuretic, such as furosemide. Diuretics have no mortality benefit and are only used for symptom relief in the setting of volume overload.

Spironolactone has been demonstrated to decrease mortality rates in patients with New York Heart Association (NYHA) functional class II to IV heart failure (dyspnea with activities of daily living). This patient has good exercise capacity and has NYHA class II heart failure. However, candidates for spironolactone therapy should already be on standard medical therapy, including an ACE inhibitor and a β-blocker.

Making no changes in this patient's treatment regimen would not be appropriate because he is not being treated with medications associated with improved outcomes in patients with systolic heart failure.

KEY POINT

- Initial treatment for patients with heart failure with reduced ejection fraction (HFrEF) includes an ACE inhibitor and a β-blocker; the β-blockers that have been shown to provide benefit in patients with HFrEF are metoprolol succinate, carvedilol, and bisoprolol.

Bibliography

Parikh R, Kadowitz PJ. A review of current therapies used in the treatment of congestive heart failure. Expert Rev Cardiovasc Ther. 2013 Sep;11(9):1171-8. [PMID: 23980607]

Item 55   Answer: A

Educational Objective: Diagnose platypnea-orthodeoxia syndrome.

The most likely diagnosis in this patient is a patent foramen ovale with right-to-left shunt. He presents with features of platypnea-orthodeoxia syndrome, characterized by positional symptoms of cyanosis and dyspnea that generally occur when the patient is sitting and resolve in the supine position. Right-to-left shunting across an atrial septal defect or patent foramen ovale may rarely cause cyanosis and dyspnea owing to deformation of the atrial septum and redirection of shunt flow that result from increased right atrial pressure in the upright position. This patient had an inferior and right ventricular myocardial infarction with associated right heart enlargement and dysfunction and clinical features of hypotension. The right heart enlargement causes annular dilatation and tricuspid regurgitation. The foramen ovale stretches and becomes patent. The preferential cyanosis is caused by the hemodynamic alterations and preferential transfer of right atrial blood across the patent foramen in the upright position.

Mitral regurgitation due to papillary muscle injury or rupture is a recognized complication after myocardial infarc-

tion; however, the presentation generally is characterized by acute dyspnea and pulmonary edema rather than platypnea-orthodeoxia. Physical examination findings include a systolic murmur at the apex that increases during expiration rather than inspiration.

Severe left ventricular systolic dysfunction generally does not cause arterial oxygen desaturation. In addition, the initial assessment of left ventricular function was normal. The clinical picture in this patient is more compatible with right ventricular dysfunction.

Ventricular septal defect is a recognized complication after transmural myocardial infarction; however, the presentation generally includes acute dyspnea and pulmonary edema rather than oxygen desaturation. The left-to-right shunt associated with the ventricular septal defect causes left heart volume overload, rather than the right heart volume overload caused by right-to-left shunting seen in this patient. Physical examination findings in patients with ventricular septal defect following myocardial infarction include a holosystolic murmur at the left sternal border that does not change with respiration.

KEY POINT

- Right-to-left shunting across an atrial septal defect or patent foramen ovale may rarely cause cyanosis and dyspnea due to deformation of the atrial septum and redirection of shunt flow that result from increased right atrial pressure in the upright position.

Bibliography

Kubler P, Gibbs H, Garrahy P. Platypnoea-orthodeoxia syndrome. Heart. 2000 Feb;83(2):221-3. [PMID: 10648502]

Item 56   Answer: A

Educational Objective: Manage heart failure with cardiac resynchronization therapy.

This patient with symptomatic heart failure and a reduced left ventricular ejection fraction with evidence of significant conduction system disease should undergo placement of a biventricular pacemaker (cardiac resynchronization therapy [CRT]). He has progressive heart failure symptoms while on appropriate medical therapy and has New York Heart Association (NYHA) functional class III symptoms. With his ejection fraction less than 35% and left bundle branch block (LBBB), he is a candidate for a biventricular pacemaker, which has been demonstrated to reduce mortality and symptoms in patients with NYHA functional class III and IV heart failure by improving cardiac hemodynamics. The 2013 American College of Cardiology Foundation/American Heart Association/Heart Rhythm Society(ACCF/AHA/HRS) guideline recommends CRT therapy in patients with an ejection fraction of 35% or below, NYHA functional class III to IV symptoms on guideline-directed medical therapy, and LBBB with QRS duration greater than or equal to 150 ms. This patient already has an implantable cardioverter-defibrillator, which is indicated for patients with NYHA functional class II to III heart failure and an ejection fraction less than 35%. Now that he has developed a LBBB and an increase in symptoms, it is reasonable to proceed with placement of a biventricular pacemaker as well.

Inotropic therapy, such as dobutamine, is reserved for patients with end-stage heart failure, either as a bridge to transplantation or for palliative care. Patients in this category often have recurrent hospitalizations for heart failure, have evidence of end-organ compromise such as worsening kidney and liver function, and have very poor exercise tolerance. Although this patient has progressive symptoms, he has not reached this stage yet, and has no indication for inotropic therapy.

The patient has no evidence of volume overload on examination and a borderline low blood pressure; therefore, increasing his diuretic dose would not be expected to improve his symptoms and may worsen them by lowering his cardiac filling pressures and cardiac output.

The patient is fairly symptomatic but has not yet had optimal therapy, as he has an indication for CRT and has not yet received it. Left ventricular assist devices (LVADs) are reserved for patients with end-stage refractory heart failure as a bridge to heart transplantation or as destination therapy in selected patients who are not candidates for transplantation. However, prior to being considered for either an LVAD or heart transplantation, a patient must be on optimal medical therapy.

KEY POINT

- Cardiac resynchronization therapy is recommended in patients with an ejection fraction of 35% or below, New York Heart Association functional class III to IV symptoms on guideline-directed medical therapy, and left bundle branch block or QRS duration of 150 ms or greater.

Bibliography

Epstein AE, DiMarco JP, Ellenbogen KA, et al; American College of Cardiology Foundation; American Heart Association Task Force on Practice Guidelines; Heart Rhythm Society. 2012 ACCF/AHA/HRS focused update incorporated into the ACCF/AHA/HRS 2008 guidelines for device-based therapy of cardiac rhythm abnormalities: a report of the American College of Cardiology Foundation/American Heart Association Task Force on Practice Guidelines and the Heart Rhythm Society. J Am Coll Cardiol. 2013 Jan 22;61(3):e6-75. [PMID: 23265327]

Item 57   Answer: E

Educational Objective: **Evaluate a patient with cardiovascular risk factors and atypical chest pain and a normal resting electrocardiogram.**

The most appropriate diagnostic test for this patient is exercise stress testing. He has an intermediate pretest probability of coronary artery disease (CAD) based on his age, sex, and symptoms. He should undergo stress testing to determine if his symptoms are related to obstructive CAD. Exercise electrocardiographic (ECG) testing is the standard stress test for CAD diagnosis in patients with a normal baseline ECG. If abnormalities limiting ST-segment analysis

are present (left bundle branch block [LBBB], left ventricular hypertrophy, paced rhythm, Wolff-Parkinson-White pattern), results may be indeterminate. This patient has none of these conditions, and therefore exercise stress testing is a reasonable option. In patients who can exercise, exercise stress is preferred to pharmacologic stress because of the functional and prognostic information exercise stress provides. Persons who can exercise have a better prognosis than those who are unable to exercise and require pharmacologic stress testing.

Among patients with resting ECG abnormalities that limit ST-segment analysis, the addition of imaging aids diagnostic accuracy and provides improvement in localizing the site and extent of ischemia. In patients with LBBB, exercise stress may result in abnormal septal motion due to conduction delay with falsely positive septal abnormalities; this abnormality is lessened with use of vasodilator (such as adenosine) stress imaging. This patient does not have ECG abnormalities that warrant adenosine myocardial imaging study and the added expense and radiation exposure that this procedure would require.

Cardiac magnetic resonance (CMR) imaging can be used to evaluate aortic pathology, pericardial diseases, and myocardial diseases, as well as to evaluate the extent of myocardial fibrosis. CMR imaging may be useful in determining the extent of myocardial infarction and potential viability. This patient is asymptomatic; therefore, CMR imaging is not indicated.

CT angiography allows determination of the presence and extent of coronary artery disease. If this intermediate-risk patient was unable to exercise or the ECG was uninterpretable, CT angiography could be performed. If, however, obstructive disease was found, the patient would then need to undergo coronary angiography to perform a percutaneous intervention, thus performing two procedures that require contrast agents and radiation exposure.

For patients unable to exercise because of physical limitations or physical deconditioning, pharmacologic stressors, such as dobutamine, can be used. These agents, which are recommended if the patient cannot achieve at least five metabolic equivalents, increase myocardial contractility and oxygen demand. This patient can exercise, and dobutamine stress echocardiography is not indicated.

KEY POINT

- Exercise electrocardiographic testing is the standard stress test for the diagnosis of coronary artery disease in the absence of conditions that limit ST-segment analysis.

Bibliography

American College of Cardiology Foundation Appropriate Use Criteria Task Force; American Society of Echocardiography; American Heart Association; American Society of Nuclear Cardiology; Heart Failure Society of America; Heart Rhythm Society; Society for Cardiovascular Angiography and Interventions; Society of Critical Care Medicine; Society of Cardiovascular Computed Tomography; Society for Cardiovascular Magnetic Resonance, Douglas PS, Garcia MJ, Haines DE, et al. ACCF/ASE/AHA/ASNC/HFSA/HRS/SCAI/SCCM/SCCT/SCMR 2011 Appropriate Use Criteria for Echocardiography. A Report of the American College of Cardiology Foundation Appropriate Use Criteria Task Force, American Society of Echocardiography, American Heart Association, American Society of Nuclear Cardiology, Heart Failure Society of America, Heart Rhythm Society, Society for Cardiovascular Angiography and Interventions, Society of Critical Care Medicine, Society of Cardiovascular Computed Tomography, and Society for Cardiovascular Magnetic Resonance Endorsed by the American College of Chest Physicians. J Am Coll Cardiol. 2011 Mar 1;57(9):1126–66. [PMID: 21349406]

Item 58 Answer: A

Educational Objective: Manage infection of an implanted electronic cardiac device.

This patient has signs and symptoms concerning for possible infection of an implanted cardiac electronic device. He should undergo laboratory evaluation including assessment of a complete blood count with differential, two peripheral blood cultures from separate phlebotomy sites, and an erythrocyte sedimentation rate to assess for the possibility of a device-related infection.

Patients with an implanted cardiac device can develop either a localized tissue infection at the implant site (pocket infection) or a systemic infection with bacteremia (for example, endocarditis). These infections can occur after initial implantation, late after implantation, or following a device battery replacement or revision. If left untreated, implanted cardiac device infections will progress to endocarditis and sepsis and ultimately death. The fatality rate for an untreated device infection approaches 75% to 100%. Antibiotic therapy alone is insufficient. Curative therapy requires antibiotic therapy and complete hardware removal.

The most common pathogens are coagulase-negative *Staphylococcus* species and *S. aureus*. Patients may present with fever or malaise; many also have local findings suggestive of infection, such as erythema or warmth at the implant site. These patients should undergo a laboratory evaluation for signs of infection. Elevated erythrocyte sedimentation rate, leukocytosis with a left shift, and anemia are suggestive of infection. All patients with possible device-related infection (with or without fever) should have a minimum of two blood cultures drawn from separate sites. Once there is suspicion for a device infection, referral to the patient's electrophysiologist or an infectious disease specialist is mandatory.

Pacemaker pocket aspiration should never be performed, as it can seed a sterile pocket and lead to infection, especially if there is superficial cellulitis without deeper tissue involvement.

Ultrasonographic examination of a pacemaker or defibrillator pocket may be helpful in patients with suspected implanted cardiac device infections. However, pocket fluid may not always represent infection, and sterile seromas are sometimes encountered. Therefore, pocket ultrasound has limited—if any—diagnostic value.

Even though the presenting symptoms of a device-related infection may be nonspecific and difficult to distinguish from other common, benign infections, delayed diagnosis may allow more significant complications to develop. Therefore, observation in a high-risk patient would not be appropriate.

KEY POINT

- Patients with possible implanted cardiac device infection (with or without fever) should have a minimum of two blood cultures drawn from separate sites.

Bibliography

Baddour LM, Cha YM, Wilson WR. Clinical practice. Infections of cardiovascular implantable electronic devices. N Engl J Med. 2012 Aug 30; 367(9):842–9. Erratum in: N Engl J Med. 2012 Oct 11; 367(15):1474. N Engl J Med. 2012 Sep 27;367(13):1272. [PMID: 22931318]

Item 59 Answer: B

Educational Objective: Manage asymptomatic moderate aortic regurgitation.

This patient with moderate aortic regurgitation should be reassessed clinically in 1 year. Patients with moderate aortic regurgitation should be evaluated on a yearly basis and echocardiography performed every 1 to 2 years.

Aortic valve replacement is indicated for symptomatic patients with chronic severe aortic regurgitation irrespective of left ventricular (LV) systolic function, asymptomatic patients with chronic severe aortic regurgitation and LV systolic dysfunction (LV ejection fraction ≤50%), and patients with chronic severe aortic regurgitation undergoing coronary artery bypass graft (CABG) or surgery on the aorta or other heart valves. This patient is not a candidate for aortic valve replacement.

Endocarditis prophylaxis is not recommended for patients with bicuspid aortic valves in the absence of another specific indication such as a prior episode of infective endocarditis, previous valve replacement, prior cardiac transplantation with valvulopathy, and certain forms of complex congenital heart disease.

Medical therapy for chronic aortic regurgitation is limited. ACE inhibitors or angiotensin receptor blockers may be used in patients with chronic severe aortic regurgitation and heart failure as well as in patients with aortic regurgitation and concomitant hypertension, but these agents, as well as dihydropyridine calcium channel blockers, have not been shown to delay surgery in asymptomatic patients without hypertension. There is no established benefit in medical therapy for this patient with moderate aortic regurgitation without other specific indications for treatment.

KEY POINT

- Asymptomatic patients with moderate aortic regurgitation should be evaluated on a yearly basis and have echocardiography performed every 1 to 2 years.

Bibliography

Helms AS, Bach DS. Heart valve disease. Prim Care. 2013 Mar;40(1):91–108. [PMID: 23402463]

Item 60   Answer: A

Educational Objective: Manage anticoagulation therapy in a pregnant woman with a mechanical valve prosthesis.

The anticoagulation regimen that will provide the greatest protection against thromboembolism in this patient is warfarin therapy. Low-dose aspirin therapy should also be continued. Women with mechanical valve prostheses carry a high risk of valve thrombosis, bleeding, and fetal morbidity and mortality during pregnancy, and the optimal anticoagulation strategy has not been established. Options include warfarin, unfractionated heparin (UFH), and low-molecular-weight heparin (LMWH). Although warfarin poses an increased risk of teratogenicity and fetal loss, it appears to be the most effective option for reducing thromboembolism risk in the mother. The current dose of warfarin (4 mg/d), used to achieve a therapeutic INR, is associated with a low risk of warfarin embryopathy and a low risk of fetal complications.

The novel oral anticoagulants, such as dabigatran, bivalirudin, rivaroxaban, and apixaban, do not adequately protect patients with mechanical valve prostheses against thromboembolism and should not be used in pregnant or nonpregnant patients with mechanical valve prostheses.

Intravenous UFH is the anticoagulant treatment of choice around the time of delivery. Intravenous UFH can also be used during the first trimester. The dose effect must be measured by activated partial thromboplastin time and the dose adjusted to a therapeutic level. Fixed-dose subcutaneous UFH may not provide adequate anticoagulation.

LMWH can be used as an anticoagulant during pregnancy, but for patients with a mechanical valve prosthesis, a weight-based regimen has been demonstrated to be inadequate. The LMWH dose must be adjusted to anti-factor Xa activity in order to provide adequate anticoagulation.

KEY POINT

- Anticoagulation strategies for pregnant women with a mechanical valve prosthesis include warfarin, dose-adjusted unfractionated heparin, and dose-adjusted low-molecular-weight heparin; of these options, warfarin poses a lesser risk of maternal thromboembolism but a greater risk of fetal embryopathy.

Bibliography

Nishimura RA, Otto CM, Bonow RO, et al; American College of Cardiology/ American Heart Association Task Force on Practice Guidelines. 2014 AHA/ACC guideline for the management of patients with valvular heart disease: executive summary: a report of the American College of Cardiology/American Heart Association Task Force on Practice Guidelines. J Am Coll Cardiol. 2014 Jun 10;63(22):2438-88. Erratum in: J Am Coll Cardiol. 2014 Jun 10;63(22):2489. [PMID: 24603192]

Item 61   Answer: D

Educational Objective: Treat a patient with thrombolytic failure following an ST-elevation myocardial infarction.

This patient with ST-elevation myocardial infarction (STEMI) should be transferred to the nearest hospital with primary percutaneous coronary intervention (PCI) capabilities for emergency PCI. Thrombolytic therapy failure, which occurs in up to 30% of patients, remains difficult to diagnose. Chest pain resolution, ST-segment elevation improvement, and reperfusion arrhythmias (most commonly an accelerated idioventricular rhythm) indicate successful thrombolysis. Although complete ST-segment elevation resolution is associated with coronary patency, it occurs in a minority of patients. Improvement in ST-segment elevation greater than 50% on an electrocardiogram (ECG) obtained 60 minutes after the administration of thrombolytic therapy is the most commonly used criterion to indicate successful reperfusion. Continued chest pain, lack of improvement in ST-segment elevation, hemodynamic instability, and the absence of reperfusion arrhythmias most likely indicate failure of thrombolytic therapy and indicate the need for rescue PCI. This patient has clear evidence of failed reperfusion or reocclusion (worsening of ST-segment elevation, persistence of symptoms) and now has signs of cardiogenic shock (low blood pressure, pulmonary edema). In patients with thrombolytic therapy failure, guidelines recommend immediate transfer for rescue PCI. In multiple trials of thrombolytic therapy failure, patients who underwent rescue PCI had a significant improvement in the rate of reinfarction when compared with those receiving conservative care, but no improvement in mortality.

The use of glycoprotein IIb/IIIa inhibitors has been tested in multiple scenarios in patients with STEMI. Based on these studies, their use has been limited owing to excessive bleeding events. In patients in whom thrombolytic therapy has failed, rescue PCI without the use of a glycoprotein IIb/IIIa inhibitor or additional thrombolytic agents is preferred.

A meta-analysis published in 2007 compared repeat thrombolytic therapy with conservative therapy in patients in whom initial thrombolytic therapy failed. This analysis showed no significant difference in mortality rates or reinfarction between the two groups, and outcomes in these groups were inferior to rescue PCI.

KEY POINT

- Patients with thrombolytic therapy failure following an ST-elevation myocardial infarction should be immediately transferred for rescue percutaneous coronary intervention.

Bibliography

Sutton AG, Campbell PG, Graham R, et al. A randomized trial of rescue angioplasty versus a conservative approach for failed fibrinolysis in ST-segment elevation myocardial infarction: the Middlesbrough Early Revascularization to Limit INfarction (MERLIN) trial. J Am Coll Cardiol. 2004 Jul 21;44(2):287-96. [PMID: 15261920]

Item 62   Answer: C

Educational Objective: Screen patients with a family history of hypertrophic cardiomyopathy for the disease at appropriate intervals.

This patient should again be screened for hypertrophic cardiomyopathy (HCM) in 5 years. All first-degree relatives of patients with HCM should undergo screening for the disorder with a comprehensive physical examination, electrocardiogram, and echocardiogram. Because HCM can manifest at any age, lifetime screening of first-degree relatives in whom the disorder has not yet been diagnosed is indicated. The recommended HCM screening intervals, which are based on clinical suspicion, patient age, family history, and participation in competitive athletics, are shown.

Recommended Hypertrophic Cardiomyopathy Screening Intervals	
Age Group	Recommendation
<12 years	Screening optional except in the following situations: (1) presence of symptoms; (2) family history of malignant ventricular tachyarrhythmias; (3) patient is competitive athlete in an intense training program; or (4) presence of other clinical suspicion of early left ventricular hypertrophy
12 to 18-21 years	Every 12 to 18 months
>18-21 years	At symptom onset or at least every 5 years (more frequently in families with malignant tachyarrhythmias or late onset)

These recommendations are for relatives of patients with HCM in whom genetic testing is negative, inconclusive, or not performed. Genetic testing of probands can be used to identify pathologic mutations, which can then be used to screen family members and, if negative, may obviate the need for continued imaging. The yield of genetic testing, which can be costly, varies according to the phenotypic expression and familial nature of HCM. Thus, referral to a cardiovascular specialist or a genetic counselor is recommended for clinical decision-making based on genetic testing in patients with HCM.

KEY POINT

- All first-degree relatives of patients with hypertrophic cardiomyopathy should undergo screening for the disorder with a comprehensive physical examination, electrocardiogram, and echocardiogram; lifetime screening of those in whom the disorder has not yet been diagnosed is indicated.

Bibliography

Gersh BJ, Maron, BJ, Bonow, RO, et al; American College of Cardiology Foundation/American Heart Association Task Force on Practice Guidelines. 2011 ACCF/AHA Guideline for the Diagnosis and Treatment of Hypertrophic Cardiomyopathy: a report of the American College of Cardiology Foundation/American Heart Association Task Force on Practice Guidelines. Developed in collaboration with the American Association for Thoracic Surgery, American Society of Echocardiography, American Society of Nuclear Cardiology, Heart Failure Society of America, Heart Rhythm Society, Society for Cardiovascular Angiography and Interventions, and Society of Thoracic Surgeons. J Am Coll Cardiol. 2011 Dec 13;58(25):e212-60. [PMID: 22075469]

Item 63   Answer: C

Educational Objective: Treat atrioventricular block complicating acute myocardial infarction.

This patient has evidence of an inferior-posterior ST-elevation myocardial infarction and should undergo urgent percutaneous coronary intervention (PCI). He is bradycardic with Mobitz type 1 second-degree heart block, also known as Wenckebach block. This type of atrioventricular block is almost always within the compact atrioventricular node (and not infra-Hisian) and in this patient is likely caused by right coronary artery occlusion. The right coronary artery supplies the atrioventricular nodal artery in 90% of patients. The most important intervention for this patient is urgent PCI and reperfusion of the infarct-related artery. Although the presence of atrioventricular block is usually transient and resolves with reperfusion, it is associated with worse prognosis and in-hospital survival.

Aminophylline increases cyclic adenosine monophosphate (cAMP) and can be used to promote atrioventricular conduction in patients with hemodynamically unstable bradycardia or advanced atrioventricular block (Mobitz type 2 second-degree or third-degree atrioventricular block) due to coronary ischemia. This patient is hemodynamically stable and his atrioventricular block is not advanced; therefore, aminophylline is not indicated.

Because the patient is not experiencing hemodynamic sequelae, low-dose dopamine infusion is not indicated. If the patient develops hemodynamically significant bradycardia, dopamine infusion could be used to stabilize him until coronary reperfusion and temporary pacing could be accomplished.

Advanced atrioventricular block in the setting of an acute coronary syndrome often requires temporary or permanent pacing. In this patient, temporary pacing is not indicated because he is hemodynamically stable and his block is not advanced. Decisions on permanent pacing should be delayed until a patient has been revascularized and stabilized to determine whether the arrhythmia persists.

KEY POINT

- Patients with acute coronary syndrome and related Mobitz type 1 second-degree atrioventricular block should undergo urgent reperfusion therapy as the treatment of choice for this conduction block.

Bibliography

Epstein AE, DiMarco JP, Ellenbogen KA, et al; American College of Cardiology/American Heart Association Task Force on Practice Guidelines (Writing Committee to Revise the ACC/AHA/NASPE 2002 Guideline Update for Implantation of Cardiac Pacemakers and Antiarrhythmia Devices); American Association for Thoracic Surgery; Society of Thoracic Surgeons. ACC/AHA/HRS 2008 Guidelines for Device-Based Therapy of Cardiac Rhythm Abnormalities: a report of the American College of Cardiology/American Heart Association Task Force on Practice Guidelines (Writing Committee to Revise the ACC/AHA/NASPE 2002 Guideline Update for Implantation of Cardiac Pacemakers and Antiarrhythmia Devices): developed in collaboration with the American Association for Thoracic Surgery and Society of Thoracic Surgeons. Circulation. 2008 May 27;117(21):e350-408. Erratum in: Circulation. 2009 Aug 4; 120(5):e34-5. [PMID: 18483207]

H **Item 64** **Answer: A**

Educational Objective: Manage intravenous lines in a patient with cyanotic congenital heart disease.

In this patient with Eisenmenger syndrome, air filters on intravenous lines are recommended to reduce the risk of paradoxical air embolism. She has clinical features of pyelonephritis, and intravenous antibiotic therapy is warranted. Patients with Eisenmenger syndrome have an intracardiac right-to-left shunt, and therefore are at risk for paradoxical air embolism. These filters can be easily and rapidly applied to any intravenous line prior to administering intravenous therapy and likely reduce the risk of air embolism. Meticulous care of intravenous lines and catheters is very important in patients with Eisenmenger syndrome owing to the potential for paradoxical embolism, which may cause stroke and debility.

There are no data to support improved survival with chronic oxygen therapy for patients with Eisenmenger syndrome and associated cyanosis. Saturation may increase minimally with oxygen therapy, but it generally does not normalize.

The hemoglobin and hematocrit levels in this patient are physiologic for a patient with Eisenmenger syndrome. Phlebotomy is not recommended.

A transthoracic echocardiogram is not recommended at this time because it is unlikely to change management in this patient who has known heart disease. The patient has features of infection, but the data suggest a urinary tract infection rather than endocarditis. If the patient presented with or develops features of endocarditis, such as a new murmur, septic emboli, or persistent bacteremia, a transesophageal echocardiogram would be favored over a transthoracic echocardiogram.

KEY POINT

- In patients with Eisenmenger syndrome, air filters and meticulous care of all intravenous lines should be instituted to prevent paradoxical air embolism.

Bibliography

Warnes CA, Williams RG, Bashore TM, et al; American College of Cardiology; American Heart Association Task Force on Practice Guidelines (Writing Committee to Develop Guidelines on the Management of Adults With Congenital Heart Disease); American Society of Echocardiography; Heart Rhythm Society; International Society for Adult Congenital Heart Disease; Society for Cardiovascular Angiography and Interventions; Society of Thoracic Surgeons. ACC/AHA 2008 guidelines for the management of adults with congenital heart disease: a report of the American College of Cardiology/American Heart Association Task Force on Practice Guidelines (Writing Committee to Develop Guidelines on the Management of Adults With Congenital Heart Disease). Developed in Collaboration With the American Society of Echocardiography, Heart Rhythm Society, International Society for Adult Congenital Heart Disease, Society for Cardiovascular Angiography and Interventions, and Society of Thoracic Surgeons. J Am Coll Cardiol. 2008 Dec 2;52(23):e143-263. [PMID: 19038677]

Item 65 **Answer: D**

Educational Objective: Manage coronary artery disease risk in an asymptomatic patient with diabetes mellitus.

This patient should continue his current therapy; no additional testing is indicated at this time. The leading cause of death in patients with diabetes mellitus is cardiovascular disease, but routine testing for coronary artery disease (CAD) in asymptomatic patients with diabetes does not reduce mortality. Aggressive treatment of cardiovascular risk factors, however, does improve outcomes and reduce mortality as seen in the Steno-2 study. In this study, intensive intervention with behavior modification and multiple pharmacologic interventions aimed at achieving hemoglobin A_{1c} levels below 6.5%, blood pressure below 130/80 mm Hg, and serum total cholesterol levels below 175 mg/dL (4.53 mmol/L) resulted in a 53% reduction of cardiovascular disease in a nearly 8-year follow-up. Continued risk factor management in this patient is, therefore, the most appropriate choice.

This patient does not need an echocardiogram. He is asymptomatic, and the murmur described is consistent with mild aortic stenosis as supported by his echocardiogram 1 year ago. He should undergo an annual clinical evaluation and echocardiography every 3 to 5 years. Echocardiography at this time in the absence of a clinical change is unnecessary.

If a screening test were to be performed prior to exercise, an exercise stress test would be the most appropriate test; exercise perfusion imaging provides no additional information. In routine screening of patients with diabetes in the DIAD study, despite 22% of patients having evidence of perfusion defects on single-photon emission CT, most of which were small, mortality rates were not changed compared with patients who did not undergo screening. The event rates were low in both groups, at about 3% over nearly 5 years.

The 2012 U.S. Preventive Services Task Force statement on screening for CAD with electrocardiography (ECG) recommended against screening with resting or exercise ECG for the prediction of CAD events in asymptomatic adults at low risk for CAD events, and stated that the evidence is insufficient to assess the balance of benefits and harms of screening in asymptomatic adults at intermediate or high risk for CAD events. The 2002 American College of Cardiology/American Heart Association (ACC/AHA) guidelines also concluded that there is no evidence to support routine testing in asymptomatic adults but concluded that it is reasonable to screen for CAD in asymptomatic patients with diabetes who plan to begin a vigorous exercise program.

KEY POINT

- Routine screening for coronary artery disease in asymptomatic patients with diabetes mellitus does not reduce mortality.

Bibliography

Gaede P, Lund-Andersen H, Parving HH, Pedersen O. Effect of a multifactorial intervention on mortality in type 2 diabetes. N Engl J Med. 2008 Feb 7;358(6):580-91. [PMID: 18256393]

Item 66 **Answer: D** **H**

Educational Objective: Manage acute limb ischemia.

The most appropriate management for this patient with an ischemic but viable extremity (severe acute limb ischemia)

CONT. is urgent angiography to define the anatomic level of occlusion and assess appropriate treatment options, which may include surgical or percutaneous revascularization or thrombolytic therapy in selected patients. He has several risk factors for atherosclerotic peripheral arterial disease (PAD), and the claudication that he has experienced for the past year has progressed to severe resting limb pain. The limb is viable as indicated by the presence of pain, slow but present capillary refill, and the presence of Doppler vascular signals. Acute ischemia can be caused by remote embolization but may also result from in-situ thrombosis. Because of this, anticoagulation is crucial once a diagnosis of acute arterial occlusion has been made by history and physical examination. The next step in management is to further evaluate the limb ischemia and plan for treatment. Digital subtraction angiography provides the most helpful information and is the preferred imaging modality for acute limb ischemia; delaying angiography could lead to limb necrosis and loss of limb functioning.

Catheter-directed thrombolytic therapy may be an option in some patients with acute limb ischemia with a viable or marginally threatened limb as an alternative to a surgical approach, particularly if the duration of acute limb ischemia is less than 1 day. However, initiating thrombolytic therapy in this patient before further evaluation of the nature of the occlusion would not be appropriate.

For a nonviable extremity, surgical amputation without angiography is indicated because of the increased risk of tissue necrosis and infection. However, this patient's foot shows evidence of viability, making immediate amputation inappropriate.

Warfarin has not been shown to be an effective therapy for managing stable PAD, and although anticoagulation is indicated in managing acute limb ischemia pending further evaluation, initiation of long-term anticoagulation with warfarin in this patient with a viable but threatened limb without further intervention would not be appropriate.

KEY POINT

- Patients with an ischemic but viable extremity on clinical examination should undergo urgent angiography to plan surgical or percutaneous revascularization.

Bibliography

Creager MA, Kaufman JA, Conte MS. Clinical practice. Acute limb ischemia. N Engl J Med. 2012 Jun 7;366(23):2198-206. [PMID: 22670905]

Item 67 Answer: D

Educational Objective: Manage asymptomatic severe mitral regurgitation with reduced left ventricular function.

Mitral valve repair is the most appropriate option for this patient with asymptomatic severe mitral regurgitation and moderate left ventricular (LV) dysfunction. Surgery is indicated for patients with symptomatic acute severe mitral regurgitation, those with symptomatic chronic severe mitral regurgitation with LV ejection fraction greater than 30%, and asymptomatic patients with chronic severe mitral regurgitation and mild to moderate LV dysfunction (ejection fraction of 30%-60% and/or LV end-systolic dimension ≥40 mm). Mitral valve repair is the operation of choice when the valve is suitable for repair and appropriate surgical skill is available and is recommended for most patients. Mitral valve replacement, especially with chordal preservation, is appropriate for patients with severe mitral regurgitation in whom the valve is not repairable or a less than optimal result would be obtained. Recently, a percutaneously placed mitral valve clip has been introduced that is placed to better approximate the edges of the anterior and posterior leaflets of the valve and may be a therapeutic option in patients who are at a prohibitive risk for mitral valve surgery.

Vasodilator therapy, such as with ACE inhibitors or angiotensin receptor blockers, has not been shown to improve outcomes in patients with severe mitral regurgitation who are asymptomatic. Additionally, vasodilator therapy may mask the development of more severe left ventricular dysfunction due to regurgitant volume. Therefore, these agents should not be used as a substitute therapy for surgery when the patient is thought to be a surgical candidate.

Mitral balloon valvuloplasty or valvotomy is indicated for patients with severe mitral stenosis in whom there is a reasonable likelihood of success and in whom there are no contraindications (such as moderate to severe mitral regurgitation or left atrial thrombus). This patient has severe mitral regurgitation, and repair, not valvotomy, is indicated.

Serial echocardiography may be helpful in follow-up of the asymptomatic patient in whom worsening of LV systolic function or increase in chamber size may help facilitate decision for surgery. This patient's LV function is compromised and intervention is indicated.

KEY POINT

- Mitral valve repair is the operation of choice for severe mitral regurgitation when the valve is suitable for repair.

Bibliography

Nishimura RA, Otto CM, Bonow RO, et al; American College of Cardiology/American Heart Association Task Force on Practice Guidelines. 2014 AHA/ACC guideline for the management of patients with valvular heart disease: executive summary: a report of the American College of Cardiology/American Heart Association Task Force on Practice Guidelines. J Am Coll Cardiol. 2014 Jun 10;63(22):2438-88. Erratum in: J Am Coll Cardiol. 2014 Jun 10;63(22):2489. [PMID: 24603192]

Item 68 Answer: C

Educational Objective: Manage Brugada syndrome.

This patient should undergo placement of an implantable cardioverter-defibrillator (ICD). He had an episode of abrupt syncope that is concerning for a cardiac etiology, specifically an arrhythmia. He has a structurally normal heart on echocardiogram, but his electrocardiogram (ECG) shows right bundle branch block and 2-mm ST-segment elevation in the precordial leads. These findings are consistent with a type 1 Brugada pattern (coved or descendant ST-segment elevation followed by negative T waves) on ECG. The presence of a type

1 Brugada pattern and symptoms (cardiac syncope) or ventricular arrhythmia is diagnostic for Brugada syndrome. Brugada syndrome can be genetically heterogeneous, but it is often caused by mutations in the SCN5a sodium channel, which are believed to cause alterations in the ventricular refractory period and are responsible for the characteristic ECG findings and predisposition to sudden cardiac death.

Because this patient with Brugada syndrome is at risk for sudden cardiac death, particularly given his recurrent episodes of near-syncope and syncope, an ICD should be implanted. Patients with precordial ST-segment abnormalities should be referred to a cardiologist or electrophysiologist. Once Brugada syndrome is diagnosed, first-degree family members should be referred to an inherited arrhythmia clinic (electrophysiology clinic specializing in genetic disorders) for counseling and screening. Patients who have a Brugada pattern but are asymptomatic often do not require ICD placement. The incidence of Brugada syndrome is higher in patients of Asian ethnicity.

Cardiac magnetic resonance (CMR) imaging would not be helpful given the normal echocardiogram and diagnosis of Brugada syndrome. CMR imaging would be helpful if occult structural heart disease was suspected, such as cardiac sarcoid, amyloidosis, or arrhythmogenic right ventricular dysplasia.

An exercise treadmill stress test can be valuable for identifying an exercise-induced arrhythmia. Brugada syndrome often presents with nocturnal arrhythmias and is usually not adrenergically driven. A stress test would not aid in this patient's diagnosis.

Tilt-table testing should be reserved for patients with recurrent syncope without known heart disease or those with heart disease in whom a cardiac cause of the syncope has been excluded. Tilt-table testing may also be helpful in evaluating patients in whom documenting neurocardiogenic syncope is important (such as in high-risk occupational settings). In this patient, the ECG is diagnostic for Brugada syndrome and tilt-table testing is not needed.

KEY POINT

- The presence of 2-mm or more coved precordial ST-segment elevation (leads V_1 through V_3) on electrocardiogram and symptoms (cardiac syncope) or ventricular arrhythmia indicates the presence of Brugada syndrome.

Bibliography

Mizusawa Y, Wilde AA. Brugada syndrome. Circ Arrythm Electrophysiol. 2012 Jun 1;5(3):606-16. [PMID: 22715240]

Item 69   Answer: C

Educational Objective: Manage end-stage heart failure with a left ventricular assist device.

This patient should be evaluated for placement of a left ventricular assist device (LVAD). He has end-stage heart failure manifested by extreme limitations of activity, multiple hos-

pitalizations, poor kidney function, diuretic dependence to maintain fluid balance, and hypotension. The two possible options for therapy in a patient with this degree of heart failure are placement of an LVAD and heart transplantation. Because of his diagnosis of disseminated prostate cancer, however, the patient is not a candidate for transplantation. LVADs are indicated either as a bridge to heart transplantation or as destination therapy in selected patients who are not candidates for transplantation. Newer LVAD devices are smaller and easier to maintain than earlier versions, making their long-term use as destination therapy possible. Although this patient might otherwise be a candidate for transplantation, his diagnosis of disseminated prostate cancer is an absolute contraindication because of the required long-term post-transplant immunosuppression. However, placement of an LVAD would be an appropriate consideration in this patient if he is expected to survive for longer than 1 year.

Other contraindications to cardiac transplantation include medical problems associated with a reduced life expectancy (rheumatologic disease, severe pulmonary disease, liver failure), fixed severe pulmonary hypertension, diabetes mellitus with end-organ manifestations, age greater than 65 to 70 years, severe peripheral arterial or cerebrovascular disease, and advanced kidney disease. Although several of these factors are also associated with poorer outcomes with LVAD use (such as advanced age and degree of comorbid disease), assist devices are a viable option for treatment in patients who are clearly not candidates for transplantation.

Metolazone inhibits sodium reabsorption in the distal tubule and may be particularly effective in inducing diuresis when used in combination with a loop diuretic in patients with volume overload who have not responded adequately to high doses of a loop diuretic. However, this patient does not have signs of volume overload (no jugular venous distention or edema) and therefore would not be expected to benefit from the addition of metolazone to his current regimen.

Home inotropic therapy is associated with a mortality rate of approximately 90% at 1 year and should be considered as a palliative care option only. Use of this therapy is associated with worsening heart failure, infection, and arrhythmias. In a patient who is a candidate for either LVAD or heart transplantation, this should not be considered as an alternative therapy. Occasionally, patients require supportive inotropic therapy until they receive a transplant. This should be managed by their transplant cardiologist.

KEY POINT

- Placement of a left ventricular assist device is an option for patients with end-stage heart failure who are not candidates for heart transplantation.

Bibliography

Garbade J, Barten MJ, Bittner HB, Mohr FW. Heart transplantation and left ventricular assist device therapy: two comparable options in end-stage heart failure? Clin Cardiol. 2013 Jul;36(7):378 82. [PMID: 23595910]

Item 70   Answer: D

Educational Objective: Prevent stroke in a patient with atrial fibrillation and chronic kidney disease.

This patient with atrial fibrillation should be prescribed dose-adjusted warfarin for stroke prevention, with a goal INR of 2 to 3. Patients with atrial fibrillation and kidney disease are at increased risk for stroke and are also at increased risk for bleeding events with oral anticoagulation. In addition to her kidney disease, the patient has three CHA$_2$DS$_2$-VASc risk factors for stroke, including her female sex (1 point), age (2 points), and the presence of hypertension (1 point). Based upon her risk profile (CHA$_2$DS$_2$-VASc score = 4), her adjusted risk of stroke is 4% per year. The presence of end-stage kidney disease is also associated with an increased risk of stroke. Accordingly, she is at moderate to high risk of stroke and requires oral anticoagulation.

In the past several years, several novel oral anticoagulants have been approved for stroke prevention in patients with nonvalvular atrial fibrillation. Dabigatran is a direct thrombin inhibitor that is dosed twice daily. Rivaroxaban is a factor Xa inhibitor dosed once daily. Apixaban is a factor Xa inhibitor that is dosed twice daily. All three agents exhibit partial clearance in the kidneys and are contraindicated in patients with end-stage kidney disease. None of the randomized controlled trials evaluating these three new agents included patients with creatinine clearance less than 30 mL/min/1.73 m^2.

Aspirin and clopidogrel (dual antiplatelet therapy) can be considered an alternative therapy for patients who cannot tolerate oral anticoagulation; however, they provide inferior stroke prevention with similar rates of bleeding when compared with dose-adjusted warfarin. The best option for stroke prevention therapy in this patient with atrial fibrillation and end-stage kidney disease at high risk for stroke is dose-adjusted warfarin.

KEY POINT

- The best option for stroke prevention therapy in a patient with atrial fibrillation and end-stage kidney disease at high risk for stroke is dose-adjusted warfarin.

Bibliography

Steinberg BA, Beckley PD, Deering TF, et al; Society of Cardiovascular Patient Care. Evaluation and management of the atrial fibrillation patient: a report from the Society of Cardiovascular Patient Care. Crit Pathw Cardiol. 2013 Sep;12(3):107-15 [PMID: 23892939]

Item 71   Answer: A

Educational Objective: Manage complicated type B aortic dissection.

The most appropriate management for this patient is emergency aortic repair. She has a complicated type B aortic dissection. Type A dissections or intramural hematomas involve the ascending aorta or aortic arch, whereas type B syndromes begin distal to the left subclavian artery. Complicated dissections include occlusion of a major aortic branch leading to end-organ ischemia, persistent severe hypertension or pain, propagation of the dissection (which may be manifested by persistent or recurrent pain), aneurysmal expansion, and rupture. This patient has new acute kidney failure because the dissection occludes the renal arteries. Emergency surgery is recommended for acute type A and complicated type B dissections; initial medical management is recommended for uncomplicated type B dissections. Because this patient has a complicated type B dissection, medical management alone would not be appropriate.

Because patients with aortic dissection have a significant prevalence of coronary artery disease, coronary angiography is sometimes performed prior to surgical intervention to allow for repair prior to or at the time of operation for treatment of the aortic dissection. However, the benefit of this approach has not been established, and the required contrast administration would be potentially harmful in this patient with acute kidney failure caused by her aortic dissection. It would therefore not be an appropriate next step in the treatment of this patient.

Although some variants of aortic dissection are associated with intramural thrombus, antithrombotic or thrombolytic therapy is contraindicated and may be potentially fatal in patients with aortic dissection. This highlights the need to exclude aortic dissection prior to initiating either therapy, which may be indicated in patients with evidence of cardiac ischemia.

KEY POINT

- Complicated type B aortic dissection is an indication for immediate aortic repair.

Bibliography

Braverman AC. Acute aortic dissection: clinician update. Circulation. 2010 Jul 13;122(2):184-8. [PMID: 20625143]

Item 72   Answer: C

Educational Objective: Treat severe asymptomatic pulmonary valve stenosis.

This patient should undergo replacement of the pulmonary valve. She has Noonan syndrome, which is an autosomal dominant disorder commonly associated with congenital cardiac lesions, one of which is pulmonary valve stenosis. The pulmonary valve is usually dysplastic in patients with Noonan syndrome and thus is not amenable to balloon intervention. This patient has severe pulmonary valve stenosis demonstrated by physical examination; features include a late-peaking palpable systolic ejection murmur located at the second left intercostal space, absence of an ejection click, and features of right ventricular pressure overload. An ejection click may be audible in patients with pulmonary valve stenosis, but as the severity progresses, the click disappears owing to loss of valve pliability. This patient's echocardiogram confirms severe pulmonary valve stenosis with a peak systolic gradient of 62 mm Hg and mean systolic gradient of 45 mm Hg. Intervention is recommended owing to the severity of obstruction despite the absence of symptoms. Surgical valve replacement is recommended given the dysplastic valve features and presence of coexisting moderate pulmonary valve regurgitation. Most patients with severe pulmonary valve stenosis are treated with balloon valvuloplasty, but this patient has a dysplastic valve related to Noonan syndrome and moderate pulmonary valve regurgitation; thus, pulmonary valve replacement is recommended.

Patients with pulmonary valve stenosis without a history of endocarditis or pulmonary valve replacement do not require endocarditis prophylaxis.

Exercise testing could help determine whether the patient has exercise limitation related to her pulmonary valve stenosis but would not change the recommendation for intervention; thus, it is not required.

Clinical observation, with continued participation in competitive sports, is not advised in patients with severe pulmonary valve stenosis regardless of symptom status because of the risk of progressive right heart failure.

KEY POINT

- In patients with severe pulmonary valve stenosis, valve intervention is recommended regardless of the presence or absence of symptoms.

Bibliography

Burch M, Sharland M, Shinebourne E, Smith G, Patton M, McKenna W. Cardiologic abnormalities in Noonan syndrome: phenotypic diagnosis and echocardiographic assessment of 118 patients. J Am Coll Cardiol. 1993 Oct;22(4):1189-92. [PMID: 8409059]

Item 73   Answer: A

Educational Objective: Manage a patient with a non–ST-elevation myocardial infarction with antiplatelet and anticoagulant medications.

This patient should be given a $P2Y_{12}$ inhibitor, such as clopidogrel, and an anticoagulant, such as the low-molecular-weight heparin enoxaparin, and be admitted to the hospital. Once the diagnosis of a non–ST-elevation myocardial infarction (NSTEMI) has been confirmed by the presence of ischemic chest pain, ST-segment depression on the electrocardiogram (ECG), and/or abnormal cardiac biomarkers, the use of antiplatelet and anticoagulant medications, antianginal medications, and cardioprotective medications is imperative. This patient was given aspirin and nitroglycerin prior to the diagnosis of NSTEMI, and he takes daily ACE inhibitor and statin medications. The additional therapies that are warranted in this situation include a $P2Y_{12}$ inhibitor (clopidogrel, prasugrel, ticagrelor), an anticoagulant (unfractionated heparin or low-molecular-weight heparin), and a β-blocker. The use of clopidogrel, in addition to aspirin, is the best-studied combination of antiplatelet medications.

In patients with an ST-elevation myocardial infarction (STEMI), reperfusion, preferably via percutaneous coronary intervention, should be performed as quickly as possible from symptom onset. This patient does not have evidence of ST-segment elevation or left bundle branch block on the initial ECG. Although an early invasive strategy (defined as within 24 hours of hospital admission) has been proved to be effective in treatment of NSTEMI, there is no evidence that earlier angiography (<6 hours or at hospital admission) offers incremental benefit to these patients.

In patients with a low TIMI risk score (0-2), indicating a low in-hospital risk of death or recurrent ischemia/infarction, predischarge stress testing may be warranted to further define a large ischemic burden and guide revascularization decisions. This patient has a TIMI risk score of 4 (≥3 traditional cardiovascular risk factors, ST-segment deviation, daily aspirin use, elevated cardiac biomarkers), placing him at intermediate risk. These patients have improved clinical outcomes with an early invasive strategy. Exercise stress testing is not appropriate and may be dangerous.

Clinical decision-making should not be affected by the results of the second set of cardiac biomarkers. The presence of an elevated troponin level drawn in the emergency department is prognostically significant and warrants hospital admission, treatment of NSTEMI, and risk stratification.

KEY POINT

- Initial therapy of non–ST-elevation myocardial infarction is medical, with antiplatelet and anticoagulant medications, antianginal medications, and cardioprotective medications; early angiography (<6 hours or at hospital admission) does not provide incremental benefit but an early invasive strategy (defined as within 24 hours of hospital admission) may improve outcomes.

Bibliography

Amsterdam EA, Wenger NK, Brindis RG, et al; ACC/AHA Task Force Members. 2014 AHA/ACC guideline for the management of patients with non–ST-elevation acute coronary syndromes: executive summary: a report of the American College of Cardiology/American Heart Association Task Force on Practice Guidelines. Circulation. 2014 Dec 3;130(25):2354-94. [PMID: 25249586]

Item 74   Answer: E

Educational Objective: Evaluate change in clinical status of a patient with mitral regurgitation.

Transthoracic echocardiography (TTE) in a patient with valvular heart disease is appropriate when there is a change in clinical symptoms. This patient has had worsening dyspnea on exertion for the past 3 weeks that may be a result of worsening mitral regurgitation. In patients with myxomatous mitral valve disease, rupture of a primary or secondary chordae may cause an acute change in the degree of mitral regurgitation and change in clinical status; this is the likely cause of this patient's worsening symptoms. Other causes of her progressive shortness of breath could also be evaluated with an echocardiogram. For example, new wall motion abnormalities could signal recent silent myocardial infarction, and changes in overall ejection fraction would prompt evaluation for new cardiomyopathies.

Exercise stress testing may be appropriate if TTE does not reveal a structural cause of her shortness of breath.

In addition to evaluating for obstructive coronary artery disease, stress echocardiography could be used to evaluate changes in mitral regurgitation and pulmonary pressures with exercise. However, a TTE at rest should be obtained before deciding whether a stress test is warranted.

This patient's mitral regurgitation increases her risk for atrial fibrillation. However, her baseline electrocardiogram demonstrates sinus rhythm, so paroxysmal atrial fibrillation as a cause of her dyspnea is less likely. In addition, she has had progressive dyspnea on exertion that has not waxed and waned, as might be expected if she was in and out of atrial fibrillation. The fact that she presents with worsening symptoms and is in sinus rhythm makes paroxysmal atrial fibrillation less likely. Therefore, 24-hour ambulatory electrocardiographic monitoring would not be the best choice for this patient.

This patient does not appear to have active asthma symptoms or changes in pulmonary status that would indicate a need for spirometry at this time.

Transesophageal echocardiography may be helpful in further defining the anatomy, particularly if surgical intervention is planned, but should not be the first diagnostic study. If the cause of the valvular disorder or degree of regurgitation is unclear from the TTE, then transesophageal echocardiography may be appropriate.

KEY POINT

- Transthoracic echocardiography in a patient with valvular heart disease is appropriate when there is a change in clinical symptoms.

Bibliography

Matulevicius SA, Rohatgi A, Das SR, et al. Appropriate use and clinical impact of transthoracic echocardiography. JAMA Intern Med. 2013 Sep 23;173(17):1600-7. [PMID: 23877630]

Item 75   Answer: A

Educational Objective: Diagnose aortic valve stenosis in an asymptomatic adult with repaired aortic coarctation.

This patient most likely has aortic valve stenosis. The systolic ejection click at the left sternal border suggests a bicuspid aortic valve. The quality and location of the systolic ejection murmur suggest associated aortic stenosis. A bicuspid aortic valve is present in more than 50% of patients with aortic coarctation, and more than 70% of patients with a bicuspid valve will require surgical intervention for a stenotic or regurgitant valve or aortic pathology over the course of a lifetime.

Ascending aortic aneurysms occur in up to 50% of patients with aortic coarctation. Aneurysms are generally clinically silent and require imaging to confirm their presence. Ascending aortic aneurysm that results in dilation of the annulus will be associated with the murmur of aortic regurgitation (diastolic murmur), not aortic valve stenosis as seen in this patient.

Mitral valve regurgitation is not an expected sequela of coarctation repair. In addition, the clinical features in patients with mitral valve regurgitation include a holosystolic murmur, heard best at the apex, that radiates to the axilla.

Recurrent aortic coarctation occurs in about 20% of patients with previous coarctation repair. Clinical features include hypertension that is difficult to control with medical therapy. This patient has hypertension that is controlled with medical therapy, which occurs in up to 75% of patients with repaired coarctation. Other features of recurrent coarctation not demonstrated in this patient include a radial artery–to–femoral artery pulse delay and a systolic murmur over the left anterior or posterior chest.

KEY POINT

- A bicuspid aortic valve is present in more than 50% of patients with aortic coarctation; more than 70% of patients with a bicuspid aortic valve will require cardiac surgical intervention for valve dysfunction or aortic pathology over the course of a lifetime.

Bibliography

Tanous D, Benson LN, Horlick EM. Coarctation of the aorta: evaluation and management. Curr Opin Cardiol. 2009 Nov;24(6):509-15. [PMID: 19667980]

Item 76   Answer: B

Educational Objective: Manage risk of sudden cardiac death in a patient with heart failure with placement of an implantable cardioverter-defibrillator.

This patient with heart failure and a low left ventricular ejection fraction should be referred for placement of an implantable cardioverter-defibrillator (ICD). For patients with an ejection fraction less than or equal to 35% and New York Heart Association (NYHA) functional class II or III heart failure on optimal medical therapy, placement of an ICD is a class I indication. Patients with new-onset heart failure should not undergo placement of an ICD because ventricular function often recovers to above 35%. This patient, however, is on appropriate medical therapy, has had heart failure for at least 6 months, and is still symptomatic. For patients with NYHA functional class IV heart failure symptoms, an ICD is not warranted unless the patient is a cardiac transplant candidate.

Cardiac resynchronization therapy (CRT) with a biventricular pacemaker to improve hemodynamic function of the heart may also be considered in patients with persistent heart failure but is reserved for patients with evidence of conduction system disease. The 2013 American College of Cardiology Foundation/American Heart Association/Heart Rhythm Society (ACCF/AHA/HRS) guideline recommends CRT in patients with an ejection fraction of 35% or below, NYHA functional class III to IV symptoms on guideline-directed medical therapy, and left bundle branch block with QRS duration greater than or equal to 150 ms. With a QRS width of 100 ms, this patient is not a candidate for a biventricular pacemaker in addition to an ICD.

Answers and Critiques

Adding an angiotensin receptor blocker to a heart failure regimen that already includes an ACE inhibitor would not be indicated in this patient as it would not provide additional benefit, and this medication combination has been shown to increase risk of hyperkalemia and kidney injury.

Because this patient's heart rate is 56/min, indicating adequate β-blockade, and his blood pressure is at a desired level, no benefit would be expected by increasing his dose of carvedilol.

Indications for mitral valve replacement, an invasive procedure that carries risks, include the presence of severe mitral regurgitation and NYHA class III or IV symptoms attributed to the valve disease. None of these are present in this patient. This patient's mitral regurgitation is "functional," meaning it is more likely to be a result of his dilated cardiomyopathy and not the underlying cause.

KEY POINT

- Implantable cardioverter-defibrillator placement is indicated for patients with heart failure and a left ventricular ejection fraction less than or equal to 35% and New York Heart Association functional class II or III heart failure while on optimal medical therapy.

Bibliography

Bardy GH, Lee KL, Mark DB, et al; Sudden Cardiac Death in Heart Failure Trial (SCD-HeFT) Investigators. Amiodarone or an implantable cardioverter-defibrillator for congestive heart failure. N Engl J Med. 2005 Jan 20;352(3):225-37. Erratum in: N Engl J Med. 2005 May 19;352(20):2146. [PMID: 15659722]

Item 77   Answer: B

Educational Objective: Treat cardiotoxicity due to chemotherapy with an anthracycline.

The doxorubicin should be discontinued indefinitely in this patient. The efficacy of anthracycline-based chemotherapy regimens for breast adenocarcinoma has been documented by multiple studies. However, doxorubicin, daunorubicin, and other anthracyclines have known cardiotoxicity, which is dependent on dosage, age, concomitant treatment with other cardiotoxic agents, chest radiation, and pre-existing cardiac disease. The incidence of cardiotoxicity for doxorubicin or daunorubicin is less than 1% for cumulative dosages of less than 400 mg/m^2 but 26% for cumulative dosages greater than or equal to 550 mg/m^2. Cardiotoxicity from anthracyclines usually develops within several months after initiation of chemotherapy, manifesting as either systolic or diastolic heart failure, although there can be a long latency period. Once heart failure is present, as in this patient, anthracyclines should be discontinued. In the absence of heart failure, anthracyclines also should be discontinued when new left ventricular dysfunction is detected. Routine surveillance with serial echocardiography is recommended in patients being treated with anthracyclines, with timing intervals based on the patient's baseline function, risk profile, dose, and clinical suspicion for toxicity. The maximum cumulative dose for these drugs

is generally limited to 450 to 500 mg/m^2, but there is considerable individual variation in doses that lead to toxic responses.

This patient developed cardiotoxicity despite a low risk (1%). Therefore, neither continuing doxorubicin nor decreasing the dose is an appropriate treatment. Additionally, because cardiotoxicity is associated with this class of agents, substituting another anthracycline for the doxorubicin, such as daunorubicin, would also not be appropriate. In this patient, anthracycline therapy must be discontinued indefinitely to reverse the cardiotoxic effects and prevent them from recurring.

ACE inhibitors are indicated in patients with asymptomatic or symptomatic systolic dysfunction. There are limited data on the use of these agents to help prevent cardiotoxicity related to chemotherapy, but their use for this indication is not routinely recommended.

KEY POINT

- Anthracyclines, such as doxorubicin, can cause cardiotoxicity in patients being treated with chemotherapy.

Bibliography

Swain SM, Whaley FS, Ewer MS. Congestive heart failure in patients treated with doxorubicin: a retrospective analysis of three trials. Cancer. 2003 Jun 1;97(11):2869-79. [PMID: 12767102]

Item 78   Answer: D

Educational Objective: Evaluate a patient with dyspnea with a history of catheter ablation for atrial fibrillation.

The most likely cause of dyspnea in this patient is pulmonary vein stenosis. He has progressive, unexplained dyspnea and a history of multiple catheter ablation procedures for atrial fibrillation. During catheter ablation of atrial fibrillation, the tissue around each of the pulmonary veins is cauterized to achieve electrical isolation and prevent ectopic foci from triggering recurrent atrial fibrillation. Following this procedure, approximately 1% to 3% of patients can develop symptomatic pulmonary vein stenosis. The risk is higher after multiple procedures, but it can occur after a single procedure. Patients present with progressive dyspnea, but more severe pulmonary vein stenosis can be accompanied by cough, hemoptysis, or chest pain. The image (shown on top of next page) depicts a three-dimensional cardiac magnetic resonance angiogram showing the pulmonary venous return to the left atrium (LA), with stenosis of a pulmonary vein at its ostium where it empties into the LA (*arrow*).

The most important step in the diagnosis of pulmonary vein stenosis is maintaining a high degree of suspicion when encountering a patient with dyspnea and prior atrial fibrillation ablation. Several diagnostic modalities can be used to make the diagnosis noninvasively, including CT angiography, magnetic resonance angiography, and nuclear lung perfusion scanning. Each method has advantages and disadvantages, and the preferred method of diagnosis often differs from institution to institution.

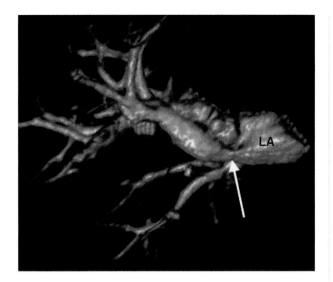

Chronic thromboembolic disease can cause progressive dyspnea, but it would be unlikely in a patient without prior venous thromboembolism and on chronic anticoagulation.

Although intermittent atrial fibrillation could cause symptoms after ablation, it is not likely to cause progressive dyspnea in the setting of sinus rhythm. Intracardiac shunting is rare after an ablation for atrial fibrillation. Although trans-septal catheterization is performed during ablation procedures, the puncture site usually seals off. The normal oxygen saturation in this patient makes the possibility of a symptomatic shunt unlikely.

Phrenic nerve injury can result from delivery of radio-frequency energy in the vicinity of the right superior pulmonary vein with bystander injury of the right phrenic nerve; however, this injury is observed immediately after ablation and is accompanied by an elevated hemi-diaphragm on chest radiograph.

KEY POINT

- Pulmonary vein stenosis is a known complication of catheter ablation of atrial fibrillation and may present with unexplained dyspnea.

Bibliography

Holmes DR Jr, Monahan KH, Packer D. Pulmonary vein stenosis complicating ablation for atrial fibrillation: clinical spectrum and interventional considerations. JACC Cardiovasc Interv. 2009 Apr;2(4):267-76. [PMID: 19463436]

Item 79   Answer: C

Educational Objective: Identify risk factors for sudden death in a patient with obstructive hypertrophic cardiomyopathy.

The patient should be treated by placement of an implantable cardioverter-defibrillator (ICD). He has asymptomatic mild obstructive hypertrophic cardiomyopathy (HCM). An essential goal in the management of patients with HCM is risk stratification and identification of patients who may benefit

from therapy with an ICD. Patients should be considered for ICD therapy if they have any of the following risk factors for sudden cardiac death: (1) massive myocardial hypertrophy (wall thickness ≥30 mm); (2) previous cardiac arrest due to ventricular arrhythmia; (3) blunted blood pressure response or hypotension during exercise; (4) unexplained syncope; (5) nonsustained ventricular tachycardia on ambulatory electrocardiography; and (6) family history of sudden death due to HCM. In patients who have ICD placement for secondary prevention of sudden death (that is, patients with prior cardiac arrest due to ventricular arrhythmia), in whom the indications for implantation are most compelling, the rate of appropriate device discharge is approximately 11% per year. For primary prevention, the annual rate of appropriate ICD discharge is approximately 4%. Although older studies from tertiary referral centers suggested an adverse prognosis for all patients with HCM, multiple contemporary investigations from relatively unselected cohorts have shown that HCM is compatible with normal longevity in most patients, particularly those without risk factors for sudden death, with the overall incidence of death ranging from 0.5% to 0.8% per year.

Septal reduction therapy, with either alcohol septal ablation or surgical myectomy, is indicated only for patients with drug-refractory, severe symptoms and not the mild symptoms that this patient has. Survival has been shown to be favorable among selected patients who undergo septal reduction therapy in experienced centers, but neither ablation nor surgical myectomy is advocated as a means of preventing sudden cardiac death.

β-Blocker therapy is reserved principally for patients with symptoms and has not been associated with reduction in risk of sudden cardiac death.

KEY POINT

- Placement of an implantable cardioverter-defibrillator is an appropriate treatment for patients with hypertrophic cardiomyopathy who have one or more risk factors for sudden cardiac death.

Bibliography

Gersh BJ, Maron BJ, Bonow RO, et al; American College of Cardiology Foundation/American Heart Association Task Force on Practice Guidelines. 2011 ACCF/AHA Guideline for the Diagnosis and Treatment of Hypertrophic Cardiomyopathy: a report of the American College of Cardiology Foundation/American Heart Association Task Force on Practice Guidelines. Developed in collaboration with the American Association for Thoracic Surgery, American Society of Echocardiography, American Society of Nuclear Cardiology, Heart Failure Society of America, Heart Rhythm Society, Society for Cardiovascular Angiography and Interventions, and Society of Thoracic Surgeons. J Am Coll Cardiol. 2011 Dec 13;58(25):e212-60. [PMID: 22075469]

Item 80   Answer: B

Educational Objective: Manage a small abdominal aortic aneurysm with surveillance.

The most appropriate management for this man with a 4.7-cm abdominal aortic aneurysm (AAA) is surveillance by abdominal ultrasonography every 6 to 12 months. Aneurysm diameter is the most important factor predisposing to rupture, with risk increasing with progressive increases in aneurysm size. For aneurysms smaller than 4.0 cm in diameter, the annual rupture risk is below 0.5%, whereas for aneurysms between 5.0 and 5.9 cm in diameter, the annual rupture risk is 3% to 15%. For AAAs with a maximum diameter less than 3.5 cm, repeat surveillance with ultrasonography may be repeated every 3 to 5 years. However, larger aneurysms require more frequent surveillance because of their tendency to expand faster than smaller aneurysms and their increased risk of rupture, with reevaluation on a 6- to 12-month basis recommended. Because this patient's aneurysm is 4.7 cm in diameter, he should undergo surveillance every 6 to 12 months.

Elective repair should be considered for AAAs of 5.5 cm in diameter in men and 5.0 cm in women, for AAAs that increase in diameter by more than 0.5 cm within a 6-month interval, and for those that are symptomatic (tenderness or abdominal or back pain).

AAA rupture has an exceedingly high mortality rate, and the risk of rupture is 0.5% to 5% annually for aneurysms between 4.0 cm and 4.9 cm in diameter. Therefore, no further management would not be appropriate in this patient with a 4.7-cm aneurysm.

KEY POINT

- An abdominal aortic aneurysm smaller than 5.5 cm in men and 5.0 cm in women is managed conservatively, with routine surveillance by abdominal ultrasonography every 6 to 12 months.

Bibliography

Chaikof EL, Brewster DC, Dalman RL, et al. SVS practice guidelines for the care of patients with an abdominal aortic aneurysm: executive summary. J Vasc Surg. 2009 Oct;50(4):880-96. [PMID: 19786241]

Item 81   Answer: B

Educational Objective: Treat a patient undergoing thrombolysis for an ST-elevation myocardial infarction with clopidogrel.

This patient who is receiving thrombolytic therapy for an ST-elevation myocardial infarction (STEMI) should be given clopidogrel, 300 mg orally. Clopidogrel is the most widely studied antiplatelet agent in patients undergoing reperfusion for STEMI. Clopidogrel is associated with improved outcomes and no apparent increase in the risk of bleeding when used with concomitant thrombolytic therapy and with primary percutaneous coronary intervention (PCI). In the CLARITY-TIMI 28 study examining clopidogrel as adjunctive therapy in patients undergoing thrombolysis, there was a 6.7% absolute risk reduction in the incidence of occluded infarct-related artery or recurrent myocardial infarction or death in patients assigned to clopidogrel when compared with placebo.

Abciximab is a platelet glycoprotein IIb/IIIa inhibitor that further inhibits platelet aggregation and impairs platelet activation. Glycoprotein IIb/IIIa inhibitors are used in patients undergoing PCI. Owing to the risk of increased bleeding with these agents, their use should be reserved for administration during PCI, rather than "up front" in the emergency department. Large studies have shown no clear mortality benefit and significantly higher rates of major bleeding in patients undergoing fibrinolysis treated with abciximab versus placebo. Use of platelet glycoprotein IIb/IIIa inhibitors in patients undergoing thrombolysis is not currently recommended.

For STEMI patients undergoing primary PCI, both prasugrel and ticagrelor have shown superior efficacy compared with clopidogrel. However, use of these agents in patients treated with thrombolytic therapy has not been well studied, and little evidence exists to recommend the use of either of these agents in patients receiving thrombolytic therapy.

KEY POINT

- Patients with ST-elevation myocardial infarction undergoing thrombolysis should be given adjunctive antiplatelet therapy with clopidogrel.

Bibliography

Sabatine MS, Cannon CP, Gibson CM, et al; CLARITY-TIMI 28 Investigators. Addition of clopidogrel to aspirin and fibrinolytic therapy for myocardial infarction with ST-segment elevation. N Engl J Med. 2005 Mar 24;352(12):1179-89. [PMID: 15758000]

Item 82   Answer: D

Educational Objective: Manage iron-deficiency anemia in a patient with cyanotic congenital heart disease.

This patient with Eisenmenger syndrome has symptomatic relative anemia, and short-course iron therapy should be initiated. Most patients with cyanosis have compensated erythrocytosis with stable hemoglobin levels. Iron deficiency and resultant microcytosis in patients with cyanosis are often caused by unnecessary phlebotomy or blood loss. Microcytes are more rigid than normal erythrocytes; thus, microcytosis increases the risk of stroke. The treatment of iron deficiency is challenging. Oral iron often causes a rapid and dramatic increase in erythrocyte mass. Therefore, administration of 1 tablet daily of ferrous sulfate or ferrous gluconate is recommended, with repeat hemoglobin assessment in 7 to 10 days. This patient's usual hemoglobin level would be in the range of 18 g/dL (180 g/L). He developed perioperative anemia that has persisted and caused dyspnea and fatigue. Once the hemoglobin and hematocrit levels begin to increase, iron therapy can be discontinued. Erythrocyte transfusion is considered only for severe symptoms.

Erythropoietin is used in patients with anemia related to kidney disease and some malignancies but is not recommended for patients with heart disease and cyanosis who develop postoperative anemia.

Data are limited regarding the efficacy of epoprostenol in patients with Eisenmenger syndrome and pulmonary hypertension. When used, oral, subcutaneous, and inhaled therapies are preferred. Intravenous epoprostenol is typically avoided because of the risk for paradoxical embolism with continuous intravenous therapy in patients with an intracardiac right-to-left shunt.

Although heart-lung transplantation is an option for end-stage cardiopulmonary disease in patients with Eisenmenger syndrome, this option is not indicated without further trial of standard medical therapy with iron.

KEY POINT

- Most patients with cyanotic heart disease have compensated erythrocytosis with stable hemoglobin levels.

Bibliography

Tay EL, Peset A, Papaphylactou M, et al. Replacement therapy for iron deficiency improves exercise capacity and quality of life in patients with cyanotic congenital heart disease and/or the Eisenmenger syndrome. Int J Cardiol. 2011 Sep 15;151(3):307-12. [PMID: 20580108]

Item 83   Answer: A

Educational Objective: Use coronary artery calcium score to clarify cardiovascular risk in an intermediate-risk patient.

The most appropriate option for this patient with intermediate cardiovascular risk is to obtain an additional factor to help clarify risk to guide therapy, such as a coronary artery calcium (CAC) score. Assessment for risk of atherosclerotic cardiovascular disease (ASCVD) is an important component of primary prevention. Several risk assessment tools for ASCVD are available, with the Framingham risk score being the most commonly used. The Pooled Cohort Equations are a new risk assessment instrument developed from multiple community-based cohorts (including the Framingham study) that includes a broader range of variables and endpoints than the Framingham score when evaluating 10-year ASCVD risk. Its use as a primary risk assessment tool was recommended in the 2013 American College of Cardiology/American Heart Association Guideline on the Assessment of Cardiovascular Risk. Using this method, a 10-year risk of ASCVD of below 5% is considered low risk, 5% to below 7.5% is classified as intermediate risk, and 7.5% or above is designated as high risk. For patients with intermediate risk, such as this patient with a risk of 6%, additional factors may be helpful in further refining risk assessment by identifying patients who may benefit from a more aggressive prevention strategy. Factors that can help further define risk include:

- CAC score greater than 300 or greater than 75% for age
- High-sensitivity C-reactive protein level (hsCRP) above 2 mg/L
- Ankle-brachial index below 0.90
- LDL cholesterol level 160 mg/dL (4.14 mmol/L) or higher or other evidence of genetic hyperlipidemia
- Family history of premature ASCVD with onset younger than 55 years in a first-degree male relative or younger than 65 years in a first-degree female relative

The results of the CAC score may help inform the individual patient-physician discussion in this intermediate-risk patient.

In this active construction worker who is asymptomatic, the pretest probability of finding ASCVD is low; because of the increased rate of false-positive test results in low-risk patients, stress testing is not recommended. The use of stress testing to diagnose ASCVD in asymptomatic persons does not reduce mortality. Appropriate risk factor modification, however, does have the potential to reduce cardiovascular risk and mortality.

This patient's blood pressure is adequately treated, and there is no evidence that further lowering of blood pressure results in decreased cardiovascular risk. Therefore, an increase in his lisinopril dosage would not be beneficial.

Although studies of the mechanisms of atherosclerosis suggest that antioxidant therapy might be protective against development of ASCVD, studies have failed to show a benefit of antioxidants as a primary prevention intervention. The use of vitamins A, C, or E, alone or in combination, is therefore not recommended to decrease cardiovascular risk.

KEY POINT

- Coronary artery calcium scoring can improve cardiovascular risk assessment in intermediate-risk patients in whom therapy may be affected by a reclassification of risk.

Bibliography

Greenland P, Alpert JS, Beller GA, et al; American College of Cardiology Foundation; American Heart Association. 2010 ACCF/AHA guideline for assessment of cardiovascular risk in asymptomatic adults: a report of the American College of Cardiology Foundation/American Heart Association Task Force on Practice Guidelines. J Am Coll Cardiol. 2010 Dec 14;56(25):e50-103. [PMID: 21144964]

Item 84   Answer: D

Educational Objective: Treat symptomatic peripheral arterial disease with a supervised exercise program.

The most appropriate management for this patient with symptomatic peripheral arterial disease is to start a supervised exercise program. Supervised exercise therapy can effectively treat claudication, with increases in pain-free walking time and maximal walking time, and is recommended as part of the initial treatment regimen for intermittent claudication. The CLEVER study demonstrated superior improvement in walking distance with supervised exercise for patients with aortoiliac disease, as compared with stent revascularization or medical therapy alone.

Cilostazol is an oral phosphodiesterase-3 inhibitor that has demonstrated increases in pain-free walking and overall walking distance in patients with claudication in randomized clinical trials, although the gains with exercise are two- to three-fold greater than with cilostazol alone. However, cilostazol is contraindicated in patients with heart failure or a left ventricular ejection fraction below 40%. This contraindication exists because cilostazol has a similar pharmacologic action to the inotropic drugs milrinone and amrinone, which demonstrated increased mortality rates with long-term use in patients with heart failure.

Patients with stable claudication progress to critical limb ischemia and limb loss at a rate of less than 5% annually. For most symptomatic patients, therefore, noninvasive therapy with exercise and medication is appropriate. If conservative therapy fails or patients have symptoms limiting their lifestyle or employment, revascularization by an endovascular or surgical approach should be considered.

KEY POINT

- Supervised exercise therapy can effectively treat claudication, with increases in pain-free walking time and maximal walking time, and is recommended as part of the initial treatment regimen for intermittent claudication.

Bibliography

Murphy TP, Cutlip DE, Regensteiner JG, et al; CLEVER Study Investigators. Supervised exercise versus primary stenting for claudication resulting from aortoiliac peripheral artery disease: six-month outcomes from the claudication: exercise versus endoluminal revascularization (CLEVER) study. Circulation. 2012 Jan 3;125(1):130-9. [PMID: 22090168]

Item 85　　Answer:　D

Educational Objective: Select proper imaging surveillance for a patient with a bicuspid aortic valve and aortopathy.

This patient with a bicuspid aortic valve should have annual transthoracic echocardiography. Bicuspid aortic valve occurs with other cardiovascular and systemic abnormalities. Specifically, ascending aortic dilation may occur in persons with a bicuspid aortic valve, in combination with aortic valve disease or as an independent condition. Previously considered a secondary event caused by abnormal aortic valve function, the aortopathy associated with a bicuspid aortic valve is now recognized to result from intrinsically abnormal connective tissue. As a result, serial evaluation of ascending aortic diameter should be performed by transthoracic echocardiography (or by CT angiography or magnetic resonance angiography if not adequately visualized by echocardiography). The frequency of surveillance depends upon aortic root and ascending aorta size. Expert consensus guidelines recommend reassessment of the aorta if the aortic root or ascending aorta dimension is greater than or equal to 4.0 cm, with the evaluation interval determined by degree and rate of aortic dilation and by family history. Annual evaluation should occur if the aortic diameter is greater than 4.5 cm. New or changing symptoms and pregnancy are indications for earlier imaging of the aorta. For this patient, in view of the similar findings on transthoracic echocardiogram and chest CT scan, serial transthoracic echocardiography is reasonable. Moreover, transthoracic echocardiography is more cost effective than both CT and cardiac magnetic resonance (CMR) imaging, and serial CT scans can result in significant cumulative doses of radiation in this young patient.

CMR imaging and multidetector CT are appropriate for further assessment of aortic pathology when transthoracic or transesophageal echocardiography is not conclusive. In this patient, CMR imaging and multidetector CT scanning are not indicated because the aortic root and ascending aorta are adequately visualized by transthoracic echocardiography. In addition, annual multidetector CT scanning would needlessly expose the patient to excessive radiation.

Transesophageal echocardiography is an invasive procedure and would be considered if transthoracic imaging was inadequate to measure aortic root size and evaluate the ascending aorta.

Because of the risk of aortic dissection and rupture, reassurance and clinical observation are inadequate follow-up for bicuspid valve–related aortopathy.

KEY POINT

- In patients with a bicuspid aortic valve, serial evaluation of ascending aortic diameter should be performed by transthoracic echocardiography (or by CT angiography or magnetic resonance angiography if not adequately visualized by echocardiography).

Bibliography

Mordi I, Tzemos N. Bicuspid aortic valve disease: a comprehensive review. Cardiol Res Pract. 2012;2012:196037. [PMID: 22685681]

Item 86　　Answer:　D

Educational Objective: Diagnose obstructive coronary artery disease in a patient with left bundle branch block.

This patient with a left bundle branch block (LBBB) on her baseline electrocardiogram (ECG) should undergo vasodilator nuclear perfusion imaging. In patients with baseline ECG abnormalities such as pre-excitation, LBBB, a paced rhythm, or baseline ST-segment depression greater than 1 mm, ECGs obtained during stress testing cannot be appropriately interpreted, and standard exercise treadmill testing is therefore not appropriate. Instead, these patients must undergo stress testing with additional imaging, such as nuclear perfusion imaging or stress echocardiography.

When myocardial perfusion imaging is used to evaluate patients with LBBB, a vasodilator study using an agent such as adenosine or dipyridamole is necessary instead of an exercise study. This is because perfusion defects that are not related to obstructive coronary artery disease (CAD) can be seen in the septum with exercise. Radiotracers are distributed with blood flow, and when the coronary arteries fill during diastole, the delay in contraction of the septum with LBBB can impair filling and create a defect in the septum in the absence of obstructive CAD. However, vasodilators produce hyperemia and a flow disparity between myocardium supplied by the stenotic vessel as compared with the unobstructed vessel that is not affected by the delay in septal contraction related to LBBB. For this reason, an exercise nuclear perfusion study would not be appropriate in this patient.

Coronary artery calcium scoring quantifies the amount of calcium in the walls of the coronary arteries and correlates well with plaque burden in the coronary arteries. It is an anatomic study with fairly high sensitivity for detecting occlusive

CAD, although the frequency of false-negative results (significant CAD with a low CAC score) is not known. Therefore, CAC scoring is more frequently used for risk stratification in patients with intermediate risk for atherosclerotic cardiovascular disease. Another anatomic study, coronary CT angiography, is an emerging technology that has high correlation with findings on invasive coronary arteriography and may be increasingly useful in evaluating for occlusive CAD.

KEY POINT

- In patients with suspected coronary artery disease with baseline electrocardiographic (ECG) abnormalities such as pre-excitation, left bundle branch block, a paced rhythm, or ST-segment depression greater than 1 mm, ECGs obtained during stress testing cannot be interpreted; therefore, stress testing with additional imaging is required.

Bibliography

Fihn SD, Gardin JM, Abrams J, et al; American College of Cardiology Foundation; American Heart Association Task Force on Practice Guidelines; American College of Physicians; American Association for Thoracic Surgery; Preventive Cardiovascular Nurses Association; Society for Cardiovascular Angiography and Interventions; Society of Thoracic Surgeons. 2012 CCF/AHA/ACP/AATS/PCNA/SCAI/STS Guideline for the diagnosis and management of patients with stable ischemic heart disease: a report of the American College of Cardiology Foundation/ American Heart Association Task Force on Practice Guidelines, and the American College of Physicians, American Association for Thoracic Surgery, Preventive Cardiovascular Nurses Association, Society for Cardiovascular Angiography and Interventions, and Society of Thoracic Surgeons. J Am Coll Cardiol. 2012 Dec 18;60(24):e44-e164. [PMID: 23182125]

Item 87   Answer: B

Educational Objective: Evaluate a woman with atypical chest pain with exercise electrocardiography.

This patient should undergo exercise electrocardiography (ECG). Although she has several risk factors for coronary artery disease (CAD), including hyperlipidemia and a family history of premature CAD, her symptoms are not typical for angina, which requires the presence of pain precipitated by exercise or emotion, a substernal location of the pain, and relief with rest or nitroglycerin. Because she has only two of the three diagnostic criteria for angina, she is classified as having atypical angina. Women in her age group with atypical angina have an intermediate pretest probability of CAD (approximately 22%). For patients with an intermediate pretest probability of disease and a normal resting ECG, exercise ECG testing is recommended as the initial test of choice.

Conventional coronary angiography identifies the location and severity of blockages and allows vascular access for percutaneous intervention. Because of the invasive nature of coronary angiography and the inherent risks of vascular complications, it should be reserved for patients with acute coronary syndrome requiring immediate intervention, lifestyle-limiting angina despite medical therapy, or high-risk criteria on noninvasive stress testing. This patient's pretest probability of CAD is intermediate, which is not high enough

to warrant immediate coronary angiography as the initial diagnostic test.

The sensitivity and specificity of noninvasive stress testing for the evaluation of chest pain are lower in women than in men. However, the routine use of exercise testing with either nuclear perfusion imaging or echocardiography to assess left ventricular regional wall motion or perfusion imaging is not recommended for women or men in the absence of baseline ECG abnormalities. Although the addition of noninvasive imaging increases diagnostic sensitivity for coronary artery disease, use of exercise nuclear perfusion testing as the initial test has not been found to reduce cardiovascular events compared with exercise ECG testing alone.

Pharmacologic stress testing with imaging is indicated for patients who are unable to exercise. In addition, patients with left bundle branch block undergoing nuclear stress testing should be administered a pharmacologic stressor even if they are able to exercise because of the potential for a false-positive test owing to a septal perfusion abnormality that may occur with exercise. Pharmacologic stress testing is not indicated because this patient is physically able to exercise and does not have a left bundle branch block.

KEY POINT

- Exercise electrocardiographic testing is recommended as the initial test of choice in patients with a normal baseline electrocardiogram and an intermediate pretest probability of coronary artery disease based on age, sex, and symptoms.

Bibliography

Qaseem A, Fihn SD, Williams S, Dallas P, Owens DK, Shekelle P; Clinical Guidelines Committee of the American College of Physicians. Diagnosis of stable ischemic heart disease: summary of a clinical practice guideline from the American College of Physicians/American College of Cardiology Foundation/American Heart Association/American Association for Thoracic Surgery/Preventive Cardiovascular Nurses Association/Society of Thoracic Surgeons. Ann Intern Med. 2012 Nov 20;157(10):729-34. [PMID: 23165664]

Item 88   Answer: E

Educational Objective: Manage aspirin use for primary prevention in a patient with diabetes mellitus and a low cardiovascular risk.

No further testing or therapy would be most appropriate in this patient. Although she has diabetes mellitus, she has no other major cardiovascular risk factors. Risk assessment for atherosclerotic cardiovascular disease (ASCVD) has traditionally been with the Framingham risk score, although the American College of Cardiology/American Heart Association Pooled Cohort Equations, a new method for assessment that includes additional variables for risk stratification, is increasingly being used. With this method, a 10-year risk of ASCVD of less than 5% is considered low risk, 5% to below 7.5% is considered intermediate risk, and 7.5% and above is designated as high risk. This patient has a calculated 10-year risk of 2.7%, making her low risk for ASCVD. Therefore, no additional testing is indicated at present.

It is reasonable to give low-dose aspirin to adults with diabetes and no previous history of vascular disease who are at increased cardiovascular risk and without increased risk for bleeding. However, aspirin should not routinely be given to patients with diabetes who are at low risk (men younger than 50 years and women younger than 60 years without other major risk factors such as hypertension or tobacco use). The risks of gastrointestinal bleeding or hemorrhagic stroke outweigh the benefits of aspirin in this low-risk patient.

Coronary artery calcium scoring is reasonable to further define cardiovascular risk in patients with intermediate risk as determined by the Pooled Cohort Equations (5% to <7.5%). However, this patient's risk of ASCVD is considered low; therefore, good adherence to lifestyle factors and monitoring of cardiovascular risk factors are most appropriate in this patient.

There is no role for routine exercise testing in an asymptomatic patient. In patients with low coronary artery disease pretest probability, false-positive results will be more common than true-positive results and may lead to unnecessary downstream testing and treatment.

Although elevated homocysteine levels are associated with cardiovascular risk, no data support the use of folic acid supplementation, which can lower homocysteine levels, to reduce the risk.

KEY POINT

- Aspirin should not routinely be given to patients with diabetes mellitus who are at low cardiovascular risk (men younger than 50 years and women younger than 60 years without other major risk factors such as hypertension or tobacco use).

Bibliography

Pignone M, Alberts MJ, Colwell JA, et al. Aspirin for primary prevention of cardiovascular events in people with diabetes: a position statement of the American Diabetes Association, a scientific statement of the American Heart Association, and an expert consensus document of the American College of Cardiology Foundation. Circulation. 2010 Jun 22;121(24):2694-701. [PMID: 20508178]

Item 89   Answer: D

Educational Objective: Treat low cardiac output in heart failure by reducing afterload.

The most appropriate additional treatment for this patient is nitroprusside. After several days of diuresis, this patient has a normal right atrial pressure (0-5 mm Hg) and pulmonary capillary wedge pressure above normal but within the acceptable range for patients with heart failure (<18 mm Hg) to provide optimal ventricular filling. These hemodynamic parameters suggest that the cardiac output is very low and is the major explanation for the patient's heart failure symptoms. Acute heart failure is typically marked by a combination of volume overload (manifested by an increased pulmonary capillary wedge pressure, usually ≥18 mm Hg) and reduced cardiac output. Part of the reason for reduced

cardiac output is a very high systemic vascular resistance, as the systemic circulation increases afterload to maintain blood pressure in the setting of low stroke volume. With correction of the volume overload state, the next step in therapy is to reduce afterload with nitroprusside.

Nitroprusside is an intravenously administered vasodilator that lowers systemic vascular resistance and, therefore, increases cardiac output. This therapy should be used only in the setting of invasive monitoring, including a right heart catheter and possibly an arterial line to closely measure systemic pressure. Counterintuitive to what would be expected, the blood pressure usually rises with nitroprusside because of the improved cardiac performance. Nitroprusside is associated with possible rebound vasoconstriction following discontinuation and potential toxicity due to its metabolism to cyanide with longer term use; therefore, therapy is generally limited to no more than 24 to 48 hours in most patients. Patients with cardiogenic shock may also be treated with an inotropic agent such as dobutamine.

Changing to continuous intravenous furosemide is not indicated because the patient has normal filling pressures manifested by the pulmonary capillary wedge pressure of 16 mm Hg and right atrial pressure of 4 mm Hg. More aggressive diuresis will not impact the principal problem, which is low cardiac output and a high systemic vascular resistance. Studies have evaluated the efficacy of continuous versus intermittent boluses of intravenous diuretics in patients hospitalized with acute heart failure. There was no difference demonstrated in patients' symptoms, kidney function, or length of stay between the two strategies. High- versus low-dose diuretics also have been evaluated. Patients taking high dosages exhibited a trend toward more diuresis and slight worsening of kidney function. Diuresis should be performed using whatever strategy is necessary to remove the fluid.

Dopamine was recently compared with nesiritide and placebo in patients with acute heart failure and mild kidney dysfunction. No benefit was demonstrated with either dopamine or nesiritide compared with placebo for either urine output or protection of kidney function. In general, the results of studies evaluating the use of inotropic therapy for the treatment of patients hospitalized with acute heart failure have been negative. For the routine care of patients hospitalized with heart failure, dopamine, dobutamine, and milrinone have not been shown to be helpful and may be associated with adverse outcomes.

Esmolol is an intravenous β-blocker. Like all β-blockers, it has some negative inotropic activity, and use of this drug might worsen the patient's hemodynamic status, not improve it.

KEY POINT

- In patients with low-output heart failure, nitroprusside can reduce afterload and increase cardiac output; nitroprusside should be used only in the setting of invasive cardiac monitoring.

Bibliography

Binanay C, Califf RM, Hasselblad V, et al; ESCAPE Investigators and ESCAPE Study Coordinators. Evaluation study of congestive heart failure and pulmonary artery catheterization effectiveness: the ESCAPE trial. JAMA. 2005 Oct 5;294(13):1625-33. [PMID: 16204662]

Item 90   Answer: A

Educational Objective: Manage liver disease resulting from constrictive pericarditis.

The patient should undergo hemodynamic cardiac catheterization. He has evidence of liver disease most likely caused by constrictive pericarditis. Patients with constrictive pericarditis can develop severe symptoms of right-sided congestion that can lead to chronic hepatic congestion and hepatopathy. When detected early, cirrhosis can be reversible if constrictive pericarditis is identified and treated in a timely manner with surgical pericardiectomy. An important clue that suggests constrictive pericarditis as a contributor to hepatopathy is an elevated jugular venous pulse, which demonstrates the presence of elevated right atrial pressures. The central venous pressure is rarely abnormal in patients with primary liver disease. A hemodynamic study with an echocardiogram is sufficient to diagnose constrictive pericarditis in most patients. For patients such as this one with an indeterminate echocardiogram, the most appropriate next step is an invasive hemodynamic study with cardiac catheterization, which provides the greatest sensitivity and specificity for the diagnosis of constrictive pericarditis.

A liver biopsy may be helpful in patients with liver disease of unknown etiology or to gauge the type and degree of liver injury or fibrosis. A liver biopsy is not performed prior to the completion of less invasive tests, such as a liver chemistry profile and ultrasonography. In this patient, the elevated central venous pressure suggests cardiac rather than primary liver disease, and cardiac catheterization with hemodynamic measurements is more likely to prove diagnostic.

B-type natriuretic peptide level is often normal or minimally elevated in patients with constrictive pericarditis despite the elevated central venous pressure. However, measurement of B-type natriuretic peptide will not establish the diagnosis of constrictive pericarditis or guide therapy.

Judicious use of loop diuretics is important in patients with constrictive pericarditis to reduce dyspnea and edema, but because higher filling pressures are needed to maintain stroke volume, overly aggressive diuresis can reduce cardiac output, causing dizziness and orthostatic hypotension.

KEY POINT

- For patients with suspected constrictive pericarditis who have an indeterminate echocardiogram, the most appropriate next step is an invasive hemodynamic study with cardiac catheterization.

Bibliography

Khandaker MH, Espinosa RE, Nishimura RA, et al. Pericardial disease: diagnosis and management. Mayo Clin Proc. 2010 Jun;85(6):572-93. [PMID: 20511488]

Item 91   Answer: D

Educational Objective: Evaluate a patient with atypical chest pain and indeterminate findings on exercise stress testing.

This patient with atypical chest pain and indeterminate results on exercise stress testing should undergo stress echocardiography. Baseline abnormalities on the resting electrocardiogram (ECG) can limit the ability to interpret the ECG during exercise. Specific abnormalities on the resting ECG preclude the use of ECG stress testing because of difficulty in accurately interpreting changes that may occur with stress. These abnormalities include the presence of left ventricular hypertrophy with repolarization abnormalities (ST-segment depressions) greater than 0.5 mm, pre-excitation, left bundle branch block, and a paced rhythm. In these settings, exercise stress testing with imaging, either with echocardiography or perfusion imaging, is required. Although patients without these exclusionary findings may undergo stress ECG, baseline changes need to be considered in interpreting the test. This patient had ST-segment depressions less than 0.5 mm at baseline; if there were no further changes with exercise testing, these findings could be interpreted as normal. However, a positive stress test is defined as greater than 1-mm ST-segment depression in two contiguous leads during exercise testing. In this patient, the 1-mm ST-segment depression that developed during exercise is a less reliable predictor of ischemia given the ST-segment baseline abnormalities. Therefore, these changes on stress testing are not definitive and her test result is considered indeterminate. She should therefore undergo repeat stress testing with imaging in order to establish a diagnosis of coronary artery disease (CAD).

The patient does not yet have a diagnosis of CAD and her hypertension is adequately treated on her current regimen; adding treatment with a β-blocker to treat myocardial ischemia would not be indicated.

Cardiac catheterization should be reserved for patients with high-risk features on exercise stress testing, such as a high-risk Duke treadmill score (below −11), hypotension, severe ST-segment depression, and early-onset angina. This patient has atypical chest pain, and cardiac catheterization should be deferred until a diagnosis of CAD is made and the extent and severity of disease are evaluated with stress imaging.

Cardiac magnetic resonance (CMR) imaging is best utilized for diagnoses of the aorta, pericardium, and myocardium, including viability and extent of myocardial fibrosis. Stress CMR imaging can be performed, but its availability is limited.

KEY POINT

- In a patient with indeterminate results on exercise stress testing, a repeat stress test with imaging should be performed to elucidate the diagnosis.

Bibliography

Fihn SD, Gardin JM, Abrams J, et al; American College of Cardiology Foundation; American Heart Association Task Force on Practice Guidelines; American College of Physicians; American Association for

Thoracic Surgery; Preventive Cardiovascular Nurses Association; Society for Cardiovascular Angiography and Interventions; Society of Thoracic Surgeons. 2012 CCF/AHA/ACP/AATS/PCNA/SCAI/STS Guideline for the diagnosis and management of patients with stable ischemic heart disease: a report of the American College of Cardiology Foundation/ American Heart Association Task Force on Practice Guidelines, and the American College of Physicians, American Association for Thoracic Surgery, Preventive Cardiovascular Nurses Association, Society for Cardiovascular Angiography and Interventions, and Society of Thoracic Surgeons. J Am Coll Cardiol. 2012 Dec 18;60(24):e44-e164. [PMID: 23182125]

Item 92   Answer: A

Educational Objective: **Manage a patient with an acute coronary syndrome with thrombolytic therapy.**

This patient should receive a thrombolytic agent such as tenecteplase and be transferred to a center capable of performing percutaneous coronary intervention (PCI). He has electrocardiographic changes consistent with an acute inferior ST-elevation myocardial infarction (STEMI). Patients with a STEMI presenting within 12 hours of symptom onset should receive reperfusion therapy with either primary PCI or thrombolysis, with PCI being the preferred intervention owing to increased efficacy. When transfer times for primary PCI exceed 120 minutes from presentation, administration of thrombolytic therapy is recommended, such as in this patient presenting to a facility without PCI capability and an inability to transport him for treatment within that time frame.

This patient has no absolute contraindications to thrombolytic therapy, which include previous intracerebral hemorrhage, a known cerebrovascular lesion (such as an arteriovenous malformation), suspected aortic dissection, active bleeding or bleeding diathesis (excluding menses), significant closed head or facial trauma within 3 months, and ischemic stroke within the past 3 months. A relative contraindication for thrombolysis is severe hypertension (defined as a systolic blood pressure >180 mm Hg); however, this patient's systolic blood pressure does not meet this threshold. Even when thrombolytic therapy is administered, treatment guidelines recommend that patients be transferred to a PCI-capable facility because of the potential for thrombolytic failure. Optimal management of patients with STEMI relies heavily upon physician recognition and rapid initiation of reperfusion therapy, with either thrombolytic therapy or PCI. Patients with an acute coronary syndrome and an electrocardiogram compatible with STEMI should be treated with reperfusion therapy without biomarker confirmation, as early biomarker results may be normal in patients with STEMI. Therefore, waiting for the results of cardiac biomarker levels would delay appropriate treatment.

The use of a glycoprotein IIb/IIIa inhibitor, such as abciximab, has not been shown to improve outcomes of patients with STEMI prior to the primary PCI procedure and should be reserved for administration in the catheterization laboratory during primary PCI.

Transfer for primary PCI is a reasonable alternative to thrombolytic therapy in the setting of absolute contraindications to thrombolytic therapy or high-risk clinical features and if an acceptable time to transfer the patient to a PCI-capable hospital can be achieved (first medical contact-to-device time of 120 minutes or less). In studies of patients transferred from a non-PCI facility for primary PCI, more than half of patients with STEMI did not undergo perfusion in 120 minutes or less. In this case, transfer time would be prolonged (>120 minutes); therefore, thrombolytic therapy is the best reperfusion strategy.

KEY POINT

- Patients with an ST-elevation myocardial infarction presenting within 12 hours of symptom onset to non-percutaneous coronary intervention (PCI)-capable hospitals should receive either primary PCI (if available in <120 minutes) or thrombolytic therapy (if primary PCI is not available within 120 minutes).

Bibliography

O'Gara PT, Kushner FG, Ascheim DD, et al; American College of Cardiology Foundation/American Heart Association Task Force on Practice Guidelines. 2013 ACCF/AHA guideline for the management of ST-elevation myocardial infarction: a report of the American College of Cardiology Foundation/American Heart Association Task Force on Practice Guidelines. Circulation. 2013 Jan 29;127(4):e362-425. Erratum in: Circulation. 2013 Dec 24;128(25):e481. [PMID: 23247304]

Item 93   Answer: A

Educational Objective: **Diagnose severe aortic regurgitation.**

This patient has aortic regurgitation. The murmur of aortic regurgitation, described as a diastolic decrescendo murmur, is heard best at the third left intercostal space and may be better heard when the patient is at end-expiration, leaning forward. Chronic aortic regurgitation has many associated findings, including widened pulse pressure, bounding carotid and peripheral pulses, and a diffuse and laterally displaced point of maximal impulse. A low-pitched rumbling diastolic murmur ("Austin Flint murmur") can accompany aortic regurgitation and is caused by premature closure of the mitral leaflets due to the regurgitant aortic flow.

The auscultatory findings for mitral stenosis include an opening snap with a low-pitched mid-diastolic murmur (often described as a rumble) that accentuates presystole and is heard best at the apex with the patient in the left lateral decubitus position. It most often occurs in patients with rheumatic valve disease and is frequently associated with atrial fibrillation.

A small patent ductus arteriosus in the adult produces an arteriovenous fistula with a continuous murmur that envelops the S_2 and is characteristically heard beneath the left clavicle. Patients with a moderate-sized patent ductus arteriosus may present with a continuous "machinery-type" murmur best heard at the left infraclavicular area and bounding pulses with a wide pulse pressure.

The sinuses of Valsalva are three aortic dilatations just above the aortic valve cusps. Two of the three sinuses are the origins of the coronary arteries. Regurgitant blood flow into the sinus structures fills the coronary arteries and assists in the closure of the aortic valve cusps. Sinus of Valsalva aneurysm is a type of aortic root aneurysm. Rupture of the aneurysm will allow flow between the sinus of Valsalva and either the right atrium or right ventricle, producing a continuous systolic and diastolic murmur heard loudest at the second left intercostal space. Clinical presentation can vary, ranging from asymptomatic to decompensated heart failure. Ruptured sinus of Valsalva aneurysm more frequently involves the left or right coronary cusps and less frequently the noncoronary cusp.

KEY POINT

- The murmur of aortic regurgitation is a diastolic decrescendo murmur heard best at the left third intercostal space; associated findings include widened pulse pressure, bounding carotid and peripheral pulses, and a diffuse and laterally displaced point of maximal impulse.

Bibliography

Choudhry NK, Etchells EE. The rational clinical examination. Does this patient have aortic regurgitation? JAMA. 1999;281(23):2231-8. [PMID: 10376577]

Item 94   Answer: B

Educational Objective: Distinguish lumbar stenosis from peripheral arterial disease.

An MRI of the lumbar spine is most likely to confirm the diagnosis in this patient. This patient's normal ankle-brachial index (ABI) bilaterally, normal distal pulses, lack of a bruit, normal skin findings, and clinical history all suggest a diagnosis other than peripheral arterial disease (PAD). Patients with pseudoclaudication (lumbar spinal stenosis) may report bilateral leg weakness associated with walking or with prolonged standing; symptoms are aggravated by prolonged standing and are relieved with bending at the waist. Nearly half of patients have absent deep tendon reflexes at the ankles, but reflexes at the knees and muscle strength are usually preserved. The American College of Physicians recommends that advanced imaging with MRI or CT should be reserved for patients with a suspected serious underlying condition or neurologic deficits, or who are candidates for invasive interventions. In the absence of these indications, back imaging is not indicated.

Measuring the exercise ABI can be useful in diagnosing PAD when the resting ABI is normal and the index of suspicion is high for PAD. This patient's history and examination findings point to a diagnosis other than PAD, so measuring the exercise ABI will not add helpful information at this time.

Segmental limb plethysmography is useful in patients with an established diagnosis of PAD to help localize the site of stenosis. In this test, blood pressures are recorded using plethysmographic cuffs placed at the upper thigh, lower thigh, calf, and ankle. A drop in systolic pressure of 20 mm Hg identifies a zone of significant disease.

An ABI greater than 1.40 is associated with calcification of the arterial wall and may occur in patients with medial calcinosis, diabetes mellitus, or end-stage kidney disease. This finding is uninterpretable and is associated with worse cardiovascular outcomes than a normal ABI; therefore, an appropriate next step after this finding is to either measure great toe pressure or calculate a toe-brachial index (systolic great toe pressure divided by systolic brachial pressure), a test that is typically performed in a vascular laboratory. This patient's ABI is normal, so measurement of the toe-brachial index is not necessary.

KEY POINT

- Patients with pseudoclaudication (lumbar spinal stenosis) may report bilateral leg weakness associated with walking or with prolonged standing; symptoms are aggravated by prolonged standing and are relieved with bending at the waist.

Bibliography

Chou R, Qaseem A, Owens DK, Shekelle P; Clinical Guidelines Committee of the American College of Physicians. Diagnostic imaging for low back pain: advice for high-value health care from the American College of Physicians. Ann Intern Med. 2011 Feb 1;154(3):181-9. Erratum in: Ann Intern Med. 2012 Jan 3;156(1 Pt 1):71. [PMID: 21282698]

Item 95   Answer: A

Educational Objective: Manage acute decompensated systolic heart failure with diuretics.

In this patient with recently diagnosed heart failure, the dosage of furosemide should be increased. She has signs of volume overload (elevated central venous pressure, an S_3, peripheral edema, weight gain).

Given the patient's relative hypotension and volume overload, increasing her diuretic dose would be more appropriate than increasing the dose of her ACE inhibitor, which might lead to low blood pressure and would not improve her volume overload.

Although there is a mortality benefit to the use of β-blockers in patients with systolic heart failure, these agents have negative inotropic activity, and initiation of β-blocker therapy is relatively contraindicated in patients with evidence of decompensated heart failure. Once the patient has been appropriately diuresed, a β-blocker can be added. Even patients with a low systolic blood pressure, once euvolemic, can often tolerate low doses of a β-blocker.

Spironolactone is an appropriate agent to add for treatment of stable patients with New York Heart Association (NYHA) functional class II to IV heart failure. This patient, however, has acute volume overload, which should be treated before initiation of this therapy. Although spironolactone has some diuretic activity, at the usual doses prescribed for patients with heart failure (12.5-25 mg/d), it would not have sufficient diuretic effect in this patient.

This patient's presentation demonstrates the importance of an early (within 7 days) post-hospital clinic visit for patients after a hospitalization for heart failure. Recognizing volume overload at a point when it can be treated on an outpatient basis is an example of the benefit of this visit. If the patient were euvolemic, adding additional therapy, such as a β-blocker or spironolactone, would be appropriate. This visit also allows the internist to reemphasize to the patient the importance of medication adherence and fluid restriction.

KEY POINT

- In patients with acute decompensated systolic heart failure, the most appropriate treatment is to increase the diuretic dosage to remove the excess fluid.

Bibliography
Felker GM, Lee KL, Bull DA, et al; NHLBI Heart Failure Clinical Research Network. Diuretic strategies in patients with acute decompensated heart failure. N Engl J Med. 2011 Mar 3;364(9):797-805. [PMID: 21366472]

Item 96   Answer: A

Educational Objective: Treat a patient with patent foramen ovale and cryptogenic stroke with aspirin.

This patient has features of a cryptogenic stroke and patent foramen ovale (PFO). Antiplatelet therapy, such as aspirin, is first-line therapy for patients with PFO and initial cryptogenic stroke. The foramen ovale usually closes within the first few weeks of life. In 25% to 30% of the population, the foramen ovale remains patent. This is usually an incidental finding.

Data are insufficient to recommend PFO device closure for secondary stroke prevention after a first stroke unless there are exceptional circumstances, such as oxygen desaturation from right-to-left shunt or thrombus trapped in the PFO, or for patients with recurrent cryptogenic stroke on warfarin therapy. Overall, the PFO device closure procedure is safe and short-term complications are rare; however, evidence of long-term follow-up and benefit is lacking. Randomized controlled studies have failed to demonstrate superiority of closure over antiplatelet therapy for secondary prevention after cryptogenic stroke. Uncertainty persists regarding the best management strategy because of limitations of current randomized controlled studies; therefore, a reasonable consideration is to encourage participation in one of the ongoing clinical trials.

Data are insufficient to support warfarin therapy for patients with PFO and initial cryptogenic stroke. Warfarin is the treatment of choice for patients with PFO and recurrent stroke or for patients with stroke and a documented hypercoagulable state.

Surgical PFO closure, including a minimally invasive approach, is another option for patients with PFO and recurrent cryptogenic stroke but the efficacy of surgical closure in these patients has been variable and randomized trials have not been performed.

KEY POINT

- Antiplatelet therapy, such as aspirin, is first-line therapy for patients with patent foramen ovale and initial cryptogenic stroke.

Bibliography
Chen L, Luo S, Yan L, Zhao W. A systematic review of closure versus medical therapy for preventing recurrent stroke in patients with patent foramen ovale and cryptogenic stroke or transient ischemic attack. J Neurol Sci. 2014 Feb 15;337(1-2):3-7. [PMID: 24300230]

Item 97   Answer: D

Educational Objective: Manage a bicuspid aortic valve in an asymptomatic adult.

The most appropriate next step in management is to repeat the echocardiogram in 1 year. This patient has a bicuspid aortic valve and is asymptomatic. Patients with a bicuspid aortic valve should undergo surveillance transthoracic echocardiogram imaging of the aortic valve, aortic root, and ascending aorta to exclude aortic valve pathology and ascending aortic aneurysm, which are commonly associated with a bicuspid aortic valve and may be independent of the degree of aortic valve disease. This patient has mild aortic valve stenosis and a slightly dilated ascending aorta. If the aortic root or ascending aortic diameter is less than 4 cm, reimaging should be done approximately every 2 years. If the aortic root or ascending aortic diameter is greater than 4 cm, reimaging should occur yearly or more often as progression of aortic dilation warrants or whenever there is a change in clinical symptoms or findings.

Aortic valve replacement is recommended in asymptomatic patients with severe aortic valve stenosis, generally defined as a valve area below 1 cm², who may be at high risk without surgery. This patient does not have severe aortic valve stenosis, so aortic valve replacement is not necessary at this time.

Surgery to repair or replace the ascending aorta in adults with a bicuspid aortic valve is recommended when the ascending aorta diameter is greater than or equal to 5.5 cm or progressive dilatation occurs at a rate of 0.5 cm per year or greater.

Medical therapy has not been shown to reduce the rate of progression of aortic dilation in patients with aortopathy associated with bicuspid aortic valve. In patients with hypertension, control of blood pressure is essential. β-Blockers and angiotensin receptor blockers have conceptual advantages to reduce the rate of aneurysm progression but have not been shown to be beneficial in clinical studies.

KEY POINT

- Patients with an asymptomatic bicuspid aortic valve should undergo surveillance transthoracic echocardiography yearly if the aortic root or ascending aortic diameter is greater than 4 cm.

Bibliography

Siu SC, Silversides CK. Bicuspid aortic valve disease. J Am Coll Cardiol. 2010 Jun 22;55(25):2789-800. [PMID: 20579534]

Item 98   Answer: A

Educational Objective: Evaluate palpitations with a loop recorder.

This patient's symptomatic episodes are intermittent and short-lived; therefore, a 30-day wearable recorder with looping memory is the best diagnostic strategy to uncover the nature of her palpitations. These recorders are worn continuously and record a continuous "loop" of heart rhythm. When the patient experiences symptoms, she can depress a button and the device captures the rhythm before, during, and after the symptoms. Loop recorders are useful for recording episodes accompanied by syncope or presyncope and for episodes that are too short to be captured by a patient-triggered event recorder.

A patient-triggered event recorder (without looping memory) is useful for recording infrequent episodes that last long enough (1-2 minutes) for the patient to hold the device to the chest and trigger it to capture the heart rhythm. A self-applied event recorder is not useful for brief episodes because the time taken to apply the monitor may be longer than the symptomatic episode.

If a patient has an abnormal cardiovascular examination or is demonstrated to have an arrhythmia, echocardiography should be performed to evaluate for the presence of structural heart disease. In this patient, however, the cardiac examination is normal, and there is no documentation of an arrhythmia at this point. Many patients with symptoms suggestive of arrhythmia are found to have causes for their symptoms that are not related to heart rhythm.

An exercise treadmill stress test would be reasonable if the episodes were precipitated by exertion or exercise, but this patient's episodes are not associated with exertion.

Given the infrequency of this patient's symptoms, 48-hour ambulatory electrocardiographic monitoring is not likely to capture the symptomatic episodes.

In patients with very infrequent or rare episodes (>30 days between episodes), an implanted loop recorder may be appropriate. These devices, which are approximately the size of a pen cap and are implanted under the skin of the chest next to the sternum, have several years of battery life. Although they are invasive, these devices have a higher diagnostic yield than other forms of outpatient heart rhythm monitoring.

KEY POINT

- A looping event recorder is useful for recording episodes of palpitations that are accompanied by syncope or presyncope and for episodes that are too short to be captured by a patient-triggered event recorder.

Bibliography

Subbiah R, Gula LJ, Klein GJ, Skanes AC, Yee R, Krahn AD. Syncope: review of monitoring modalities. Curr Cardiol Rev. 2008 Feb;4(1):41-8. [PMID: 19924276]

Item 99   Answer: D

Educational Objective: Treat native valve infective endocarditis complicated by heart block.

The patient should undergo aortic valve replacement now. Although he is hemodynamically stable and does not require pacemaker support, the presence of a new conduction defect confirms extension of the infection into the perivalvular tissues as suggested by echocardiography. When this occurs, the effectiveness of cure with antibiotics alone is decreased significantly, and early surgical intervention is indicated. Other indications for early surgery in native valve infective endocarditis include valve stenosis or regurgitation resulting in heart failure; left-sided endocarditis caused by *Staphylococcus aureus*, fungal, or other highly resistant organisms; endocarditis complicated by annular or aortic abscess; and endocarditis with persistent bacteremia or fever lasting longer than 5 to 7 days after starting antibiotic therapy. Additionally, early surgery is reasonable in patients with infective endocarditis who have recurrent emboli and persistent vegetations on antibiotic therapy, and may be considered in patients with native valve endocarditis who have mobile vegetations greater than 10 mm in length.

Duration of antibiotic therapy in patients with native valve infective endocarditis is generally 4 to 6 weeks, based upon the specific organism, the site of infection, and any associated complications. Generally, 6-week treatment regimens are used in patients with more virulent or highly resistant organisms and those with cardiac or extracardiac infectious complications. Prolonged treatment for 3 months as therapy for this patient would not be appropriate, even with surgical intervention, and would not be indicated in other patients with native valve endocarditis except in certain situations.

Delaying intervention for 6 weeks of antibiotic therapy or treating with antibiotics alone without surgery would not likely adequately address this patient's endocarditis-related complications. In addition, this approach may result in further decompensation of the patient's clinical status and an increased operative risk for intervention at a later time.

Key to management of patients with infective endocarditis requiring surgery is a multidisciplinary approach involving the internist, cardiologist, infectious disease specialist, and cardiac surgeon.

KEY POINT

- The presence of a conduction block is an indication for surgical therapy in patients with native valve infective endocarditis.

Bibliography

Nishimura RA, Otto CM, Bonow RO, et al; American College of Cardiology/American Heart Association Task Force on Practice Guidelines. 2014 AHA/ACC guideline for the management of patients with valvular heart disease: executive summary: a report of the American College of Cardiology/American Heart Association Task Force on Practice Guidelines. J Am Coll Cardiol. 2014 Jun 10;63(22):2438-88. Erratum in: J Am Coll Cardiol. 2014 Jun 10;63(22):2489. [PMID: 24603192]

Item 100   Answer: A

Educational Objective: Treat an acute episode of supraventricular tachycardia.

This patient should be given adenosine. She has hemodynamically stable narrow-complex tachycardia consistent with supraventricular tachycardia. The rhythm is regular and no obvious P waves are visible; therefore, atrioventricular nodal reciprocating tachycardia (AVNRT) is the most likely cause. AVNRT accounts for up to two thirds of cases of supraventricular tachycardia. Patients often report neck pulsations, which are caused by simultaneous contraction of the atria and ventricles. Because the patient failed to terminate her tachycardia with vagal maneuvers, adenosine should be administered. Adenosine is highly effective at termination of nodal-dependent rhythms and can help identify the underlying etiology. For example, continued atrial activity (P waves) during atrioventricular block can help identify atrial flutter and atrial tachycardia. Patients given adenosine should be on a cardiac monitor with a running rhythm strip on paper to document the results. Prior to giving adenosine, patients should be warned that they may experience nausea, flushing, chest pain, or a sense of dread. Patients with bronchospastic lung disease should not receive adenosine.

Although amiodarone would be effective for terminating this patient's arrhythmia, it has many long-term risks, including thyroid, liver, pulmonary, and neurologic toxicity. In this young patient, amiodarone would not be an appropriate option.

Cardioversion is not indicated because the patient is hemodynamically stable, and pharmacologic attempts at cardioversion, such as adenosine, have not been attempted.

Ibutilide is an intravenous Vaughan-Williams class III antiarrhythmic drug FDA approved for pharmacologic cardioversion of atrial fibrillation. The patient has regular supraventricular tachycardia, not atrial fibrillation.

KEY POINT

- Patients with hemodynamically tolerated supraventricular tachycardia refractory to vagal maneuvers should be given adenosine.

Bibliography

Link MS. Clinical practice. Evaluation and initial treatment of supraventricular tachycardia. N Engl J Med. 2012 Oct 11;367(15):1438-48. [PMID: 23050527]

Item 101   Answer: C

Educational Objective: Manage dual antiplatelet therapy in a patient who had a non–ST-elevation myocardial infarction treated with a bare metal stent.

A full year of clopidogrel therapy is indicated in this patient who has sustained a non–ST-elevation myocardial infarction (NSTEMI). Clopidogrel added to aspirin improves outcomes after hospitalization in patients with NSTEMI regardless of the in-hospital treatment approach. Current recommendations from the American College of Cardiology and the American Heart Association state that all patients with an acute coronary syndrome (unstable angina, NSTEMI, or ST-elevation myocardial infarction) treated medically or with a stent (bare metal stent or drug-eluting stent) should be given $P2Y_{12}$ inhibitor therapy (for example, clopidogrel, prasugrel, or ticagrelor) in addition to aspirin for at least 12 months.

Patients who receive a stent in the absence of an acute coronary syndrome (that is, for stable angina pectoris) also require dual antiplatelet therapy with aspirin and clopidogrel until endothelialization of the stent is completed and the risk for acute stent thrombosis decreases. For a bare metal stent placed under these circumstances, clopidogrel should be continued for at least 1 month; for a drug-eluting stent, clopidogrel should be continued for at least 1 year. There is no indication for dual antiplatelet therapy for less than 1 month. Neither ticagrelor nor prasugrel has been studied extensively in patients undergoing coronary stent implantation for stable angina pectoris; therefore, these patients should be treated with clopidogrel in addition to aspirin.

KEY POINT

- Patients with an acute coronary syndrome should be treated with dual antiplatelet therapy (aspirin and a $P2Y_{12}$ inhibitor) for 1 year regardless of initial treatment approach.

Bibliography

2012 Writing Committee Members, Jneid H, Anderson JL, Wright RS, et al; American College of Cardiology Foundation; American Heart Association Task Force on Practice Guidelines. 2012 ACCF/AHA focused update of the guideline for the management of patients with unstable angina/Non-ST-elevation myocardial infarction (updating the 2007 guideline and replacing the 2011 focused update): a report of the American College of Cardiology Foundation/American Heart Association Task Force on practice guidelines. Circulation. 2012 Aug 14;126(7):875-910. [PMID: 22800849]

Item 102   Answer: A

Educational Objective: Recognize late complications in a cardiac transplant patient.

This patient should undergo coronary angiography. He underwent heart transplantation 10 years ago and presents with exertional dyspnea. The two most common causes of dyspnea in post–cardiac transplant patients are rejection and cardiac allograft vasculopathy. The prevalence of cardiac allograft vasculopathy is approximately 50% by year 5 post-transplant and is the most common cause of mortality in patients after the first year post-transplant. Because the transplanted heart is denervated at the time of transplant, vasculopathy and subsequent ischemia may occur without the classic symptoms of angina. Therefore, this diagnosis must be suspected in long-term transplant patients presenting with symptoms compatible with ischemia without chest pain. In this patient with exertional dyspnea 10 years after transplantation, the most likely cause is cardiac allograft vasculopathy, and therefore proceeding to coronary angiography to confirm the diagnosis is the appropriate next step.

Dobutamine stress echocardiography would be a reasonable option in lower-risk patients (such as those with a relatively recent coronary angiography study).

If the patient had undergone heart transplantation within the past year, the suspicion for rejection would be high. However, the incidence of rejection after the first year is low unless patients are not compliant with their immuno-suppressive medications. Therefore, endomyocardial biopsy to evaluate for rejection is not the most appropriate step.

Because of the patient's significant history of tobacco use, pulmonary function testing might be a reasonable con-sideration for evaluation of possible underlying lung disease. However, the rapid onset of respiratory symptoms in a pre-viously asymptomatic patient who is currently a nonsmoker would make this diagnosis less likely, and testing would not be appropriate before excluding a cardiac cause.

The transplanted heart is denervated, and without the normal vagal tone, a normal heart rate for transplant patients is between 90/min and 110/min. Because sinus tachycardia may also be present in patients with pulmonary embolism, it may be more difficult to assess tachycardia as a possible presenting sign in patients who are post-transplant. How-ever, this patient is not at increased risk for pulmonary embolism, and his heart rate of 102/min is not unusual and should not increase suspicion for this diagnosis. Therefore, a ventilation-perfusion lung scan to test for this possibility would not be an appropriate next step.

KEY POINT

- The most common cause of reduced left ventricular function in heart transplant patients after the first year is cardiac allograft vasculopathy.

Bibliography

Toyoda Y, Guy TS, Kashem A. Present status and future perspectives of heart transplantation. Circ J. 2013;77(5):1097-110. [PMID: 23614963]

Item 103   Answer: C

Educational Objective: Manage a patient with an implantable cardioverter-defibrillator undergoing surgery.

In this patient with an implantable cardioverter-defibrillator (ICD) with planned shoulder surgery, her ICD should be reprogrammed immediately before the procedure to asyn-chronous pacing with disabling of tachycardia detection and shocking function.

In any patient with a cardiac implanted electronic device, three fundamental questions must be answered in order to appropriately determine perioperative device man-agement. First, what type of device does the patient have (for example, pacemaker versus defibrillator)? Second, is the patient pacemaker dependent? Third, will the surgery be performed with instruments that result in electromagnetic interference in the vicinity of the device or its leads (for example, electrocautery)?

There is often confusion about pacemakers and defibrillators. An ICD is a pacemaker with extra capabil-ities (detection and treatment of a ventricular tachycar-dia or ventricular fibrillation). Management of the pacing and defibrillator functions may differ in specific clinical situations. For example, this patient can be considered pacemaker dependent given her history of complete heart block and atrioventricular sequential pacing on her elec-trocardiogram, requiring continued pacemaker function during surgery. However, her shoulder surgery will be in close proximity to her device and will increase the likeli-hood of electromagnetic interference that could alter both the pacing and defibrillator functions of her device. There-fore, in order to ensure adequate pacing and avoidance of shocks caused by electrical interference associated with instruments used during surgery, the device should be reprogrammed before the procedure.

Programming the device to asynchronous mode (DOO) will allow continued pacing of the atrium and ventricle but without the device sensing the cardiac response, thereby avoiding suppression of pacing due to electrical interference that the device might interpret as an elevated heart rate (that is, oversensing). Disabling the shock function will eliminate false detection of a tachyarrhythmia due to electrical inter-ference. However, not all patients with pacemaker depen-dence require asynchronous pacing during surgery, and guidelines for device management before, during, and after surgery continue to evolve. Because of this, it is advisable to consult with the patient's outpatient electrophysiologist in advance of surgery.

Disabling the shock function of an ICD is possible by applying an external magnetic field to the device. The change in function associated with the application of a magnet to an ICD differs from doing so to a pacemaker. Magnet application induces asynchronous pacing (pac-ing regardless of what is sensed) in pacemakers, whereas magnet application in ICDs disables the shocking function of the device without changing pacing programming. In this patient, although disabling the shocking function is appropriate, doing so will not change the device to an asynchronous mode.

Devices often need to be interrogated after surgery; however, this option is incorrect because reprogramming is needed in this patient before she can proceed to surgery. In any patient whose device is reprogrammed before surgery, the device should be interrogated after surgery and con-firmed to be "active."

Advising against surgery is incorrect. Patients with implanted cardiac devices can safely undergo surgery pro-vided the correct precautions are taken. Patients with acute arrhythmias may require stabilization, but in general, an implanted cardiac device in and of itself is not a contraindi-cation to surgery or invasive procedures.

In summary, this patient is pacemaker dependent, has an ICD, and is having surgery in the vicinity of her device. Therefore, the patient's ICD requires reprogramming to an asynchronous mode, disabling of the tachytherapies, and appropriate device interrogation and reprogramming after the surgery.

Answers and Critiques

KEY POINT

- Patients with an implantable cardioverter-defibrillator who are pacemaker dependent often require reprogramming of their device before surgery.

Bibliography

Crossley GH, Poole JE, Rozner MA, et al. The Heart Rhythm Society (HRS)/American Society of Anesthesiologists (ASA) Expert Consensus Statement on the perioperative management of patients with implantable defibrillators, pacemakers and arrhythmia monitors: facilities and patient management. This document was developed as a joint project with the American Society of Anesthesiologists (AS), and in collaboration with the American Heart Association (AHA), and the Society of Thoracic Surgeons (STS). Heart Rhythm. 2011 Jul;8(7):1114-54. [PMID: 21722856]

Item 104   Answer: B

Educational Objective: Diagnose ostium primum atrial septal defect.

The most likely diagnosis is ostium primum atrial septal defect (ASD). The patient has clinical features of an ASD, presenting with dyspnea, previous atrial fibrillation, and features of volume overload of the right heart with elevation of the central venous pressure and a right ventricular lift. A systolic murmur at the base results from increased flow across the right ventricular outflow tract from the left-to-right shunt. Fixed splitting of the S_2 throughout the cardiac cycle is a characteristic clinical feature of ASD. The apical systolic murmur is from mitral regurgitation and is related to the mitral valve cleft. The electrocardiogram demonstrates left axis deviation, first-degree atrioventricular block, and interventricular conduction delay. This combination of findings, including fixed splitting of S_2, mitral regurgitation murmur, and left axis deviation on the electrocardiogram, are most consistent with an ostium primum ASD.

Patients with coronary sinus ASD have features of right heart volume overload but do not have mitral valve disease and thus will not have a murmur of mitral regurgitation. The electrocardiogram may be normal or demonstrate first-degree atrioventricular block and incomplete right bundle branch block.

Patients with ostium secundum ASD have features of right heart volume overload but do not have mitral valve disease and thus will not have a murmur of mitral regurgitation. The electrocardiogram may be normal or demonstrate first-degree atrioventricular block and incomplete right bundle branch block. Left axis deviation on the electrocardiogram is not found in patients with an ostium secundum ASD.

Patients with patent foramen ovale have a normal echocardiogram and physical examination. These patients are also generally asymptomatic.

Patients with sinus venosus ASD have features of right heart volume overload but do not have mitral valve disease and thus will not have a murmur of mitral regurgitation. The electrocardiogram may be normal or demonstrate first-degree atrioventricular block and incomplete right bundle branch block.

KEY POINT

- Ostium primum atrial septal defect is characterized by the combination of fixed splitting of the S_2, a mitral regurgitation murmur, and left axis deviation on the electrocardiogram.

Bibliography

Warnes CA, Williams RG, Bashore TM, et al; American College of Cardiology; American Heart Association Task Force on Practice Guidelines (Writing Committee to Develop Guidelines on the Management of Adults With Congenital Heart Disease); American Society of Echocardiography; Heart Rhythm Society; International Society for Adult Congenital Heart Disease; Society for Cardiovascular Angiography and Interventions; Society of Thoracic Surgeons. ACC/AHA 2008 guidelines for the management of adults with congenital heart disease: a report of the American College of Cardiology/American Heart Association Task Force on Practice Guidelines (Writing Committee to Develop Guidelines on the Management of Adults With Congenital Heart Disease). Developed in Collaboration With the American Society of Echocardiography, Heart Rhythm Society, International Society for Adult Congenital Heart Disease, Society for Cardiovascular Angiography and Interventions, and Society of Thoracic Surgeons. J Am Coll Cardiol. 2008 Dec 2;52(23):e143-263. [PMID: 19038677]

Item 105   Answer: A   H

Educational Objective: Manage ventricular septal defect complicating myocardial infarction.

This patient has developed a clinically significant ventricular septal defect (VSD) and is in cardiogenic shock; he requires emergency surgery to repair the defect. VSD manifests as hemodynamic compromise in the setting of a new holosystolic murmur 3 to 7 days after an initial myocardial infarction (MI). Although surgical mortality is high, urgent cardiac surgery (coronary artery bypass grafting and VSD patch repair) offers the only chance of survival for patients with large post-infarction VSDs, especially in the presence of cardiogenic shock. There is no consensus on the optimal timing of surgery as early surgical repair is difficult because of infarcted myocardium, which is often friable and makes surgical closure of the septal defect difficult. There have been several reports of successful percutaneous closure of VSDs, but anatomy of the VSD and clinical expertise limit widespread use of this procedure in all patients.

Acute ventricular free wall rupture also occurs 3 to 7 days after MI and has a high mortality rate. Patients most commonly present with pericardial tamponade (due to hemopericardium), pulseless electrical activity, and death. Emergent pericardiocentesis and subsequent surgical reconstruction can improve survival. The echocardiographic findings in this patient did not reveal pericardial effusion or tamponade, and his presentation is consistent with VSD.

This patient has an occluded left anterior descending artery and persistent ST-segment elevation; however, the presence of hemodynamic compromise and echocardiographic evidence of VSD requires emergency cardiac surgery. Although coronary artery bypass grafting is usually performed during an attempted repair of the septal defect, percutaneous coronary intervention of the left anterior

H
CONT.

descending artery is not indicated once the VSD has been diagnosed.

The performance of right heart catheterization may aid in the diagnosis of VSD, and the use of a vasopressor such as dopamine may help initially stabilize the patient. However, this patient has a severe hemodynamic impairment and requires emergency cardiac surgery.

KEY POINT

- Urgent cardiac surgery offers the only chance of survival for patients with large postinfarction ventricular septal defects, especially in the presence of cardiogenic shock.

Bibliography

Van de Werf F, Bax J, Betriu, A, et al; ESC Committee for Practice Guidelines (CPG). Management of acute myocardial infarction in patients presenting with persistent ST-segment elevation: the Task Force on the Management of ST-Segment Elevation Acute Myocardial Infarction of the European Society of Cardiology. Eur Heart J. 2008 Dec;29(23):2909-45. [PMID: 19004841]

Item 106   Answer: A

Educational Objective: Treat a black patient with heart failure with hydralazine and isosorbide dinitrate in addition to usual therapy.

This patient should have hydralazine and isosorbide dinitrate added to her medication regimen for the treatment of her heart failure. She has New York Heart Association (NYHA) functional class III heart failure and is black. Hydralazine and isosorbide dinitrate have been demonstrated to improve symptoms and reduce mortality in patients who are black and who are already on maximal therapy with NYHA class III or IV heart failure symptoms. Adverse effects of this therapy include peripheral edema and headaches, but this regimen should be attempted in these patients.

Optimal therapy for patients with heart failure includes treatment with an ACE inhibitor, β-blocker, and an aldosterone antagonist. The addition of an angiotensin receptor blocker, such as losartan, to this combination is generally not recommended, primarily because of concern for hyperkalemia. Additionally, no benefit to this treatment regimen has been documented. It would therefore not be appropriate in this patient.

In patients with heart failure, warfarin treatment is appropriate only in those with another indication, such as atrial fibrillation meeting CHA_2DS_2-VASc criteria, but not with heart failure alone. The routine treatment of patients with heart failure with warfarin is not indicated.

Cardiac resynchronization therapy (CRT) may be an effective therapy in patients with heart failure and a prolonged QRS duration indicating dyssynchrony. Indications include a left ventricular ejection fraction of 35% or less in patients in sinus rhythm, with a left bundle branch block, and with a QRS duration of 150 ms or greater in whom moderate to severe symptoms (NYHA class III or IV) are present despite optimal medical therapy. Because this patient does not have evidence of dyssynchrony or an ejection fraction of 35% or less, she is not a candidate for treatment.

KEY POINT

- Hydralazine and isosorbide dinitrate improve symptoms and reduce mortality in patients with New York Heart Association class III or IV heart failure symptoms who are black and are already on maximal therapy.

Bibliography

Flack JM, Sica DA, Bakris G, et al; International Society on Hypertension in Blacks. Management of high blood pressure in Blacks: an update of the International Society on Hypertension in Blacks consensus statement. Hypertension. 2010 Nov;56(5):780-800. [PMID: 20921433]

Item 107   Answer: D   **H**

Educational Objective: Evaluate for suspected perivalvular abscess in a patient with infective endocarditis.

This patient should undergo transesophageal echocardiography (TEE). He has evidence of a new conduction defect on electrocardiogram suggesting a possible perivalvular abscess complicating *Staphylococcus aureus* infective endocarditis. Perivalvular abscesses may be present in 30% to 40% of patients with infective endocarditis, and the risk may be further increased in those with a bicuspid aortic valve. The diagnosis should be considered in patients with persistent bacteremia, fever, or evidence of conduction system disorders who are being treated with appropriate antibiotic therapy. TEE has a high sensitivity and specificity for identifying perivalvular extension of infection and is the diagnostic study of choice when a perivalvular abscess is suspected.

Cardiac CT has not been extensively studied for use in diagnosing myocardial infection and is not typically used for this purpose. Cardiac magnetic resonance (CMR) imaging, however, is effective in identifying intramyocardial infection, although it is a more complex technology that may have limited availability in some areas. CMR imaging is often used in situations in which a perivalvular abscess is suspected but transesophageal echocardiography is equivocal.

Evidence of a conduction system disorder may be the only indicator of a perivalvular abscess in a patient otherwise responding clinically to treatment for infective endocarditis, as in this patient. Because of the significance of this possible complication, failure to further evaluate conduction system abnormalities in this setting would be inappropriate.

Although transthoracic echocardiography is effective for initial evaluation for endocarditis and assessing for potential complications once endocarditis has been diagnosed (such as valvular or left ventricular dysfunction), TEE is significantly more sensitive for detecting perivalvular abscess because of the closer proximity of the ultrasound probe to the valve structures. It is therefore preferred to transthoracic echocardiography if this diagnosis is a consideration.

KEY POINT

- Transesophageal echocardiography is the diagnostic study of choice in patients with a possible perivalvular abscess complicating infective endocarditis.

Bibliography

American College of Cardiology Foundation Appropriate Use Criteria Task Force; American Society of Echocardiography; American Heart Association; American Society of Nuclear Cardiology; Heart Failure Society of America; Heart Rhythm Society; Society for Cardiovascular Angiography and Interventions; Society of Critical Care Medicine; Society of Cardiovascular Computed Tomography; Society for Cardiovascular Magnetic Resonance, Douglas PS, Garcia MJ, Haines DE, et al. ACCF/ASE/AHA/ASNC/HFSA/HRS/SCAI/SCCM/SCCT/SCMR 2011 Appropriate Use Criteria for Echocardiography. A Report of the American College of Cardiology Foundation Appropriate Use Criteria Task Force, American Society of Echocardiography, American Heart Association, American Society of Nuclear Cardiology, Heart Failure Society of America, Heart Rhythm Society, Society for Cardiovascular Angiography and Interventions, Society of Critical Care Medicine, Society of Cardiovascular Computed Tomography, and Society for Cardiovascular Magnetic Resonance Endorsed by the American College of Chest Physicians. J Am Coll Cardiol. 2011 Mar 1;57(9):1126–66. [PMID: 21349406]

Item 108   Answer: B

Educational Objective: Diagnose upper extremity peripheral arterial disease.

Measurement of systolic blood pressure in both arms is indicated in this patient at high risk for atherosclerotic cardiovascular disease (ASCVD) who likely has upper extremity peripheral arterial disease (PAD) as the cause of his symptoms. His extremity symptoms are consistent with impaired arterial blood flow with exertion causing claudication in the left arm, and his associated neurologic symptoms suggest the subclavian steal syndrome. In subclavian steal, a stenosis in the left subclavian artery proximal to the take-off of the vertebral artery results in retrograde blood flow from the central nervous system to the arm, resulting in neurologic symptoms. A hallmark feature of upper extremity PAD on physical examination is a difference in systolic blood pressures between the arms, with a differential of greater than 15 mm Hg being typical. Differences in the distal pulses (upstroke and duration) may also be noted when comparing the upper extremities, and a bruit detected over the subclavian artery may be present. Noninvasive vascular testing with Doppler ultrasonography may be confirmatory. Upper extremity PAD, whether symptomatic or asymptomatic, is a marker for significant ASCVD and is associated with an increased risk for future cardiovascular disease. Therefore, primary treatment is aggressive therapy for ASCVD, including antiplatelet therapy. Treatment for clinically symptomatic upper extremity PAD, as in this patient, may include angioplasty with stenting or surgical bypass.

The ankle-brachial index is used to assess for lower extremity PAD and might be abnormal in this patient with likely ASCVD, although this test would not be helpful in evaluating his upper extremity symptoms.

Pulsus paradoxus is an exaggerated drop in systolic blood pressure (>10 mm Hg) during inspiration and may be present in patients with severe pericardial disease (tampon-

ade and occasionally constrictive pericarditis), asthma, and COPD. This patient, however, does not have a history suggestive of these disorders, and evaluation for pulsus paradoxus would not be diagnostically helpful.

Thoracic outlet maneuvers are used to evaluate for neurovascular impingement at the point where the upper extremity neurovascular bundle exits the thoracic cavity. Although thoracic outlet syndrome could be responsible for his vascular symptoms, the obstruction occurring with this syndrome is distal to the vertebral artery and would not explain his accompanying neurologic symptoms.

KEY POINT

- A hallmark feature of upper extremity peripheral arterial disease on physical examination is a difference in systolic blood pressures between the arms (typically >15 mm Hg).

Bibliography

Clark CE, Taylor RS, Shore AC, Ukoumunne OC, Campbell JL. Association of a difference in systolic blood pressure between arms with vascular disease and mortality: a systematic review and meta-analysis. Lancet. 2012 Mar 10;379(9819):905–14. Erratum in: Lancet. 2012 Jul 21;380(9838):218. [PMID: 22293369]

Item 109   Answer: D

Educational Objective: Manage first-degree atrioventricular block accompanied by bifascicular block.

No intervention is indicated. This octogenarian has first-degree atrioventricular (AV) block (PR interval >200 ms), right bundle branch block, and left posterior fascicular block. The combination of first-degree AV block and bifascicular block is often referred to as "trifascicular block," although this term is not correct because true trifascicular block would imply complete AV block. There is no indication for pacing in patients with first-degree AV block and bifascicular block who have no symptoms due to bradycardia. The risk of this type of block progressing to complete heart block is less than 2% to 3% per year.

The patient is asymptomatic, has no evidence of left ventricular dysfunction, and no clinical evidence of ischemia. Therefore, stress testing, including adenosine perfusion imaging, is not indicated. Because right coronary artery ischemia can cause paroxysms of bradycardia, stress testing for ischemia may be indicated in patients with paroxysmal bradycardia or clinical findings suggestive of ischemia, neither of which is present in this patient. In patients in whom symptomatic bradycardia is a concern, treadmill stress testing may be helpful in evaluating whether there is an appropriate chronotropic response to exercise.

Permanent pacing is only indicated in two clinical situations. First, pacemakers are indicated in patients with symptomatic bradycardia in the absence of a reversible cause. Second, pacemakers are indicated in patients with evidence of AV conduction disturbances that have a high likelihood of progression to complete heart block or life-threatening sudden asystole. Second-degree Mobitz II block, alternating bundle branch block, atrial fibrillation with pauses greater than 5 seconds, and complete heart block are all indications for permanent pacing. This patient has none of these conditions, and neither dual-chamber nor single-chamber pacing is indicated.

KEY POINT

- Asymptomatic first-degree atrioventricular block with bifascicular block does not require pacemaker implantation.

Bibliography

Epstein AE, DiMarco JP, Ellenbogen KA, et al; American College of Cardiology/American Heart Association Task Force on Practice Guidelines (Writing Committee to Revise the ACC/AHA/NASPE 2002 Guideline Update for Implantation of Cardiac Pacemakers and Antiarrhythmia Devices); American Association for Thoracic Surgery; Society of Thoracic Surgeons. ACC/AHA/HRS 2008 Guidelines for Device-Based Therapy of Cardiac Rhythm Abnormalities: a report of the American College of Cardiology/American Heart Association Task Force on Practice Guidelines (Writing Committee to Revise the ACC/AHA/NASPE 2002 Guideline Update for Implantation of Cardiac Pacemakers and Antiarrhythmia Devices): developed in collaboration with the American Association for Thoracic Surgery and Society of Thoracic Surgeons. Circulation. 2008 May 27;117(21):e350-408. Erratum in: Circulation. 2009 Aug 4; 120(5):e34-5. [PMID: 18483207]

Item 110   Answer: D

Educational Objective: Manage secondary risk reduction in a patient with established coronary artery disease.

The intervention that offers the greatest cardiovascular risk reduction for this patient is to start an ACE inhibitor for secondary prevention after myocardial infarction (MI) and to reduce systolic blood pressure. ACE inhibitors have been shown to decrease both cardiovascular and all-cause mortality in patients with chronic ischemic heart disease, especially in those patients with prior MI, left ventricular systolic dysfunction, or heart failure. Guidelines from the American College of Physicians/American College of Cardiology Foundation/American Heart Association recommend a treatment goal of 140/90 mm Hg or below in patients with stable ischemic coronary heart disease. Although previous guidelines recommended treatment to reduce blood pressure to below 130/80 mm Hg, there is limited evidence to show a benefit of doing so, with the potential for adverse consequences owing to overtreatment of blood pressure in these patients. The 2014 Eighth Joint National Commission (JNC-8) report does not provide specific recommendations for treatment of patients with established atherosclerotic disease, although the recommended threshold for treatment for all patients younger than 60 years is also 140/90 mm Hg. Therefore, this patient would be expected to benefit from therapy to decrease her blood pressure to at least 140/90 mm Hg or below.

While there is observational evidence from the GISSI (Gruppo Italiano per lo Studio della Sopravvivenza nell'Infarto Miocardico) Prevention study that patients with prior MI who take fish oil have a 20% reduction in mortality rate, the current American College of Cardiology/American Heart Association guidelines do not currently provide recommendations for use of fish oil after MI. Fish oil is effective in reducing triglyceride levels; however, this patient's triglyceride levels are normal.

Recently released guidelines recommend treatment of patients with established atherosclerotic disease with a high-intensity statin with a goal of lowering the LDL cholesterol level to less than 50% of the baseline level but without treatment to a specific LDL cholesterol level. As this patient has had the expected decrease in LDL cholesterol level on her present regimen, the addition of another agent for managing dyslipidemia, such as niacin, would not be appropriate.

Although moderate alcohol consumption (approximately one to three drinks daily) is associated with a lower risk of coronary heart disease, excessive alcohol intake accounts for approximately 4% of cases of dilated cardiomyopathy. However, reducing this patient's current level of alcohol consumption will not reduce her risk of a future cardiovascular event.

KEY POINT

- Patients with prior myocardial infarction should receive an ACE inhibitor for secondary cardiovascular prevention.

Bibliography

Qaseem A, Fihn SD, Dallas P, Williams S, Owens DK, Shekelle P; Clinical Guidelines Committee of the American College of Physicians. Management of stable ischemic heart disease: summary of a clinical practice guideline from the American College of Physicians/American College of Cardiology Foundation/American Heart Association/American Association for Thoracic Surgery/Preventive Cardiovascular Nurses Association/Society of Thoracic Surgeons. Ann Intern Med. 2012 Nov 20;157(10):735-43. [PMID: 23165665]

Item 111   Answer: A

Educational Objective: Manage revascularization in a patient with an acute coronary syndrome with a high TIMI risk score and multivessel disease.

This patient should undergo coronary artery bypass graft (CABG) surgery. In patients with a non–ST-elevation acute coronary syndrome (unstable angina or non–ST-elevation myocardial infarction), the TIMI risk score is used to determine whether a conservative strategy or an early invasive strategy is warranted. This patient has several TIMI risk factors, including aspirin use in the past week, ST-segment deviation, elevated biomarkers, more than three traditional coronary artery disease (CAD) risk factors, and documented CAD with greater than or equal to 50% diameter stenosis; therefore, an early invasive strategy is warranted. In this patient, an oral P2Y$_{12}$ inhibitor (clopidogrel, prasugrel, ticagrelor) was not administered, but if this had been given, the surgery should be delayed 5 days to allow discontinuation and excretion of the antiplatelet medication.

Intra-aortic balloon pump placement may be considered for patients with recurrent cardiac ischemia and poor left ventricular function. However, although this patient had recurrent chest pain during hospitalization, his symptoms improved with intravenous nitroglycerin and medical therapy, and he

CONT.

has remained hemodynamically stable. Therefore, intra-aortic balloon pump placement is not indicated.

Because this patient has multivessel disease and a reduced left ventricular ejection fraction, he should undergo CABG rather than percutaneous coronary intervention.

In patients with left main coronary artery stenosis, depressed left ventricular function, and an acute coronary syndrome, the optimal treatment strategy includes revascularization rather than medical therapy.

KEY POINT

- Patients with multivessel coronary disease and a reduced left ventricular ejection fraction should undergo coronary artery bypass graft surgery rather than percutaneous coronary intervention.

Bibliography

Amsterdam EA, Wenger NK, Brindis RG, et al; ACC/AHA Task Force Members. 2014 AHA/ACC guideline for the management of patients with non-ST-elevation acute coronary syndromes: executive summary: a report of the American College of Cardiology/American Heart Association Task Force on Practice Guidelines. Circulation. 2014 Dec 23;130(25):2354-94. [PMID: 25249586]

Item 112   Answer: C

Educational Objective: Treat a patient with severe calcific aortic stenosis and aortic regurgitation with surgical valve replacement.

This patient should undergo surgical aortic valve replacement. Surgical aortic valve replacement is the only treatment of aortic stenosis associated with a survival benefit and durable symptom relief. Surgical aortic valve replacement is the treatment of choice for most patients with symptomatic severe aortic stenosis and is associated with low mortality rates for patients younger than 70 years (1%-3%).

Aortic valve repair is an option in a limited number of adult patients with aortic valve disease. In general, it is restricted to patients with aortic regurgitation and anatomically favorable aortic valve and root anatomy and can range from simple cusp plication to complex valve-sparing aortic root replacement. This patient has severe calcific aortic stenosis and a valve that is unlikely to be amenable to repair.

Balloon valvuloplasty, although important in the treatment of pediatric patients with severe aortic stenosis, has a more limited role in adults, either as a bridge to definitive treatment, to differentiate dyspnea symptoms in high-risk patients with comorbid conditions such as COPD, or to treat patients with calcific aortic stenosis with hemodynamic instability or decompensation. While balloon valvuloplasty is a potential consideration for this patient, the presence of significant aortic regurgitation is a contraindication. Improvement in aortic valve area from this procedure is modest, and many patients have residual severe aortic stenosis immediately after valvuloplasty. Balloon valvuloplasty would not be the best option for this patient.

Transcatheter aortic valve replacement (TAVR) is indicated for patients with severe symptomatic aortic stenosis who are considered unsuitable for conventional surgery because of severe comorbidities. Candidates for TAVR must be carefully selected. Surgical risk should be assessed objectively, such as by using the Society of Thoracic Surgeons adult cardiac risk score (STS score) (http://riskcalc.sts.org/STSWebRiskCalc273/de.aspx). Patients with an STS risk score of greater than or equal to 8% may be candidates for TAVR. In addition, TAVR is not approved in patients with concomitant valve disease (such as significant aortic regurgitation or mitral valve disease) and a bicuspid aortic valve. This patient has a bicuspid aortic valve and moderate aortic regurgitation; therefore, she would not be a candidate for TAVR.

KEY POINT

- Surgical aortic valve replacement is the treatment of choice for most patients with symptomatic severe aortic stenosis and is associated with low mortality rates for patients younger than 70 years (1%-3%).

Bibliography

Lindman BR, Bonow RO, Otto CM. Current management of calcific aortic stenosis. Circ Res. 2013 Jul 5;113(2):223-37. [PMID: 23833296]

Item 113   Answer: D

Educational Objective: Diagnose a left atrial myxoma.

This patient most likely has a myxoma that is causing her symptoms and clinical findings. Left atrial myxomas are the most common benign tumors of the heart. These lesions can cause constitutional symptoms, such as fatigue, dyspnea, fever, and weight loss, related to tumor cytokine production; systemic embolization from either tumor fragments or associated thrombi may cause neurologic symptoms or other systemic sequelae. Left atrial myxomas most commonly appear as a mass arising from the atrial septum; the mass can involve the mitral valve intermittently to cause a "tumor plop" that may clinically mimic mitral stenosis. Myxomas may occur as part of the Carney complex, which is an autosomal dominant disorder associated with pigmentation abnormalities (such as blue nevi), schwannomas, and endocrine tumors.

Metastatic adenocarcinoma with cardiac involvement can manifest from direct invasion or hematogenous spread, with symptoms and signs dependent on the site of involvement. Metastatic adenocarcinoma with cardiac involvement, although common in patients with this tumor type (15% of patient at autopsy), would be less likely in this patient given the isolated anatomic location and recent negative malignancy screening results.

Angiosarcomas are malignant tumors that can occur in the atria but are less common than myxomas and typically infiltrate the myocardium, which is normal in this patient.

Lipomas typically are located in the subendocardium, not the atrium, and rarely cause symptoms.

Papillary fibroelastomas, like myxomas, can be mobile with a pedunculated stalk. However, they most commonly arise on left-sided cardiac valves and the left ventricular outflow tract.

KEY POINT

- The most common benign tumors of the heart, left atrial myxomas can cause constitutional symptoms, such as fatigue, dyspnea, fever, and weight loss, related to tumor cytokine production and neurologic symptoms related to systemic embolization from either tumor fragments or associated thrombi.

Bibliography

Shapiro LM. Cardiac tumours: diagnosis and management. Heart. 2001 Feb;85(2):218-22. [PMID: 11156679]

Item 114   Answer: B

Educational Objective: Manage acute pericarditis on an outpatient basis.

This patient should receive clinical follow-up without hospital admission or further diagnostic testing to monitor her response to therapy, evaluate for possible complications, and assess the timing for tapering her medications. Slow tapering over 2 to 4 weeks after initial presentation with improvement in symptoms is usually performed to reduce the risk of recurrent inflammation.

The vast majority of patients with acute pericarditis, including the patient presented, can be managed medically on an outpatient basis. For a subset of patients, high-risk features of acute pericarditis may be present and warrant hospitalization for treatment and monitoring for possible complications; these include fever, leukocytosis, acute trauma, abnormal cardiac biomarkers, an immunocompromised host, oral anticoagulant use, large pericardial effusions, or evidence of cardiac tamponade.

CT can be used to show pericardial thickening in patients with acute pericarditis. However, this finding would not change the diagnosis or appropriate management strategy in this patient.

Medical therapy with anti-inflammatory agents is appropriate for acute pericarditis. However, glucocorticoids are reserved for patients who do not respond to NSAIDs, such as ibuprofen, aspirin, and indomethacin, none of which has been tried yet in this patient. Glucocorticoid therapy may also increase the risk of recurrent pericarditis and should only be considered in highly selected patients with refractory pericarditis.

Pericardiocentesis is indicated only for patients with tamponade or for those in whom the analysis of pericardial fluid can be of assistance in diagnosis and management. Signs of tamponade are not present in this patient whose inferior vena cava is normal in size on echocardiography, whose Doppler ultrasound shows minimal change in mitral inflow with respiration, and whose bedside maneuvers reveal no pulsus paradoxus.

KEY POINT

- Patients with acute pericarditis who do not have high-risk features (fever, leukocytosis, acute trauma, abnormal cardiac biomarkers, immunocompromise, oral anticoagulant use, large pericardial effusions, or evidence of cardiac tamponade) can be managed medically on an outpatient basis with close clinical follow-up.

Bibliography

Imazio M, Brucato A, Cemin R, et al; ICAP Investigators. A randomized trial of colchicine for acute pericarditis. N Engl J Med. 2013 Oct 17;369(16):1522-8. [PMID: 23992557]

Item 115   Answer: C

Educational Objective: Manage a patient with Wolff-Parkinson-White syndrome with syncope.

This patient should undergo an electrophysiology study. He has evidence of pre-excitation on his electrocardiogram with a history of palpitations and syncope. The slurring of the QRS complex (delta wave) represents early ventricular depolarization owing to conduction over the accessory pathway (bypass tract). The presence of a delta wave and symptoms of tachycardia are consistent with Wolff-Parkinson-White syndrome. The episodes could be caused by supraventricular tachycardia (orthodromic or antidromic reciprocating tachycardia) or pre-excited atrial fibrillation. The presence of syncope suggests that these episodes are hemodynamically significant. Identification of syncope in a patient with Wolff-Parkinson-White syndrome should prompt referral to a cardiologist or electrophysiologist.

An electrophysiology study would allow diagnosis of the cause of this patient's palpitations and allow risk stratification for risk of sudden cardiac death. The electrophysiology procedure also affords the opportunity to ablate the accessory pathway and potentially cure his arrhythmia. Stress testing can be an appropriate method for risk stratification in patients with asymptomatic pre-excitation; however, this patient clearly has symptoms and therefore should undergo invasive testing and ablation.

Antiarrhythmic drug therapy is not indicated in this patient because the type and mechanism of the arrhythmia are not known. Catheter ablation is preferred in young persons with Wolff-Parkinson-White syndrome in order to avoid lifelong use of potentially toxic medications. Antiarrhythmic agents are reserved for second-line therapy, particularly in patients with accessory pathways located close to the atrioventricular (AV) node.

Metoprolol and diltiazem are AV nodal blockers and may be unsafe if the patient has anterograde conduction down the accessory pathway during atrial fibrillation. These drugs can block the AV node and promote rapid 1:1 conduction from the atrium to the ventricle during atrial fibrillation and thus induce ventricular fibrillation. AV nodal blockers are contraindicated in patients with pre-excited atrial fibrillation, such as this patient.

KEY POINT

- Identification of syncope in a patient with pre-excitation should prompt referral to a cardiologist or electrophysiologist.

Bibliography

Delacrétaz E. Clinical practice. Supraventricular tachycardia. N Engl J Med. 2006 Mar 9;354(10):1039-51. [PMID: 16525141]

Item 116   Answer: C

Educational Objective: Consider reversible causes in the evaluation of heart failure.

The most appropriate diagnostic test to perform in this young patient with new-onset heart failure is to obtain thyroid studies. This patient exhibits signs and symptoms consistent with a diagnosis of hyperthyroidism, including tachycardia, a hyperdynamic precordium, palpitations, weight loss, and loose stools. Hyperthyroidism is a well-described, reversible cause of heart failure due to cardiac overstimulation by excess thyroid hormone that resembles sympathetic stimulation. Hyperthyroidism causes an increase in heart rate and myocardial contractility; systemic vascular resistance often decreases and may result in a widened pulse pressure. Hypothyroidism is also a known cause of heart failure, although it would be less likely in this patient with symptoms more consistent with excess thyroid hormone. Because thyroid function abnormalities are a potentially reversible cause of heart failure, assessment of thyroid function should be considered in patients with new-onset heart failure and clinical findings suggestive of thyroid dysfunction.

Evaluation of unusual causes of heart failure should not be performed routinely but should be pursued when there are suggestions of specific diseases by history or physical examination. The patient has no signs or symptoms suggesting a rheumatologic disorder, and routine screening with an antinuclear antibody level is not indicated. Similarly, this patient does not have a history of flu-like symptoms suggesting a viral etiology, making the potential yield of viral titers quite low. Furthermore, directed treatment options in the presence of positive viral titers are quite limited.

Endomyocardial biopsy is rarely indicated in the evaluation of acute heart failure as it is invasive and is unlikely to be helpful in identifying a reversible cause. It may be considered in patients whose heart failure is unresponsive to medical therapy or is associated with ventricular arrhythmias or conduction block in order to evaluate for giant cell myocarditis.

KEY POINT

- Evaluation of unusual causes of heart failure should not be performed routinely but should be performed when there are suggestions of specific diseases by history or physical examination findings.

Bibliography

Fermann GJ, Collins SP. Initial management of patients with acute heart failure. Heart Fail Clin. 2013 Jul;9(3):291-301, vi. [PMID: 23809416]

Item 117   Answer: B

Educational Objective: Appropriately perform surveillance imaging in a patient with Marfan syndrome and aortic root dilation.

This patient with Marfan syndrome should undergo surveillance imaging annually. Dilation of the ascending aorta is a systemic feature of Marfan syndrome, and the most life-threatening complication of Marfan syndrome is aortic aneurysm, which can lead to an acute aortic syndrome (aortic dissection, rupture, or both). Accordingly, examination of the ascending aorta and heart valves is mandatory in patients with Marfan syndrome. The severity of aortic disease is in relation to the extent of aortic dilation, the length of the dilated segment, and the location of aortic involvement. Most patients with Marfan syndrome present with enlargement of the ascending aorta; therefore, serial examination is focused mainly on assessing this portion of aorta. American College of Cardiology Foundation/American Heart Association guidelines recommend follow-up imaging 6 months after diagnosis, with annual surveillance thereafter if the aortic root is less than 4.5 cm in diameter and otherwise stable. This threshold is lower than for patients with an aortic aneurysm due to other causes because of the tendency for complications in patients with Marfan syndrome with an aortic root diameter above this level. If the aortic root diameter is 4.5 cm or greater or if the aortic root diameter shows significant growth from baseline, more frequent imaging of the aorta should be considered.

Imaging of the aortic root in patients with Marfan syndrome is usually performed with transthoracic ultrasound because it is able to accurately evaluate this portion of the aorta and is noninvasive. However, for aneurysms above the aortic root, CT or MRI is preferred as they more accurately measure the aortic dimensions in that region.

KEY POINT

- In patients with Marfan syndrome and aortic root dilation, surveillance imaging should be performed 6 months after diagnosis and annually thereafter if the aortic size remains stable.

Bibliography

Hiratzka LF, Bakris GL, Beckman JA, et al; American College of Cardiology Foundation/American Heart Association Task Force on Practice Guidelines; American Association for Thoracic Surgery; American College of Radiology; American Stroke Association; Society of Cardiovascular Anesthesiologists; Society for Cardiovascular Angiography and Interventions; Society of Interventional Radiology; Society of Thoracic Surgeons; Society for Vascular Medicine. 2010 ACCF/AHA/AATS/ACR/ASA/SCA/SCAI/SIR/STS/SVM guidelines for the diagnosis and management of patients with Thoracic Aortic Disease: a report of the American College of Cardiology Foundation/American Heart Association Task Force on Practice Guidelines, American Association for Thoracic Surgery, American College of Radiology, American Stroke Association, Society of Cardiovascular Anesthesiologists, Society for Cardiovascular Angiography and Interventions, Society of Interventional Radiology, Society of Thoracic Surgeons, and Society for Vascular Medicine. Circulation. 2010 Apr 6;121(13):e266-369. Erratum in: Circulation. 2010 Jul 27;122(4):e410. [PMID: 20233780]

Item 118   Answer: B

Educational Objective: Manage a patient with a high-risk score on exercise treadmill testing with cardiac catheterization.

This patient's exercise electrocardiographic (ECG) stress testing results indicate that he has coronary artery disease (CAD), and his Duke treadmill score (-11.5) indicates the presence of high-risk disease. He should undergo cardiac catheterization for diagnosis and possibly revascularization.

Exercise ECG stress testing can be used for the diagnosis of CAD (as in this patient), to evaluate adequacy of medical therapy in patients with known CAD, and to evaluate functional status. When used to evaluate chest pain, the test is considered diagnostic of obstructive CAD (>70% obstruction) if there is greater than 1-mm ST-segment depression with exercise in two contiguous leads. The findings in this patient are consistent with occlusive coronary disease as the cause of his exertional chest pain.

In addition to diagnosis, a positive treadmill study can be used to further risk stratify obstructive CAD. The Duke treadmill score is one method and is calculated as follows: Exercise time in minutes - (5 × ST-segment depression) - (4 × angina score). (Angina score: 0 = asymptomatic; 1 = nonlimiting angina; 2 = exercise-limiting angina.) Scores below -11 are high risk, and those above 5 are low risk. Patients with high-risk scores are likely to have left main or proximal left anterior descending (LAD) artery disease. Other markers of a high-risk exercise study that would be suggestive of proximal LAD artery disease or multi-vessel disease would include a drop in blood pressure with exercise or severe ST-segment depression. Based on his high-risk Duke treadmill score, this patient should be further evaluated with coronary arteriography.

Although this patient should be treated with medical therapy including aspirin, a β-blocker, and a statin, he should also undergo cardiac catheterization because of the high likelihood of severe obstructive CAD.

The use of imaging, such as stress echocardiography or myocardial perfusion imaging, can localize ischemia to a vascular territory and can be helpful to determine affected vascular territory prior to revascularization. Stress testing with imaging can also be helpful in making the diagnosis of CAD in patients with equivocal exercise stress tests or those in whom there is a higher likelihood of a false-positive exercise stress test. However, because

of this patient's high-risk ECG stress test, he should undergo catheterization for a definitive diagnosis and possible revascularization. There would be no benefit to a noninvasive imaging test prior to or instead of that intervention.

KEY POINT

- Cardiac catheterization is indicated in patients with a positive electrocardiographic stress test and findings indicative of high-risk coronary artery disease.

Bibliography

Mark DB, Hlatky MA, Harrell FE Jr, Lee KL, Califf RM, Pryor DB. Exercise treadmill score for predicting prognosis in coronary artery disease. Ann Intern Med. 1987 Jun;106(6):793-800. [PMID: 3579066]

Item 119   Answer: C

Educational Objective: Diagnose peripartum cardiomyopathy.

The most likely diagnosis in this woman who gave birth 2 weeks ago is peripartum cardiomyopathy. Peripartum cardiomyopathy is left ventricular systolic dysfunction identified toward the end of pregnancy or in the months following delivery in the absence of another identifiable cause. This occurs with increased frequency in women with a history of preeclampsia. Patients may be asymptomatic or present with features of heart failure. Prompt initiation of medical therapy is recommended for women with peripartum cardiomyopathy and includes an ACE inhibitor or an angiotensin receptor blocker (after delivery), β-blockers, digoxin, hydralazine, nitrates, and diuretics.

Pulmonary embolism can occur postpartum, particularly if prolonged bed rest is required in the peripartum period. Although both pulmonary embolism and heart failure frequently are marked by dyspnea, this patient's presentation is more indicative of heart failure, with pulmonary congestion and elevated central venous pressure.

Most patients with ischemic cardiomyopathy have symptomatic coronary artery disease, abnormal electrocardiographic findings demonstrating previous myocardial infarction, or regional hypokinesis on echocardiography. These findings are absent in this patient.

Stress-induced cardiomyopathy (takotsubo cardiomyopathy) is characterized by transient cardiac dysfunction with ventricular apical ballooning, usually triggered by intense emotional or physical stress, although in several published cases, no trigger was identifiable. The presenting clinical picture may mimic an acute coronary syndrome, with chest pain, mildly elevated cardiac enzyme levels, and electrocardiographic changes consistent with ischemia. The patient's clinical presentation is not consistent with stress cardiomyopathy.

Answers and Critiques

KEY POINT

- Peripartum cardiomyopathy is left ventricular systolic dysfunction identified toward the end of pregnancy or in the months following delivery in the absence of another identifiable cause.

Bibliography

Sliwa K, Hilfiker-Kleiner D, Petrie MC, et al; Heart Failure Association of the European Society of Cardiology Working Group on Peripartum Cardiomyopathy. Current state of knowledge on aetiology, diagnosis, management, and therapy of peripartum cardiomyopathy: a position statement from the Heart Failure Association of the European Society of Cardiology Working Group on peripartum cardiomyopathy. Eur J Heart Fail. 2010 Aug;12(8):767-78. [PMID: 20675664]

Item 120   Answer: C

Educational Objective: Manage severe symptomatic mitral stenosis.

This patient has severe symptomatic mitral stenosis with a valve that by description appears amenable to percutaneous balloon mitral valvuloplasty (PBMV). Classifying mitral stenosis as moderate or severe can be difficult owing to variance in heart rate and forward flow on transmitral gradient. As such, mean gradients are no longer included in the severity criteria. However, the mean gradient is usually greater than 5 mm Hg to 10 mm Hg in severe mitral stenosis, and the mitral valve area is usually less than 1.5 cm^2 in severe mitral stenosis and 1.0 cm^2 or less in very severe mitral stenosis.

PBMV is indicated for symptomatic patients (New York Heart Association [NYHA] functional class II, III, or IV) with severe mitral stenosis and valve morphology favorable for PBMV in the absence of left atrial thrombus or moderate to severe mitral regurgitation. Valve morphology is evaluated by assessing the degree of valvular calcification, valve thickening, degree of leaflet restriction, and extent of subchordal thickening. The most common cause of mitral stenosis is rheumatic heart disease, in which valve inflammation leads to progressive degenerative changes including leaflet thickening, calcification, and impaired valve function, as seen in this patient.

Given that this patient has severe symptomatic mitral stenosis and that there are no obvious contraindications to therapy, a conservative approach would not be appropriate.

Mitral valve replacement is indicated in patients with symptomatic (NYHA functional class III–IV) severe mitral stenosis when PBMV is unavailable or contraindicated or valve morphology is unfavorable.

Generally, rheumatic mitral valve disease is not as amenable to surgical repair as that from degenerative causes, such as myxomatous mitral valve disease. Moreover, the percutaneous option is preferable in a patient when available.

KEY POINT

- Percutaneous balloon mitral valvuloplasty is the preferred treatment for severe symptomatic mitral stenosis.

Bibliography

Nishimura RA, Otto CM, Bonow RO, et al; American College of Cardiology/American Heart Association Task Force on Practice Guidelines. 2014 AHA/ACC guideline for the management of patients with valvular heart disease: executive summary: a report of the American College of Cardiology/American Heart Association Task Force on Practice Guidelines. J Am Coll Cardiol. 2014 Jun 10;63(22):2438-88. Erratum in: J Am Coll Cardiol. 2014 Jun 10;63(22):2489. [PMID: 24603192]

Index

A
NAME AND ADDRESS (Please complete.)

Last Name   First Name   Middle Initial

Address

Address cont.

City   State   ZIP Code

Country

Email address

ACP®
American College of Physicians
Leading Internal Medicine, Improving Lives

Medical Knowledge Self-Assessment Program® 17

TO EARN *AMA PRA CATEGORY 1 CREDITS™* YOU MUST:

1. Answer all questions.
2. Score a minimum of 50% correct.

TO EARN *FREE* INSTANTANEOUS *AMA PRA CATEGORY 1 CREDITS™* ONLINE:

1. Answer all of your questions.
2. Go to **mksap.acponline.org** and enter your ACP Online username and password to access an online answer sheet.
3. Enter your answers.
4. You can also enter your answers directly at **mksap.acponline.org** without first using this answer sheet.

To Submit Your Answer Sheet by Mail or FAX for a $15 Administrative Fee per Answer Sheet:

1. Answer all of your questions and calculate your score.
2. Complete boxes A-F.
3. Complete payment information.
4. Send the answer sheet and payment information to ACP, using the FAX number/address listed below.

B
Order Number
(Use the Order Number on your MKSAP materials packing slip.)

C
ACP ID Number
(Refer to packing slip in your MKSAP materials for your ACP ID Number.)

COMPLETE FORM BELOW ONLY IF YOU SUBMIT BY MAIL OR FAX

Last Name   First Name   MI

Payment Information. Must remit in US funds, drawn on a US bank.

The processing fee for each paper answer sheet is $15.

☐ Check, made payable to ACP, enclosed

Charge to   ☐ **VISA**   ☐ **MasterCard**   ☐ **AMERICAN EXPRESS**   ☐ **DISCOVER**

Card Number _____

Expiration Date _____/_____
       MM   YY

Security code (3 or 4 digit #s) _____

Signature _____

Fax to: 215-351-2799

Mail to:
Member and Customer Service
American College of Physicians
190 N. Independence Mall West
Philadelphia, PA 19106-1572

1 Ⓐ Ⓑ Ⓒ Ⓓ Ⓔ
2 Ⓐ Ⓑ Ⓒ Ⓓ Ⓔ
3 Ⓐ Ⓑ Ⓒ Ⓓ Ⓔ
4 Ⓐ Ⓑ Ⓒ Ⓓ Ⓔ
5 Ⓐ Ⓑ Ⓒ Ⓓ Ⓔ

6 Ⓐ Ⓑ Ⓒ Ⓓ Ⓔ
7 Ⓐ Ⓑ Ⓒ Ⓓ Ⓔ
8 Ⓐ Ⓑ Ⓒ Ⓓ Ⓔ
9 Ⓐ Ⓑ Ⓒ Ⓓ Ⓔ
10 Ⓐ Ⓑ Ⓒ Ⓓ Ⓔ

11 Ⓐ Ⓑ Ⓒ Ⓓ Ⓔ
12 Ⓐ Ⓑ Ⓒ Ⓓ Ⓔ
13 Ⓐ Ⓑ Ⓒ Ⓓ Ⓔ
14 Ⓐ Ⓑ Ⓒ Ⓓ Ⓔ
15 Ⓐ Ⓑ Ⓒ Ⓓ Ⓔ

16 Ⓐ Ⓑ Ⓒ Ⓓ Ⓔ
17 Ⓐ Ⓑ Ⓒ Ⓓ Ⓔ
18 Ⓐ Ⓑ Ⓒ Ⓓ Ⓔ
19 Ⓐ Ⓑ Ⓒ Ⓓ Ⓔ
20 Ⓐ Ⓑ Ⓒ Ⓓ Ⓔ

21 Ⓐ Ⓑ Ⓒ Ⓓ Ⓔ
22 Ⓐ Ⓑ Ⓒ Ⓓ Ⓔ
23 Ⓐ Ⓑ Ⓒ Ⓓ Ⓔ
24 Ⓐ Ⓑ Ⓒ Ⓓ Ⓔ
25 Ⓐ Ⓑ Ⓒ Ⓓ Ⓔ

26 Ⓐ Ⓑ Ⓒ Ⓓ Ⓔ
27 Ⓐ Ⓑ Ⓒ Ⓓ Ⓔ
28 Ⓐ Ⓑ Ⓒ Ⓓ Ⓔ
29 Ⓐ Ⓑ Ⓒ Ⓓ Ⓔ
30 Ⓐ Ⓑ Ⓒ Ⓓ Ⓔ

31 Ⓐ Ⓑ Ⓒ Ⓓ Ⓔ
32 Ⓐ Ⓑ Ⓒ Ⓓ Ⓔ
33 Ⓐ Ⓑ Ⓒ Ⓓ Ⓔ
34 Ⓐ Ⓑ Ⓒ Ⓓ Ⓔ
35 Ⓐ Ⓑ Ⓒ Ⓓ Ⓔ

36 Ⓐ Ⓑ Ⓒ Ⓓ Ⓔ
37 Ⓐ Ⓑ Ⓒ Ⓓ Ⓔ
38 Ⓐ Ⓑ Ⓒ Ⓓ Ⓔ
39 Ⓐ Ⓑ Ⓒ Ⓓ Ⓔ
40 Ⓐ Ⓑ Ⓒ Ⓓ Ⓔ

41 Ⓐ Ⓑ Ⓒ Ⓓ Ⓔ
42 Ⓐ Ⓑ Ⓒ Ⓓ Ⓔ
43 Ⓐ Ⓑ Ⓒ Ⓓ Ⓔ
44 Ⓐ Ⓑ Ⓒ Ⓓ Ⓔ
45 Ⓐ Ⓑ Ⓒ Ⓓ Ⓔ

46 Ⓐ Ⓑ Ⓒ Ⓓ Ⓔ
47 Ⓐ Ⓑ Ⓒ Ⓓ Ⓔ
48 Ⓐ Ⓑ Ⓒ Ⓓ Ⓔ
49 Ⓐ Ⓑ Ⓒ Ⓓ Ⓔ
50 Ⓐ Ⓑ Ⓒ Ⓓ Ⓔ

51 Ⓐ Ⓑ Ⓒ Ⓓ Ⓔ
52 Ⓐ Ⓑ Ⓒ Ⓓ Ⓔ
53 Ⓐ Ⓑ Ⓒ Ⓓ Ⓔ
54 Ⓐ Ⓑ Ⓒ Ⓓ Ⓔ
55 Ⓐ Ⓑ Ⓒ Ⓓ Ⓔ

56 Ⓐ Ⓑ Ⓒ Ⓓ Ⓔ
57 Ⓐ Ⓑ Ⓒ Ⓓ Ⓔ
58 Ⓐ Ⓑ Ⓒ Ⓓ Ⓔ
59 Ⓐ Ⓑ Ⓒ Ⓓ Ⓔ
60 Ⓐ Ⓑ Ⓒ Ⓓ Ⓔ

61 Ⓐ Ⓑ Ⓒ Ⓓ Ⓔ
62 Ⓐ Ⓑ Ⓒ Ⓓ Ⓔ
63 Ⓐ Ⓑ Ⓒ Ⓓ Ⓔ
64 Ⓐ Ⓑ Ⓒ Ⓓ Ⓔ
65 Ⓐ Ⓑ Ⓒ Ⓓ Ⓔ

66 Ⓐ Ⓑ Ⓒ Ⓓ Ⓔ
67 Ⓐ Ⓑ Ⓒ Ⓓ Ⓔ
68 Ⓐ Ⓑ Ⓒ Ⓓ Ⓔ
69 Ⓐ Ⓑ Ⓒ Ⓓ Ⓔ
70 Ⓐ Ⓑ Ⓒ Ⓓ Ⓔ

71 Ⓐ Ⓑ Ⓒ Ⓓ Ⓔ
72 Ⓐ Ⓑ Ⓒ Ⓓ Ⓔ
73 Ⓐ Ⓑ Ⓒ Ⓓ Ⓔ
74 Ⓐ Ⓑ Ⓒ Ⓓ Ⓔ
75 Ⓐ Ⓑ Ⓒ Ⓓ Ⓔ

76 Ⓐ Ⓑ Ⓒ Ⓓ Ⓔ
77 Ⓐ Ⓑ Ⓒ Ⓓ Ⓔ
78 Ⓐ Ⓑ Ⓒ Ⓓ Ⓔ
79 Ⓐ Ⓑ Ⓒ Ⓓ Ⓔ
80 Ⓐ Ⓑ Ⓒ Ⓓ Ⓔ

81 Ⓐ Ⓑ Ⓒ Ⓓ Ⓔ
82 Ⓐ Ⓑ Ⓒ Ⓓ Ⓔ
83 Ⓐ Ⓑ Ⓒ Ⓓ Ⓔ
84 Ⓐ Ⓑ Ⓒ Ⓓ Ⓔ
85 Ⓐ Ⓑ Ⓒ Ⓓ Ⓔ

86 Ⓐ Ⓑ Ⓒ Ⓓ Ⓔ
87 Ⓐ Ⓑ Ⓒ Ⓓ Ⓔ
88 Ⓐ Ⓑ Ⓒ Ⓓ Ⓔ
89 Ⓐ Ⓑ Ⓒ Ⓓ Ⓔ
90 Ⓐ Ⓑ Ⓒ Ⓓ Ⓔ

91 Ⓐ Ⓑ Ⓒ Ⓓ Ⓔ
92 Ⓐ Ⓑ Ⓒ Ⓓ Ⓔ
93 Ⓐ Ⓑ Ⓒ Ⓓ Ⓔ
94 Ⓐ Ⓑ Ⓒ Ⓓ Ⓔ
95 Ⓐ Ⓑ Ⓒ Ⓓ Ⓔ

96 Ⓐ Ⓑ Ⓒ Ⓓ Ⓔ
97 Ⓐ Ⓑ Ⓒ Ⓓ Ⓔ
98 Ⓐ Ⓑ Ⓒ Ⓓ Ⓔ
99 Ⓐ Ⓑ Ⓒ Ⓓ Ⓔ
100 Ⓐ Ⓑ Ⓒ Ⓓ Ⓔ

101 Ⓐ Ⓑ Ⓒ Ⓓ Ⓔ
102 Ⓐ Ⓑ Ⓒ Ⓓ Ⓔ
103 Ⓐ Ⓑ Ⓒ Ⓓ Ⓔ
104 Ⓐ Ⓑ Ⓒ Ⓓ Ⓔ
105 Ⓐ Ⓑ Ⓒ Ⓓ Ⓔ

106 Ⓐ Ⓑ Ⓒ Ⓓ Ⓔ
107 Ⓐ Ⓑ Ⓒ Ⓓ Ⓔ
108 Ⓐ Ⓑ Ⓒ Ⓓ Ⓔ
109 Ⓐ Ⓑ Ⓒ Ⓓ Ⓔ
110 Ⓐ Ⓑ Ⓒ Ⓓ Ⓔ

111 Ⓐ Ⓑ Ⓒ Ⓓ Ⓔ
112 Ⓐ Ⓑ Ⓒ Ⓓ Ⓔ
113 Ⓐ Ⓑ Ⓒ Ⓓ Ⓔ
114 Ⓐ Ⓑ Ⓒ Ⓓ Ⓔ
115 Ⓐ Ⓑ Ⓒ Ⓓ Ⓔ

116 Ⓐ Ⓑ Ⓒ Ⓓ Ⓔ
117 Ⓐ Ⓑ Ⓒ Ⓓ Ⓔ
118 Ⓐ Ⓑ Ⓒ Ⓓ Ⓔ
119 Ⓐ Ⓑ Ⓒ Ⓓ Ⓔ
120 Ⓐ Ⓑ Ⓒ Ⓓ Ⓔ

121 Ⓐ Ⓑ Ⓒ Ⓓ Ⓔ
122 Ⓐ Ⓑ Ⓒ Ⓓ Ⓔ
123 Ⓐ Ⓑ Ⓒ Ⓓ Ⓔ
124 Ⓐ Ⓑ Ⓒ Ⓓ Ⓔ
125 Ⓐ Ⓑ Ⓒ Ⓓ Ⓔ

126 Ⓐ Ⓑ Ⓒ Ⓓ Ⓔ
127 Ⓐ Ⓑ Ⓒ Ⓓ Ⓔ
128 Ⓐ Ⓑ Ⓒ Ⓓ Ⓔ
129 Ⓐ Ⓑ Ⓒ Ⓓ Ⓔ
130 Ⓐ Ⓑ Ⓒ Ⓓ Ⓔ

131 Ⓐ Ⓑ Ⓒ Ⓓ Ⓔ
132 Ⓐ Ⓑ Ⓒ Ⓓ Ⓔ
133 Ⓐ Ⓑ Ⓒ Ⓓ Ⓔ
134 Ⓐ Ⓑ Ⓒ Ⓓ Ⓔ
135 Ⓐ Ⓑ Ⓒ Ⓓ Ⓔ

136 Ⓐ Ⓑ Ⓒ Ⓓ Ⓔ
137 Ⓐ Ⓑ Ⓒ Ⓓ Ⓔ
138 Ⓐ Ⓑ Ⓒ Ⓓ Ⓔ
139 Ⓐ Ⓑ Ⓒ Ⓓ Ⓔ
140 Ⓐ Ⓑ Ⓒ Ⓓ Ⓔ

141 Ⓐ Ⓑ Ⓒ Ⓓ Ⓔ
142 Ⓐ Ⓑ Ⓒ Ⓓ Ⓔ
143 Ⓐ Ⓑ Ⓒ Ⓓ Ⓔ
144 Ⓐ Ⓑ Ⓒ Ⓓ Ⓔ
145 Ⓐ Ⓑ Ⓒ Ⓓ Ⓔ

146 Ⓐ Ⓑ Ⓒ Ⓓ Ⓔ
147 Ⓐ Ⓑ Ⓒ Ⓓ Ⓔ
148 Ⓐ Ⓑ Ⓒ Ⓓ Ⓔ
149 Ⓐ Ⓑ Ⓒ Ⓓ Ⓔ
150 Ⓐ Ⓑ Ⓒ Ⓓ Ⓔ

151 Ⓐ Ⓑ Ⓒ Ⓓ Ⓔ
152 Ⓐ Ⓑ Ⓒ Ⓓ Ⓔ
153 Ⓐ Ⓑ Ⓒ Ⓓ Ⓔ
154 Ⓐ Ⓑ Ⓒ Ⓓ Ⓔ
155 Ⓐ Ⓑ Ⓒ Ⓓ Ⓔ

156 Ⓐ Ⓑ Ⓒ Ⓓ Ⓔ
157 Ⓐ Ⓑ Ⓒ Ⓓ Ⓔ
158 Ⓐ Ⓑ Ⓒ Ⓓ Ⓔ
159 Ⓐ Ⓑ Ⓒ Ⓓ Ⓔ
160 Ⓐ Ⓑ Ⓒ Ⓓ Ⓔ

161 Ⓐ Ⓑ Ⓒ Ⓓ Ⓔ
162 Ⓐ Ⓑ Ⓒ Ⓓ Ⓔ
163 Ⓐ Ⓑ Ⓒ Ⓓ Ⓔ
164 Ⓐ Ⓑ Ⓒ Ⓓ Ⓔ
165 Ⓐ Ⓑ Ⓒ Ⓓ Ⓔ

166 Ⓐ Ⓑ Ⓒ Ⓓ Ⓔ
167 Ⓐ Ⓑ Ⓒ Ⓓ Ⓔ
168 Ⓐ Ⓑ Ⓒ Ⓓ Ⓔ
169 Ⓐ Ⓑ Ⓒ Ⓓ Ⓔ
170 Ⓐ Ⓑ Ⓒ Ⓓ Ⓔ

171 Ⓐ Ⓑ Ⓒ Ⓓ Ⓔ
172 Ⓐ Ⓑ Ⓒ Ⓓ Ⓔ
173 Ⓐ Ⓑ Ⓒ Ⓓ Ⓔ
174 Ⓐ Ⓑ Ⓒ Ⓓ Ⓔ
175 Ⓐ Ⓑ Ⓒ Ⓓ Ⓔ

176 Ⓐ Ⓑ Ⓒ Ⓓ Ⓔ
177 Ⓐ Ⓑ Ⓒ Ⓓ Ⓔ
178 Ⓐ Ⓑ Ⓒ Ⓓ Ⓔ
179 Ⓐ Ⓑ Ⓒ Ⓓ Ⓔ
180 Ⓐ Ⓑ Ⓒ Ⓓ Ⓔ